Pediatric Psychooncology

Pediatric Psychooncology

Psychological Perspectives on
Children with Cancer

EDITED BY

David J. Bearison

Raymond K. Mulhern

New York   Oxford
OXFORD UNIVERSITY PRESS
1994

Oxford University Press

Oxford New York Toronto
Delhi Bombay Calcutta Madras Karachi
Kuala Lumpur Singapore Hong Kong Tokyo
Nairobi Dar es Salaam Cape Town
Melbourne Auckland Madrid

and associated companies in
Berlin Ibadan

Library of Congress Cataloging-in-Publication Data
Pediatric psychooncology ; psychological perspectives on children with
cancer / edited by David J. Bearison and Raymond K. Mulhern.
p. cm. Includes bibliographical references and index.
ISBN 0-19-507931-0
1. Tumors in children—Psychological aspects.
I. Bearison, David J. II. Mulhern. Raymond K.
[DNLM: 1. Neoplasms—psychology.
2. Neoplasms—in infancy & childhood. 3. Child Psychology.
QZ 200 P3705 1994]
RC281.C4P445 1994
618.92′994′0019—dc20
DNLM/DLC
for Library of Congress 93-15993

2 4 6 8 9 7 5 3 1

Printed in the United States of America
on acid-free paper

To my wife, Linda

D.J.B.

To my parents, Alice Mary and Ray Sr.

R.K.M.

Foreword

BY DONALD PINKEL

My experience with the psychology of pediatric cancer began in July 1951, during the first month of pediatric internship. I made the diagnosis of acute leukemia in a preschooler and went to a professor of child psychiatry to secure his help in telling the child's parents. He was helpful to me, but there was no easing the pain the parents faced with no prospect for cure. Perhaps it was for this reason that psychologists and psychiatrists took little interest in children with cancer until late in the 1960s when the introduction of combination chemotherapy and its coordination with surgery and radiotherapy measurably improved the chance for cure.

Another significant personal experience occurred in 1955 when I was a fellow at an institution where children and adolescents with leukemia were not told their diagnosis. A boy with acute leukemia in temporary remission asked me out of the blue if he was going to die. I said, "Why do you ask?" He replied that his schoolmates had told him he had leukemia and was going to die soon, but he couldn't understand why his parents and his doctor would not have told him if this were true. It may be difficult for a contemporary physician or psychologist to appreciate, but the mere suggestion that we tell children and adolescents their diagnosis and prognosis generated severe anger among professionals well into the 1960s. The publication of the landmark paper, "Who's Afraid of Death on a Leukemia Ward" (Vernick & Karon, 1965), was a breakthrough that opened the way to truthfulness with our children, illustrating the power of the printed word to succeed when reasoning aloud failed.

A third interesting personal experience occurred in 1970. Pediatricians and hematologists generally agreed that leukemia was incurable with contemporary treatment methods; mental health professionals dealing with children with leukemia were largely focused on death and dying. But it had become apparent to some of us that a substantial proportion of children might be cured of leukemia by a "total therapy" strategy using already available agents. When we stated these observations, there was considerable emotional resentment expressed by many of our colleagues, as if a sacred tomb was being unsealed. When George Marten, Sam Pitner, and Sileen Soni first applied for support to study the neuropsychological consequences of acute leukemia and its therapy, the granting agency deferred decision pending a site visit. The site visitors had only one question: "Do children survive acute leukemia?" Amazed to see the survivors, the visitors quickly resolved their skepticism, financial support began, and the path was cleared for the extensive research that ensued on the psychology of pediatric cancer survivors.

Psychology has several roles in the care of children with cancer and their families. Among them is the assessment of patients and their families to determine their psychosocial frames of reference, which is useful knowledge in providing effective and efficient care. Another role is assisting the children and their families to develop coping skills for the myriad problems posed by the diagnosis and treatment. Counseling the entire family, whose ties are severely stressed by the experience of having a child with cancer, is also important. Additionally, it is well demonstrated that school adjustment and vocational success can be promoted by psychometric testing to identify learning deficits consequent to cancer and its treatment. A significant, although often awkward function is helping other members of the health-care team reinforce their skills in coping with their own feelings as well as those of the children and the families.

However, the most important role of pediatric psychooncologists is to conduct scientific investigations with children with cancer. Beliefs, sentiments, opinions, and theories need to be replaced by hypotheses and tested by well-designed and rigorously conducted experiments that, while respecting the individual dignity and best interests of each child, lead to definitive conclusions on which to base practices. For the reality is that the vast majority of children with cancer receive their treatment outside major pediatric cancer centers and without the availability of psychological services. They are managed primarily by pediatricians and nurses who depend for their guidance on principles and methods of treatment developed and tested in major centers. Just as they need chemotherapy guidelines for treatment of cancer, they also require mental health guidelines readily applicable in practice to ensure the best "total care" of the children. Psychologists working in major centers best serve children with cancer by testing concepts and methods and developing knowledge that can be readily applied in medical practice outside the centers. It is preferable that they perceive their patient-care activities primarily as model systems for developing and testing hypotheses and techniques rather than just professional practices or educational exercises.

I am grateful to the editors for the opportunity to prepare a foreword for this volume and hope that it will define and promote research that will continue to benefit all children with cancer.

Reference

Vernick, V., & Karon, M. (1965). Who's afraid of death on a leukemia ward? *American Journal of Diseases of Children, 109,* 393–397.

Foreword

BY GERALD P. KOOCHER

More than two decades ago, before the advent of modern cancer treatment, most children diagnosed with cancer died. Such deaths were rapid and painful. Very few mental health professionals were actively writing about their work with the families of these children. This may have been because of the high personal and emotional costs of working with dying children and their families under these circumstances, but the stresses were magnified by the ambience of concealment common in that era. The reality of impending death was not an acceptable topic of open conversation.

One reflection of the ambience of the times was a paper in the prestigious *New England Journal of Medicine* that argued in favor of a kind of benign lying to such patients (Evans & Edin, 1968). Mental health professionals generally preferred a more open approach, but the oncologists on the front lines, at a time when there was little medical hope, viewed this with apparent dismay. In place of open and frank discussion of death with the fatally ill child, the authors argued in favor of shielding the child from fears of death. They reasoned that, although such fears were well-founded, they could not be dissipated by discussion. It was suggested that children with leukemia be told that they had "anemia and tired blood." If children asked directly whether they had cancer or leukemia, the physician was advised to, "characterize it as an anemia that is rather like leukemia, but one that responds to treatment" (p. 139).

The years that followed saw dramatic changes in the care of children with cancer. Pediatric oncologists around the country, including the authors of the aforementioned article, changed their views about sharing information which reflected the new hope that chemotherapy offered their patients. This shift in attitude was a metaphor for the transformation in the field to follow. The ability to adapt to changing psychological needs as a function of new developments in cancer therapy and an awareness of the psychological aspects of cancer treatment became crucial elements in patient care at oncology treatment centers.

Today, remission is easily induced for the vast majority of newly diagnosed children with acute lymphoblastic leukemia (ALL), the most common type of cancer in childhood, and more than 70 percent of such patients can be expected to survive at least 5 years. ALL is considered a frequently curable disease. This evolution was accompanied by an explosion of contributions by mental health professionals, which focused on topics ranging from the psychological adaptation of the patient and family, consultation and liaison work with medical teams, management of medical side effects, to psychosocial consequences of long-term survival. The new realities of stressful but effective treatments present the mental health community with a challenge—the need to help families cope with what has become a chronic life-threatening illness, as opposed to an acutely fatal one.

This volume provides both a chronicle and a forecast with respect to psychosocial care of the child with cancer. It teaches the reader how we have arrived, where we are now, and where we should consider going as people who care about the psychological well-being of children with cancer. More important, it provides a wonderful illustration of the full range of psychosocial interventions that are possible in addressing the problems involved in the treatment of a complex life-threatening illness.

Reference

Evans, A. E., & Edin, S. (1968). If a child must die. . . . *New England Journal of Medicine, 278,* 138–142.

Acknowledgments

An edited book of this kind obviously is a collaborative effort, and we want to acknowledge the authors of the chapters for their diligence in preparing their manuscripts as well as for their continuing contributions to this emerging field of study which we have come to refer to as psychooncology. We very much appreciate the opportunity to work with Joan Bossert, our editor at Oxford University Press, who immediately recognized the need for a book that would bring together the diverse studies in this area and thereby advance this field of study.

We also are grateful for the opportunities to work with pediatric oncologists, nurses, and social workers who are at the forefront of advancing new approaches in pediatric oncology that recognize both the medical and the psychological needs of the children they treat and their families. The Mount Sinai Medical Center in New York and St. Jude Children's Research Hospital in Memphis are exemplary institutions in promoting this enlightened approach to patient care. Our knowledge and experience in this field is enhanced by our participation in the Pediatric Oncology Group (POG), a national consortium of research hospitals supported by the National Cancer Institute for the purpose of advancing interinstitutional research in pediatric oncology. The increasing recognition that POG and its affiliate, the Children's Cancer Group (CCG), afford psychologists not only provides a forum for the fermentation of new ideas, but it supports and enhances the professional role of psychologists among pediatric oncologists.

We wish to acknowledge our students, who, by their research and inquiries, provide the impetus for us to continually try to stay just one step ahead of them. Our greatest appreciation goes to all the children with cancer who we have come to know in our clinical practice and research. Without their ever having to tell us, we know that they understand and appreciate our efforts and that they, in their own ways, share our struggle to reduce the pain and suffering of all children who have cancer.

New York   D. J. B.
Memphis   R. K. M.
July 1993

Contents

Contributors

David J. Bearison, Ph.D. Ph.D. Program in Developmental Psychology, The Graduate School and University Center of the City University of New York and Division of Pediatric Hematology/Oncology, Department of Pediatrics, Mount Sinai Medical Center and Mount Sinai School of Medicine

Paul J. Carpenter, Ph.D. Behavioral Medicine Unit of the Cancer Center, University of Rochester Medical Center

Linda Granowetter, M.D. Division of Pediatric Hematology/Oncology, Department of Pediatrics, Mount Sinai Medical Center and Mount Sinai School of Medicine

Anne E. Kazak, Ph.D. University of Pennsylvania School of Medicine and Division of Oncology, The Children's Hospital of Philadelphia

Gerald P. Koocher, Ph.D. Department of Psychiatry, The Children's Hospital Medical Center and Harvard Medical School

Mary Jo Kupst, Ph.D. Department of Pediatrics, Medical College of Wisconsin and Midwest Children's Cancer Center

Carla S. LeVant, MSW Behavioral Medicine Unit of the Cancer Center, University of Rochester Medical Center

Ida M. Martinson, R.N., Ph.D. Department of Family Health Care Nursing, University of California at San Francisco School of Nursing

Raymond K. Mulhern, Ph.D. Division of Psychology, St. Jude Children's Research Hospital and Department of Pediatrics, University of Tennessee College of Medicine

Danai Papadatou, Ph.D. School of Nursing, University of Athens, Athens, Greece

Sean Phipps, Ph.D. Division of Psychology, St. Jude Children's Research Hospital and Department of Pediatrics, University of Tennessee College of Medicine

Donald Pinkel, M.D. Section of Leukemia/Lymphoma, Division of Pediatrics, University of Texas M. D. Anderson Cancer Center

Lonnie Zeltzer, M.D. Department of Pediatrics, University of California at Los Angeles School of Medicine

Pediatric Psychooncology

Introduction

DAVID J. BEARISON AND RAYMUND K. MULHERN

As Granowetter states in Chapter 1 of this volume, cancer in children is a relatively rare disease, and yet it is the largest nonaccidental cause of death of children between the ages of 2 and 16 years. Six thousand children each year in the United States are diagnosed with cancer and, because of remarkable cure rates that have been achieved in the past 20 to 30 years, one out of every thousand adults in the United States today is a survivor of childhood cancer. In the past 30 years the cure rate for children who have acute lymphoblastic leukemia (ALL), the most common form of childhood cancer, has increased from 0 to 70 percent.

Ironically, as the practice of pediatric oncology continues to advance and prognoses continue to improve, the course of treatment for children with poor prognoses becomes more biologically aggressive, more stressful, and more uncertain. Even for those children who cannot be cured, new treatments have prolonged survival with active disease and consequently have complicated the dying process. For those children who are cured, there are the lingering uncertainties of having undergone medical regimens whose adverse late effects are not yet fully understood. Moreover, there are the families and friends of children who have cancer who are profoundly affected by the experience. Consequently, the field of pediatric oncology today encompasses more than strictly medical concerns. The conditions of treatment, survivorship, and dying have become the concerns of social scientists and health-care practitioners, including psychologists, psychiatrists, child life specialists, behavioral pediatricians, social workers, physical therapists, medical ethicists, and pediatric oncology nurses.

Pediatric health psychologists have responded to these concerns. They have sought means to improve the quality of life for children who have cancer and to work with physicians to advance medical regimens that reflect the biological as well as the behavioral aspects of pediatric oncology. They have sought to promote healthier ways by which society can deal with children who have cancer and their families. They have developed and provided interventions that help children and their families cope with the fears, uncertainties, anger, and frustrations of having cancer, including the management of pain and medical side effects. They have advocated and suggested means of open communication and informed consent from children about treatments and their effects. They have considered the consequences of long-term survival and have helped families bereaved by the loss of children who failed to survive. In all of these efforts, psychologists have relied on a growing body of theoretical and applied research that advances new ways of understanding behavioral and neurological functions in relation to chronic and life-threatening illnesses.

Twenty or thirty years ago there were few psychologists working with children who had cancer and their families. Their role as members of treatment teams was largely peripheral. Behavioral research in pediatric cancer was limited to a few studies of coping, anticipatory grieving, and mourning. However, once it became evident that childhood cancer was no longer a prescription for death and that dismal prognoses were becoming more the exception than the norm, opportunities arose at an astonishing rate for psychologists to enter pediatric oncology, both as health-care providers and as basic and applied researchers. Accordingly, the role of psychologists and psychological research in the care and treatment of pediatric cancer patients assumed increasing importance.

Today, psychologists are core members of treatment teams and collaborate with pediatric oncologists in research studies. In addition, findings from psychological studies help define some of the critical aspects of medical decisions and biomedical research. Thus there is today a substantial body of clinical and empirical findings from psychological research in pediatric oncology. For example, as Kupst notes in Chapter 2 in this volume, more than 200 studies of coping with and adjusting to childhood cancer have been published since the 1960s, and issues of coping and adjustment are only one area studied by psychologists. The number of psychological studies in pediatric oncology has been found to be "disproportionate in terms of the number of children affected by cancer compared with other diseases" (Eiser, 1990, p. 88), and this is testimony to both the commitment of investigators to this area of inquiry and the urgency to learn more about psychosocial aspects of childhood cancer.

Psychological studies in pediatric oncology are reported in an increasing number of specialized scientific journals in both medicine and psychology. These journals include *The Journal of Pediatric Psychology, The Journal of Applied Developmental Psychology, Medical and Pediatric Oncology, The American Journal of the Diseases of Children, The American Journal of Pediatric Hematology/Oncology, The American Journal of Psychiatry, The American Journal of Orthopsychiatry, The Journal of Nervous and Mental Diseases, Archives of Disease in Children, The Journal of Behavioral Medicine, Pediatrics, The Journal of Health Psychology, The Journal of Developmental and Behavioral Pediatrics, The Journal of Consulting and Clinical Psychology, The Journal of Clinical Psychology, The Journal of Pediatric Oncology Nursing, The Journal of Psychosomatic Research, The Journal of Nervous and Mental Diseases, Oncology, The New England Journal of Medicine, The Journal of Child Psychology and Psychiatry, Can-*

cer, *The Journal of Clinical Oncology, The Journal of Pediatrics, The Journal of Psycho-Social Oncology,* and *Psycho-Oncology.* It is no longer practical for those of us involved in pediatric oncology to keep abreast of psychological findings published in so many diverse sources. Consequently, there is a need for a book that integrates state-of-the-art research findings and their conclusions. Current books in pediatric oncology (e.g., Pizzo & Poplack, 1989) and books that focus solely on the psychological aspects of oncology (e.g., Holland, 1989) devote only a small section to psychological issues pertinent to children who have cancer. The present volume addresses a range of psychological issues pertaining to the practice of pediatric oncology and is written for a broad audience with interests in psychological research and the care of children with cancer.

The organization of this book has been delineated according to the major topics of psychological research in pediatric cancer. Each topic encompasses a substantial body of research that not only has theoretical and applied significance but also raises further issues and the need for continuing research. Each chapter is written by a nationally recognized investigator in his or her respective area of inquiry, and each contextually defines the research area, discusses theoretical and methodological concerns of the area, critically reviews and integrates research findings in the area, and discusses unresolved research issues and suggests future research. The authors and their topics are not meant to delimit the scope of psychological research in pediatric cancer. Rather, the chapters illustrate what we consider to be the most important topics and issues which are currently supported by sufficient empirical research to allow useful generalization of findings to the clinical setting. Beyond sharing the current state of knowledge, our primary objective is to further advance the state of knowledge in pediatric psychooncology and to consider how it might generalize to other populations of children with chronic life-threatening illnesses.

Chapter 1 offers a concise yet comprehensive discussion of the medical aspects of pediatric cancer, which will be valuable to readers with little or no background in biomedical sciences and medical practice. Granowetter, a pediatric oncologist, discusses the etiology, clinical symptoms, diagnostic procedures, and different kinds of treatments of childhood cancers. She then discusses the characteristics and late effects of the most common kinds of pediatric malignancies, including leukemias, brain tumors, lymphomas, and bone tumors. This chapter will help those who are relatively unfamiliar with medical issues in pediatric oncology to better appreciate the nature of this disease and establish a context for the discussion of psychological issues in the following chapters.

How children who have cancer and their families cope with and adjust to the experience is considered in Chapter 2 by Kupst, a pediatric health psychologist. She discusses the problems in defining adequate coping and adjustment reactions given the continuing uncertainties and life-threatening conditions of childhood cancers. She critically reviews the major "paradigmatic models" that serve as theoretical contexts for coping research and considers such findings in terms of adaptive and maladaptive coping strategies as well as the correlates of healthy adjustment.

Problems associated with pain and symptom management among children undergoing treatment for cancer is a major area of concern for clinicians. In Chapter 3, Zeltzer, a pediatrician, discusses methods of assessing and treating chemotherapy-induced nausea and vomiting, pain secondary to invasive procedures, and other distressing symptoms. She also reviews methods of evaluating individual differences among pediatric cancer patients in their vulnerability to pain symptoms, managing children's procedure-related pain and distress according to the needs of the individual child, and relationships between children's acute and chronic pain reactions.

A significant and growing problem in pediatric oncology is the alarming rates of medication noncompliance. Among adolescent oncology patients, it has been found that as many as 60 percent are not compliant, and this has been shown to have critical implications for their survival. Bearison, a developmental and clinical psychologist, discusses the varieties of noncompliance in pediatric oncology and reviews findings on noncompliance and factors that place children at risk for noncompliance relative to demographic, biomedical, and psychosocial variables. He also considers the need for new ways of intervening in order to promote compliance among pediatric cancer patients.

The dramatic improvements in treating childhood cancers also have occasioned a variety of treatment-related toxicities. None are more significant than neuropsychological late effects caused by pathological changes in children's central nervous systems that are secondary to cancer and/or its treatment and that affect children's intellectual abilities and their cognitive development. Mulhern, a pediatric psychologist, discusses the evidence for neuropsychological deficits associated with the treatment of pediatric acute lymphoblastic leukemia and brain tumors, the two most prevalent forms of childhood malignancy. Critical factors determining neuropsychological function such as age at treatment and radiation therapy are discussed in terms of modifying medical management, and remedial and rehabilitative programs are considered.

Childhood cancer is a family crisis that poses a range of stressors and demands that affect the entire family. Carpenter, a pediatric psychologist, and LeVant, a pediatric social worker, critically review, from a family systems orientation, studies of how siblings of pediatric cancer patients cope with and adapt to this crisis and the kinds of family-focused interventions that can help them.

An increasingly important means of treating many kinds of pediatric malignancies is the process of bone marrow transplantation (BMT), a particularly arduous and psychologically stressful procedure. According to Phipps, a pediatric psychologist, medical advances in this high-risk procedure have been so rapid that there is a "gap in our understanding of the psychological sequelae of the procedure." Psychological issues related to this method of treatment include patients' responses to aversive preparatory treatment regimens and the prolonged restrictions of protective isolation, unique compliance issues, behavioral reactions to pharmacological effects, special intervention techniques, evaluations of and interventions with sibling donors, stress among caregivers, informed consent, ethical and legal considerations, and late effects of BMT treatment.

Survival of cancer presents a new series of challenges and uncertainties, and while most childhood cancer survivors sooner or later are able to adjust to these conditions, there is a subset that have difficulty adjusting. Kazak, a pediatric psychologist, considers the particular challenges of survivorship including cognitive sequelae, treatment-related late effects, social and emotional adjustment, and family relations. She also considers the need for more innovative theories to better understand the impact of surviving cancer for children relative to issues presented by other kinds of trauma and survival.

The care of children who are dying of cancer and their bereaved families is a growing concern both in this country and in others. Martinson, a pediatric nurse who initiated home care for children dying of cancer in 1972, and Papadatou, a clinical psychologist working with dying children and their families in Greece, discuss the pediatric hospice movement from a historical perspective and identify issues that have to be considered when offering palliative care to a child dying of cancer, including the needs of the caregivers. They also consider the need to formulate new ways of studying death and dying in order to enhance the quality of living for children dying of cancer and provide greater support for their families.

Given that a primary purpose of this book is to advance our current state of knowledge in pediatric psychooncology, it is fitting that we conclude with a chapter addressing future directions for research and practice in this area. In chapter 10 Mulhern and Bearison consider the implications of findings discussed in the previous chapters with the aim of identifying unifying themes and reaching conclusions. They also discuss emerging areas of psychological research in the field of pediatric oncology that, although promising, are not yet sufficiently developed in terms of an empirical base to warrant separate chapter topics yet show promise of further contributing to the treatment and welfare of children who have cancer.

References

Eiser, C. (1990). Psychological effects of chronic disease. *Journal of Child Psychology and Psychiatry, 31,* 85–98.

Holland, J. (1989). *Handbook of psychooncology.* New York: Oxford University Press.

Pizzo, P. A., & Poplack, D. G. (Eds.). (1989). *Principles and practice of pediatric oncology.* Philadelphia: Lippincott.

1

Pediatric Oncology:
A Medical Overview

LINDA GRANOWETTER

Pediatric oncology is a broad field, encompassing a variety of malignancies with varying medical consequences, treatment plans, and prognoses. The purpose of this chapter is to present basic medical information about childhood cancer so that the reader may better appreciate the psychosocial issues presented later in the book. An overview of the characteristics, manifestations, and current thought regarding etiology is presented: information about establishing a diagnosis and explaining the diagnosis and treatment plans to the family is presented; and the course and general principles of cancer treatment are discussed. Some of the more common forms of childhood cancer are then considered. The chapter ends with a summary of late effects of treatment.

Characteristics of Childhood Cancer

Pediatric cancers are rare, accounting for less than 2 percent of all malignancies. Yet cancer is the second leading cause of death in children. In the United States about 6,550 new cases of cancer in children under 15 years of age occur yearly (Young, Ries, Silverberg, Horm, & Miller, 1986). The risk of developing cancer between birth and age 15 is about 1 in 600. Advances in the treatment of childhood cancer have resulted in overall cure rates of 60 percent. Thus 1 of each 1000 adults at age 20 is a survivor of childhood cancer (Meadows, Krejmas, & Belasco, 1980). The most common form of childhood cancer is leukemia, followed by brain tumor, and then lymphoma (cancer of the lymph glands). Other typical childhood cancers are Wilms' tumor (a cancer of the kidney), neuroblastoma (a tumor of sympathetic nervous tissue), and a variety of solid tumors involving muscle (rhabdomyosarcoma), bone, the eye (retinoblastoma), ovarian and germ cell tumors, and the liver. Table 1.1 summarizes the incidence of childhood cancers. The age of onset of cancer varies with the specific disease. For example, bone tumors occur most often in the second decade of life; in contrast, Wilms' tumor and neuroblastoma most commonly occur in children of 2 to 3 years of age. These differences suggest that the former tumors may be related in part to postnatal events (although genetic influence may still be important), whereas tumors which occur in the very young are more likely related to genetic and prenatal influences (Mulvihill, 1989).

Cancer is abnormal, uncontrolled proliferation of cells, which can occur in any organ system of the body. On the level of the individual cell, cancer is a genetic defect. Cancer occurs when a cell's genetic instructions allow growth without normal control mechanisms; thus the cell produces aberrant progeny when and where it should not. This is not to say, however, that cancer is a genetic disease in the sense of heritability, for except in very rare cases cancer is neither inherited nor caused by an obvious genetic defect manifested in other normal tissues. Advances in understanding the molecular mechanisms of cancer indicate that acquired cellular genetic defects are responsible, at least in part, for many if not all cancers (Yunis, 1986). The rare childhood cancers which are heritable, such as bilateral retinoblastoma or cancers associated with consistent chromosomal abnormalities of the tumor cells, will help elucidate the mechanisms causing cancer at the molecular level. Nonetheless, the "why" of cancer for most individuals remains an unanswered question. The etiology of most childhood cancers is most likely due to a complex interaction between environmental factors and genetic susceptibility and will vary in specifics among the different forms of cancer.

Etiology

Research into the etiology of childhood cancers is hampered by the limitations of retrospective studies, most often case control studies based on questionnaires.

Table 1.1. Estimated Number of New Cancers in Children under 15 Years of Age, United States, 1985

Site	Number
Leukemias	2,000
Brain and nervous system	1,230
Lymphomas	780
Neuroblastoma	525
Soft tissues	420
Kidney	410
Bone	320
Retinoblastoma	200
Other	665
Total, all sites	6,550

Source: Adapted from Young, Ries, Silverberg, Horm, & Miller (1986), Cancer Incidence, Survival, and Mortality for Children Younger than Age 15 Years. *Cancer, 58,* 598–602

Case control studies match each patient to demographically similar but well individuals in an attempt to define factors which differ and thus might contribute to the genesis of the illness. The rarity of childhood cancer makes prospective studies following cohorts of healthy children virtually impossible. For many adult cancers, there are clear environmental and behavioral associations, such as between smoking and lung cancer. In pediatric malignancy there is rarely clear evidence for environmental cause; however, there are genetic and multisystem disorders that are associated with increased risk of cancer during childhood.

There is an increased risk of cancer associated with inherited diseases such as Bloom's syndrome, ataxia-telangiectasia, and Fanconi's anemia; these are illnesses characterized by abnormalities of the system that repairs DNA (the genetic machinery) after the routine damage which occurs in life (Miller, 1967). Certain cancers, particularly lymphomas, are associated with genetic (Weinberg & Parkman, 1989) and acquired immunodeficiency, for example, AIDS (Rubenstein, 1986). Some genetic diseases such as neurofibromatosis are associated with an increased risk of cancer, specifically tumors of the visual pathways, sarcomas, and leukemias (Cohen & Rothner, 1989). Down's syndrome is associated with an increased risk of cancer, particularly leukemia (Miller, 1970).

Research into environmental exposures and pediatric cancer yields conflicting results. There are studies linking increased risk of childhood cancer to prenatal exposure to ionizing radiation (Harvey, Boice, Honbeyman, & Flannery, 1985), to proximity to nuclear power installations and electromagnetic fields (Savitz, John & Kleckner, 1990), to certain parental occupations such as work in the petroleum industry (Savitz & Chen, 1990), to older maternal age at birth (Kaye et al., 1991), and to a variety of other environmental exposures (Greenberg & Shuster, 1985). Some cancers are clearly linked to toxic agents; for example, myeloid leukemia may occur after benzene exposure (Vigliani & Sarta, 1964), but most childhood cases of myeloid leukemia have no known cause. It has been hypothesized that childhood leukemia is a consequence of a rare reaction to a yet to be identified virus, based on epidemiologic observations (Kinlen, Clarke, & Hudson, 1990). The contribution of any of these causes to the overall incidence of childhood cancers remains uncertain.

Studies have demonstrated an increased incidence of cancer in first-order family members of patients with cancer (Draper, Heaf, & Kennier-Wilson, 1977). However, the magnitude of this risk remains very small. For example, if the risk of acute lymphoblastic leukemia is 4 in 100,000 children under age 15 each year, even a twofold to fourfold increased risk would still result in a very remote risk to a sibling. Thus siblings and family members should not be unduly alarmed. There are, however, rare instances in which the risk to a family member is significant. For example, in identical twins, the concordance for leukemia is near 100 percent for leukemia in early infancy (Miller, 1971) yet only 25 percent for leukemia later in childhood (Macahon & Levy, 1964). The Li-Fraumeni cancer family syndrome is a very rare disorder characterized by familial clustering of cases of sarcoma, breast cancer at a young age, and bone, brain, laryngeal, and adrenocortical cancers (Li & Fraumeni 1982). A mutation in an inherited gene, called the p53 gene, has been associated with this syndrome (Malkin et al., 1990). The implications of the presence of this or other heritable gene mutations in the etiology of adult and childhood cancers is not known at this time, and it is likely that this marker is associated with limited numbers of childhood cancers. The risk of second malignancies in patients successfully treated for childhood cancer may be related to genetic predisposition. The social, psychological, and ethical implications of informing individuals of genetic markers for cancer risk are enormous and will require further investigation (Lerman, Rimer, & Engstrom 1991).

Clinical Manifestations of Childhood Cancer

The manifestations of cancer relate to its organ of origin. For example, the leukemias comprise a group of cancers of the bone marrow which manifest as disorders of blood cell production such as anemia, bleeding, or tendency to infection and fever. Children with leukemia may also experience bone pain due to expansion of the bone marrow filled with leukemia cells. In contrast, solid tumors are tumors which occur in an organ system or soft tissue and cause harm by excessive local growth or by metastasis. Brain tumors, for example, cause symptoms based on the specific site of the tumor. There may be headache and vomiting, changes in personality or cognitive function or motor control, or other neurologic changes. Other solid tumors may present as a growth ("mass"), which may be visible or may cause pain or some change in function. Solid tumors also may cause vague systemic symptoms such as malaise, weight loss, and fever. Physicians suspect cancer when there is a constellation of symptoms that suggest the diagnosis.

The time between the onset of symptoms and the diagnosis of cancer varies among the specific cancer types and ranges from days to many months. Delay in diagnosis may occur because pediatric cancers are rare and perhaps not considered early by the general pediatrician. There is some evidence that cancer is diagnosed more frequently in the pediatric emergency room (compared to a primary practitioner's office) than would be expected (Jaffe, Fleischer, & Grosflam, 1985). Parental or patient denial of symptoms or of the possible diagnosis may also be a factor. There may be a wide gap in the time between the onset of symptoms and diagnosis, varying among the different tumors. For example, the lag time between onset of symptoms and diagnosis is greater in brain tumors than in leukemia (Flores, Williams, Bell, O'Brien, & Ragab, 1986). Investigations to understand the reasons for delay in diagnosis of childhood cancer are under way. Although much is made of a delay in diagnosis as a major determinant of outcome, most pediatric tumors grow relatively rapidly and thus are diagnosed relatively promptly. For the majority of pediatric tumors, the prognosis is forged more by the biologic behavior of the tumor than the promptness of diagnosis.

Diagnostic Studies

Once cancer is suspected, the child must undergo a variety of interventions to determine the specific diagnosis and extent of disease. The examinations required are tailored to the suspected illness. For the leukemias, the initial diagnostic test is a blood count, followed by examination of the bone marrow, the place where blood is formed. In contrast, imaging studies, such as X-rays and computed to-mography (CT) scans, demonstrate a mass or tumor; however, biopsy of the tumor tissue is required for definitive diagnosis. After a specific diagnosis is made, im-aging studies and occasionally biopsy of areas where the tumor is known to spread are required to determine if the tumor has metastasized. Some solid tumors are considered either localized or nonlocalized. Others are "staged" by a system in which Stage I refers to the most localized and Stage IV the most advanced stage. Staging systems are used to estimate prognosis, to determine appropriate treatment plans, and to allow investigators to compare the results among different treat-ment regimens.

The bone marrow aspirate and biopsy procedures are required to unequivocally diagnose leukemia and determine the type of leukemia. Bone marrow aspirates and biopsies require the insertion of a needle into a marrow-bearing bone, most often the hip bone in the back. Depending on the age and tolerance of the patient, the procedure may be done with injections of local anesthesia only, with local anesthesia and some form of heavy sedation, or even under general anesthesia. Little more than a teaspoon of bone marrow is removed and examined. The proce-dure is completed in minutes, after which the bone marrow aspirate is examined under the microscope, and a diagnosis usually is made within hours. To clearly define the subtype of leukemia, more sophisticated studies are often required and results from these studies may not be available for 1 to 2 days. Such studies include analysis of the chromosomes of the tumor and immunological tests which define the origin of the leukemic cell. A bone marrow biopsy is sent to the pathol-ogy laboratory, and results may not be available for 1 to 2 days. A second proce-dure, called a lumbar puncture, or spinal tap, is required to determine if the leuke-mia has spread to the central nervous system. This test requires the insertion of a needle between the backbones in the lower back to remove about a teaspoon of spinal fluid, which surrounds the spinal cord and is in continuity with the fluid that normally bathes the brain. Bone marrow aspirates are performed intermittently throughout the course of treatment to evaluate the state of the disease; lumbar punctures are done intermittently to evaluate and to give medicine directly into the spinal fluid. Bone marrow and spinal fluid tests cause pain, and coping with these procedures is an important part of treatment for most patients.

For solid tumors a variety of tests which image the area of involvement and possible areas of metastasis are required. Simple X-rays of involved areas are often the first step. CT scans or magnetic resonance images (MRIs) are used to obtain detailed pictures, in all planes, of the areas in question. These studies may be uncomfortable and frightening for a child, because they require lying still on a hard table, in an enclosed space, for as long as 2 hours. Often young children require sedation before these examinations are completed. Nuclear medicine stud-ies may also be necessary; these require the intravenous injection of radioactive material, which is picked up by areas of tumor. An hour to several days after injection, images are made which may identify areas of spread. These procedures are not painful, nor is the radiation level dangerous to the patient or family mem-bers, but the studies do require the patient to be still for up to an hour; thus sedation may be required.

Once a solid tumor is suspected on the basis of the imaging studies, the next step is a biopsy or, if appropriate, removal of the tumor. Generally this is done under general anesthesia by a surgeon in the operating room. However, under certain circumstances a needle biopsy may be done. The results of a biopsy occasionally are available immediately, but often the pathologist requires 1 to 2 days to make a diagnosis. Sometimes, particularly with a very rare tumor, up to a week is required to make a definitive diagnosis. Unavoidable delay is not injurious to the patient; however, delay is distressing to patients and parents. Bone marrow aspirates and biopsies and lumbar punctures may be required to determine if the tumor has spread to these areas. Imaging studies are repeated periodically throughout the course of treatment and in follow-up to determine if the disease is under control.

Discussing the Diagnosis and Treatment Plan with Families

Once a diagnosis of cancer is made, the family must be told the diagnosis, the treatment plan, and the prognosis. Generally, the pediatric oncologist discusses the diagnosis and treatment in the company of the oncology team, which may include a specialized nurse, social worker, psychologist, and pediatric physician. After the parents are informed, the team meets with the child as well. Occasionally with an older adolescent the oncology team and the parents and patient are told the diagnosis and implications at the same time. The diagnostic conference is stressful because the family must absorb a great deal of information at a time of emotional turmoil. Since most pediatric cancers are treated at centers participating in national studies, the parents must give signed informed consent to participate in investigational programs, which may require them to hear details of treatment that are extremely difficult to understand. Bioethicists have suggested that in order to avoid coercion and obtain true informed consent from parents and assent from patients, sufficient time to recover from the emotional shock of receiving a diagnosis of cancer is necessary (Leikin, 1985). However, this extra time is rarely possible because of the urgency to start definitive treatment. Further research regarding the best ways to obtain appropriate informed consent in a timely fashion would be valuable to treating physicians.

National Groups and Clinical Trials

In the United States, the majority of children with cancer are treated at institutions associated with national consortiums which study treatment programs for childhood cancer. Because pediatric cancers are rare, cooperative groups were formed in the 1960s to develop organized systems of studying cancer. Today the major groups are the Pediatric Oncology Group (POG) and the Children's Cancer Group (CCG). Most pediatric oncologists agree that the major advances in pediatric cancer result from the organized national trials performed by these groups. Sometimes "studies" are offered which include no investigational treatments but ask participants to allow investigators to submit data to the study group's central office. Most studies, however, include either some investigational medicines or new schedules or uses of standard medicines. Many studies require randomization between what is considered standard therapy and newer study plans. Most national clinical trials for newly diagnosed children are termed Phase III trials, in which the chemotherapeutic medicines to be used have shown efficacy in the cancer to be studied; it is the details of therapy, including length of treatment, schedules of treatment, and comparisons among medicines all known to be useful, which are being tested. Newly diagnosed patients are less frequently offered therapy with investigational medications because it would be unethical to use unproven methods before offering established medicines. Parents and patients often misunderstand these Phase III clinical trials and mistakenly assume they are being offered medications without known efficacy or even placebo trials.

Investigational medications are studied in Phase I and II trials. These studies are offered only to patients who have already received treatment and have relapsed, to those who have not responded to standard treatment, or to those whose tumor has a very poor prognosis with standard therapy. Phase II studies are designed to determine if a new, investigational medicine is useful in the treatment of a particular cancer. Phase I studies are to determine the appropriate doses and side effects of new drugs which have been tested in laboratories, in animal models, and in adults.

Families facing a new diagnosis of cancer may not readily comprehend why physicians who care for children with cancer often refer to treatment programs as studies and themselves as investigators. The physicians may find the explanations extremely constraining, particularly when the goal is to quickly treat a sick child. It may be difficult for parents and patients to accept the idea of studies, particularly randomized trials. A detailed informed consent document, required at the time of initial diagnosis, is daunting to the lay person. Yet the majority of families do accept participation in appropriate national therapeutic trials. Reasons why families and physicians decline participation in national trials are being studied in order to optimize enrollment in clinical trials. Children's ability to comprehend and consent or assent to treatment programs have also been studied, but there is a relative paucity of literature in this area (Fletcher, van Eys, & Dorn 1989).

Schedules of Treatment and Natural History of Cancer

After diagnosis, treatment is started as soon as feasible. Cancer is invariably fatal if untreated. The goal is to obtain a remission; for almost all pediatric patients remission is a realistic goal. Further therapy to consolidate and maintain remission until planned treatment is finished follows. Fortunately, most children with cancer respond to initial therapy, but disease progression in the face of apparently appropriate therapy may occur; this usually portends a poor outcome. Relapse is the recurrence of disease during or after therapy. In general no relapse is good; however, most cancers will respond to treatment for relapse and some patients may be cured after relapse. Death due to relapsed disease or as a consequence of therapy complications occurs in about 40 percent of all childhood cancer patients. Thus for too many children death must be considered part of the natural history of cancer.

Treatment Plan for Leukemia

The initial phase of treatment is called *induction,* indicating that treatment is planned to induce a remission or obtain a state of no obvious disease. *Remission* is defined as having a blood count appropriate for the treatment received, a normal bone marrow, and a spinal fluid which shows no leukemia cells. Remission implies that although there is no obvious disease, microscopic disease still exists; thus further treatment is required. For virtually all childhood cancers, the natural history of the illness has demonstrated that this is so. Most leukemia treatment plans include *consolidation* treatment, which means that more treatment is used to consolidate the remission. Consolidation therapy generally includes specific treatment designed to prevent the occurrence of central nervous system (CNS) disease. Thereafter, *maintenance* treatment continues for 2 to 3 years. *Relapse* is the reappearance of leukemia in the blood, bone marrow, or nonmarrow (extramedullary) site such as CNS or less commonly the testicles, or other sites. In general, relapse is ominous. Although some patients will survive relapse when treated aggressively, the majority of patients with leukemia who relapse eventually succumb to the disease. *Cure* is defined as the absence of leukemia, off treatment, for a period of time based on the natural history of the disease. For example, a child free of leukemia for 4 years after initial completion of therapy is generally considered cured because later relapses are rare.

Treatment Plan for Solid Tumors

No evidence of disease (NED) or remission for a solid tumor means that no tumor is present on physical examination and imaging studies. Often a biopsy confirms remission, but this is not always necessary. For solid tumors, therapy includes local control and systemic treatment. Local control is the eradication of the tumor in its initial site; systemic therapy is treatment to prevent metastases. Local control with a complete surgical resection of tumor may be the initial therapy. If the tumor is not or cannot be removed totally, the next step is treatment designed to decrease the tumor size and to prevent spread or decrease the size of metastases if they exist, before attempting definitive local control with surgery or radiation. For most solid tumors, surgery and/or radiation is required for local control. After local control is accomplished, maintenance chemotherapy is resumed to obliterate micrometastases.

Some tumors require as much as 2 years of therapy while others are treated for as little as several months. The length of treatment is determined by the natural history of the tumor and results from experience treating previous patients. The goal of therapy is to eradicate all tumor, visible and microscopic, so that when treatment is complete the patient remains in remission. Cure is defined as it is for the leukemias: there is no evidence of disease off therapy for a time long enough to ensure the rarity of relapse for the tumor in question.

Pain Control during All Phases of Treatment

Control of the symptoms of cancer is a critical part of pediatric oncology practice. Pain is often a part of the symptomatology which brings the patient to the physician. During the diagnostic phase, standard pain control measures are usually effective. As soon as the cancer is under control, the need for analgesia is usually decreased. In a prospective study of children with cancer who presented with pain, a National Cancer Institute study documented that pain persisted for a median of 10 days once appropriate treatment commenced (Miser, McCalla, Dothage, Wesley, & Miser, 1987). Pain may recur as a consequence of specific procedures, such as procedures to draw blood, diagnostic procedures, treatment itself, and surgical interventions. In studies of children with cancer, 50 percent of inpatients and 25 percent of outpatients experience pain; however, this is primarily treatment-related pain and thus shortlived (Miser, Dothage, Wesley, & Miser, 1987).

When children relapse, pain as a consequence of the cancer itself may be a significant problem. The availability of a variety of oral and intravenous pain medicines and an array of methods to deliver analgesia, which include self-administered oral medication, home infusion pumps, pumps designed for patient self-dosage, and even the ability to deliver pain medications directly to the site of pain by specially placed catheters, would lead one to believe appropriate pain control can always be accomplished promptly. Unfortunately, this is not the case and continuing research into this aspect of supportive care should not be ignored by physicians and psychologists. The ability of medical caregivers to evaluate pain and prescribe adequate analgesia has been shown to be inadequate in several studies (Twycross, 1984). Although pediatric oncologists seem to believe this is more true of those caring for adult cancer patients, there is little factual evidence to support this contention (Schechter, Allen, & Hanson, 1986). The ability to offer appropriate pain control methods for the different phases of therapy is essential in caring for people with cancer (Levy, 1985). These issues are discussed in greater depth by Zeltzer (Chapter 3, this volume).

Death and Dying

About 40 percent of children with cancer will eventually die as a consequence of treatment complications or the cancer itself. When death comes suddenly, as an unexpected complication, or early in the course of treatment, issues arise regarding trust and communication between the family and the treatment team. Sudden unexpected death is relatively rare with current levels of medical supportive care; few children die of "toxic deaths" during initial therapy. However, during aggressive treatment for relapse or very poor prognosis disease, higher toxic death rates are expected.

Death more frequently occurs after medical treatments have been ineffective and it is clear to the physicians that the child has entered a "terminal" phase.

Physicians, parents, and the child may perceive the child's future very differently during this phase. Parents may express a desire to use extraordinary means to prolong life when physicians see this as futile, or the reverse may be true. There is no simple way to determine when treatment is "enough," for example, which child and family should seek investigational care or heroic care and which child should receive only supportive palliative care. In the ideal situation, the family, physician, and patient talk openly about all options and come to a plan agreeable to all; sadly, this is not always the case. In one study detailing the results of a program of family conferences about a child's failure to respond to standard treatment for cancer, of 43 patients between the ages of 6 and 20 years, 14 chose further chemotherapy (investigational agents) and 28 chose supportive care; children at all ages seemed to be active participants in decision making (Nitschke et al., 1982). The physician's involvement in the child's death must be motivated by a desire to avoid unnecessary pain and suffering, yet this is not always simple to accomplish. Physicians and families have varying levels of denial and physicians and families may want to explore experimental treatments for differing reasons. Research examining the motivations, emotional outcomes, and ethics of these issues is important.

It is often assumed that the best place for a child to die is in the home; however, all options such as hospital care and home or institutional hospice care must also be considered. The physician and other medical caregivers have a strong influence over the parents' and child's desires regarding palliative care for a dying child. There is little research which informs caregivers about the best place and way to die in order to minimize long-term family suffering, but that which is published seems to support home care (Martinson et al., 1986) or hospice care (Corr & Corr, 1985). Further research in this area is needed (see Martinson, Chapter 9, this volume).

Modalities of Therapy

There are three primary modalities of treatment available to eradicate cancer: chemotherapy, surgery, and radiation therapy. Most leukemias are treated only with chemotherapy, although radiation therapy may also be used. Most solid tumors require combined modality therapy, that is, chemotherapy used in combination with surgery and radiation therapy or both. Bone marrow transplantation involves aggressive treatment with chemotherapy and/or radiation.

Chemotherapy

The backbone of most cancer treatment programs is chemotherapy, because medication given systemically can fight the cancer at the site of its origin and throughout the body. Most chemotherapeutic agents work by preventing division or growth of rapidly growing cells. Some chemotherapy is given by vein, some by mouth, or some by injection into a muscle or directly into the spinal fluid. Unfortunately, the effects of most treatments now in use are not completely selective; therefore, there are unavoidable side effects on normal tissues. The most common side effects are temporary low blood counts, which result in susceptibility to infection, bleeding tendency, and anemia; blood transfusion is often necessary. New medications called hematopoietic growth factors (e.g., G-CSF) are often given after chemotherapy because these agents partly ameliorate the bone marrow suppression, but virtually all patients still experience abnormal blood counts during the course of therapy. Reversible hair loss associated with many chemotherapy agents is a side effect with significant psychological and social impact. Nausea and vomiting are significant effects; however, new antiemetics have dramatically lessened the severity of nausea and vomiting for most patients. Many medicines also cause malaise, mouth sores, or changes in appetite or ability to eat. Short- and long-term damage to internal organs, particularly the heart, kidneys, and liver, may occur despite optimal monitoring of therapy.

The treatment team works with the patients and family to help them understand and cope with side effects. It is important to remember that these are potential side effects and most patients experience only some side effects, although almost all experience hair loss. The most serious side effects are relatively rare with close patient monitoring. Late side effects of chemotherapy are discussed in the final section of this chapter.

Radiation Therapy

Treatment with radiation is required when surgery and/or chemotherapy cannot completely remove the tumor, when apparent complete removal is known to be associated with relapses, or when the obvious tumor is removed but the pathologist documents residual microscopic tumor. For a very few tumors, radiation or radiation and surgery are the only treatment modalities required.

Planning for radiation usually requires two sessions of several hours' duration, called simulation and verification. Most radiation treatments are a form of external beam radiation, which means that the radiation is delivered from a machine to the patient, outside the body. This treatment is generally given on a schedule of 5 days a week for 2 to 6 weeks depending on the tumor type and site of the tumor. The treatment itself generally takes only minutes, and it is not painful. Radiation must be delivered to a completely still patient; thus strong sedation or anesthesia may be required for very young children.

During the course of radiotherapy a variety of effects, including reddening and irritation of the skin areas receiving radiation, loss of appetite, and malaise, may occur. Other specific effects are related to the site of tumor. For example, if the abdomen is irradiated, diarrhea may ensue; if the head is irradiated, headache may occur. Radiation in high doses will prevent normal growth of the areas irradiated and may be associated with secondary malignancies. Thus in pediatric oncology radiation therapy principles include giving radiation only when required for cure and use of the lowest effective total doses.

Recent investigations are designed to determine if radiation given in smaller doses more often (e.g., twice a day instead of once a day) is associated with fewer side effects. Occasionally it is appropriate to institute brachytherapy, which is radiation therapy delivered by placing radioactive material directly into a tumor site, usually in the form of radioactive "seeds," which are later removed. Recent advances in radiation therapy also include the use of "gamma knife" radiation, which is radiation that is very sharply focused by laser and may have particular application in the treatment of some brain tumors.

Surgery

Despite responses to chemotherapy and radiation therapy, surgery to remove solid tumors is required for cure of many tumor types. Most brain tumors and primary bone tumors require removal of all or most of the primary tumor or residual tumor after initial therapy. Sometimes it is appropriate to perform surgery immediately. This is commonly the case in brain tumors. Most often, after initial diagnostic surgery, chemotherapy and radiation therapy are instituted to control or shrink the tumor and facilitate definitive surgery.

Surgical advances in the field of pediatric oncology have helped increase cure rates and preserve normal function and growth. For example, in the past bone tumors of the extremities were most often treated with amputation. Today, most patients are treated with limb-sparing surgery, complex surgery designed to remove tumor and preserve the extremity. Many patients and parents feel that removing the cancer by surgery is the single most important aspect of treatment. Although the role of surgery cannot be underestimated, for most pediatric cancers surgery alone would result in extremely poor cure rates owing to the presence of micrometastases at diagnosis.

Bone Marrow Transplantation

Bone marrow transplantation (BMT) is often an appropriate modality of therapy for the leukemias, in which the bone marrow must be ablated because it is the origin of the cancer. Bone marrow transplantation may also be used in the treatment of solid tumors, in order to give intensive doses of chemotherapy and/or radiation therapy which would not otherwise be tolerated. Bone marrow transplantation refers to transplantation of the marrow, that is, the cells which are capable of forming blood and not the bone itself. Thus the actual transplant is not a surgical procedure, but it is a transfusion of bone marrow.

Before bone marrow transplantation, chemotherapy (often with radiation therapy) is given in doses so high that normal bone marrow function would not recover, resulting in death, without the transfusion of marrow replacement. After the patient receives the required bone marrow ablative treatment, the replacement bone marrow is given to the patient intravenously. The donated marrow enters by vein but then finds its way to the bone marrow and repopulates the marrow with the cells necessary to regenerate all the blood-forming elements. After the bone marrow is infused, the patient will not have normal bone marrow function for 3 to 6 weeks. During this period, the patient is at extremely high risk of infection or other complications such as bleeding. To minimize the possibility of infection, the patient remains in protective isolation for as long as is required for a safe level of bone marrow function to return. There is a significant risk of death to the patient from the complications of prolonged lack of marrow function and from the intensity of therapy.

The source of marrow for transplantation may be a donor or the patient, from whom marrow is collected during a remission. Allogeneic transplantation refers to a BMT from a nontwin donor. The most common donor is a matched sibling donor; however, a partially matched donor or matched unrelated donor (called a MUD) may be used. Allogeneic transplants are preferred in any form of cancer which involves the bone marrow, such as leukemia. Each sibling has a one in four chance of having the appropriate matched bone marrow. Parents virtually never are a complete match because the patient's genetic material comes from both parents, although occasionally a parent is an appropriate partially matched donor. Because of the enormous diversity of bone marrow tissue types and the necessity for closely matched bone marrow, matched unrelated donors are rare. However, the development of large population-based bone marrow registries may make MUD transplants more available in the future. In general, the most closely matched transplants are safer, thus sibling transplants are always preferred over partially matched donors or MUD transplants. Syngeneic transplants—transplants from an identical twin—are obviously rare. Autologous transplants are those in which some of the patient's own bone marrow is stored prior to the intensive therapy and then returned after the therapy. In certain diseases, such as some forms of leukemia and neuroblastoma, the patient's bone marrow may be removed, treated with chemotherapy or other methods to remove tumor outside the body, then stored and returned to the patient after intensive chemotherapy and radiation therapy given to the patient.

Marrow is obtained from the donor under general anesthesia. The procedure is the same as a bone marrow aspirate described previously, but much more bone marrow is removed, prolonging the procedure so that the donor must be anesthetized. The risk to the donor is the risk of general anesthesia, a variable amount of back pain for a few days after the procedure, and occasionally a red blood cell blood transfusion required after the procedure. If transfusion is anticipated, the donor may store blood prior to the procedure for reinfusion later.

An important complication of the use of allogeneic, partially mismatched, or MUD transplantation is the occurrence of graft versus host disease (GVHD). GVHD is a reaction of the donor's immune cells to certain recipient tissue which is seen as foreign. GVHD may be acute, chronic, or both; it may be mild or severe enough to result in death. GVHD is more likely in older patients and recipients, and in MUD or partially matched marrow transplants. Common manifestations of GVHD are rash, diarrhea, liver disease, dry skin, arthritis, poor immune function, and other organ damage. Treatment of severe GVHD is improving, yet it is still challenging for patient and physician. Ironically, in the leukemias it has been noted that the incidence of GVHD is inversely related to relapse after transplantation. Thus mild to moderate GVHD may be a desired consequence of allogeneic transplantation for leukemia, as the transplanted marrow graft also fights the leukemia.

The psychological issues relating to transplantation are numerous. Important issues include patients, parents, and siblings coping with and understanding the procedure, isolation during the procedure, and neuropsychological sequelae. These issues are discussed at length by Phipps (Chapter 7, this volume).

Discussion of the Most Common Pediatric Malignancies
Acute Lymphoblastic Leukemia

Acute lymphoblastic leukemia (ALL) is the most common pediatric malignancy, with an incidence of about 4 per 100,000 children under age 15 per year in the United States. The peak incidence of ALL is between ages 3 and 6, although it may occur at any age. ALL is more common in whites compared to nonwhites, and its incidence in males is greater than in females (Poplack, 1989). ALL is a cancer of the bone marrow, specifically the white blood cells called lymphoblasts. Abnormal lymphoblasts proliferate in the bone marrow, causing a failure of production of the other normal bone marrow elements. Children with ALL come to medical attention because of symptoms such as unexplained persistent fever, infection, bone pain, easy bruising, bleeding, or enlargement of lymph nodes, liver, or spleen. The duration of symptoms usually ranges from weeks to a few days.

Reviews of treatment regimens for ALL demonstrate that treatment will result in cure for 50 to 70 percent of patients (Niemayer, Hitchcock-Bryan, & Sallan, 1985). The differences in survival rates among clinical trials are due both to differences in treatment and differences among the patients included in the trials. It has been established that certain criteria will predict outcome. For example, children between ages 1 and 10 with low white blood cell counts at diagnosis have the best prognosis and are considered to have standard- or low-risk ALL; those younger than 1 year, older than 10 years, or with higher white blood cell counts have high-risk ALL. In addition, a variety of laboratory parameters are used to assign patients to risk groups. Current treatment programs treat children with high-risk ALL more intensely than those with standard-risk ALL. With appropriate treatment strategies, the differences in outcome between standard- and high-risk groups is lessened; for example, a recent trial demonstrates relapse-free survivals of 86 percent; $\pm$ 4 percent and 71 percent; $\pm$ 3 percent for standard- and high-risk groups, respectively (Clavell et al., 1986). The most recent projections are overall survivals of greater than 70 percent for children under 10 years of age at diagnosis (Bleyer, 1990).

Initial induction treatment requires combinations of three to five medications. Over 90 percent of patients will enter remission after induction; 95 to 98 percent of standard-risk patients will obtain remission. Most treatment regimens include consolidation therapy for 1 to 2 months, followed by maintenance therapy for a 2- to 3-year treatment program.

In most centers, the initial induction period of therapy takes place in the hospital. Once the patient is in remission, therapy continues on an outpatient basis with intermittent admissions to the hospital for the expected infectious complications or for administration of medications which require hospital observation. Every attempt is made to have the child enjoy as normal a life as possible. Virtually all children with ALL in remission are encouraged, for example, to attend school and participate in age-appropriate activities.

ALL has a propensity to invade the central nervous system (CNS). This is partly because systemic chemotherapy does not always reach the nervous system. Thus treatment to protect the CNS is required. Before this fact was recognized, at least 50 percent of children treated for ALL would relapse in the spinal fluid (Evans, Gilbert, & Zandstra, 1970). Radiation therapy to the head (cranium) and/or spine was instituted to decrease the incidence of CNS relapse, and it did so markedly (Bleyer & Poplack, 1985). However, significant neuropsychological sequelae may occur after CNS radiation, particularly in young children (see Mulhern, Chapter 5, this volume). Current CNS preventive therapy may take the form of multiple injections of medication into the spinal fluid alone, with or without medications that enter the CNS when given systemically. Some centers reserve radiation therapy to the CNS for patients who relapse despite initial therapy and some centers still use radiation therapy during the consolidation phase for patients in high-risk groups for CNS relapse. With current treatment plans, 5 to 10 percent of patients have CNS relapses (Bleyer, 1988). The long-term sequelae of radiation therapy, intrathecal chemotherapy, and systemic chemotherapy which enters the CNS are being studied, and the relative risks and benefits among the differing treatment regimens must be compared in order to determine the most effective and least harmful therapy.

Relapse of leukemia in the bone marrow after appropriate therapy is ominous. The majority of children who relapse will enter a second remission; unfortunately most will relapse again and eventually succumb to leukemia (Butturini, Rivera, Bortin, & Gale, 1987). Thus the goal is to optimize initial therapy. Patients who relapse undergo chemotherapy to obtain a second remission. Most patients at second remission who have an appropriate bone marrow donor match are referred for bone marrow transplantation, as most investigators believe transplantation offers the best outlook for cure despite the immediate risks of the procedure. Relapse isolated to sites other than the bone marrow, such as the CNS or the testicles, is also serious. However, 50 percent of patients relapsing in sites other than bone marrow will survive with chemotherapy and/or radiation (Bleyer, 1990).

Acute Nonlymphoblastic Leukemia

Acute nonlymphoblastic leukemia (ANLL), including acute myeloid leukemia, is a group of hematologic cancers affecting blood-forming cells other than lymphoblasts. The symptoms of ANLL are similar to ALL. ANLL, however, is one-quarter as common as ALL. Unlike ALL, the peak incidence of ANLL is stable until adolescence and then increases during the second decade. There are no significant racial or gender differences in the incidence of ANLL. The outlook for ANLL is not as sanguine as that for ALL. With chemotherapy alone, the chance of remission is between 70 and 85 percent and the chance for long-term survival is about 35 percent (Gaynon, 1992). Because of the poor outlook with chemotherapy alone, bone marrow transplantation in first remission is advocated for patients with matched sibling donors. With allogeneic marrow transplantation, the survival rate is 50 to 70 percent of those who enter remission after initial chemotherapy. Prospective randomized trials comparing autologous transplantation, using the patient's own marrow after remission is obtained and treated outside the body, to chemotherapy are under way.

Remission induction therapy for ANLL is very intensive. Patients are often hospitalized for the entire 5 to 8 weeks of induction therapy. Consolidation therapy generally takes 4 to 8 weeks. If a transplant is undertaken, it is done after consolidation. If chemotherapy alone is planned, continued chemotherapy is generally given for up to 6 months. Prolonged maintenance therapy has not been shown to be of benefit in ANLL in most series performed in the United States.

Brain Tumors

Brain tumors are a heterogeneous group of tumors, occurring in about 2.5 children per 100,000 each year. There is a slight male predominance in incidence. In childhood, the peak age for brain tumors is between 3 and 9 years, but these tumors may occur at any time. Symptoms of brain tumors vary with the tumor's site of origin and may include headache, often due to increased intracranial pressure; visual changes, particularly double vision; vomiting; difficulty in balance or coordination; or unexplained cognitive or neurologic deficits.

The primary treatment of most brain tumors is surgical resection. The goal of surgery is to remove as much tumor as possible without sacrificing function to an undue extent. Some brain tumors, for example, those in the brain stem, cannot be removed because of their vital location; others are treated successfully with surgery alone. Advances in neurosurgical techniques, including microsurgery and the use of lasers, have substantially decreased the morbidity and mortality from surgery for brain tumor patients. Nonetheless, many brain tumors cannot be completely removed without significant neurologic insult and most have a propensity to recur despite apparent complete removal. For these, radiation has been the most important element of therapy after surgery. In the last decade, chemotherapy has been proven to be an effective adjunctive treatment in many forms of brain tumor. Thus for most tumors surgery, radiation, and chemotherapy are used in combination. As radiation therapy for brain tumors requires relatively high total doses of radiation, the neuropsychological sequelae of radiation may be severe, particularly in children under 3 years of age. Recent treatment programs employ chemotherapy after surgery in order to delay administration of radiation as long as possible in the youngest children. Because these chemotherapy treatment plans generally have been effective, some treatment studies using surgery and chemotherapy alone have been initiated at some centers for the youngest children.

The outlook for a child with a brain tumor varies considerably with the histologic subtype of tumor, the location of the tumor, and the degree of spread of the tumor in the central nervous system at the time of diagnosis. Children with tumors classified as low-grade astrocytomas which occur in the cerebral hemispheres have a 5-year survival of about 70 percent, yet a child with a similar tumor arising in the brain stem has a 15 to 20 percent survival at 5 years (Duffner, Cohen, & Freeman, 1985).

The Lymphomas

Non-Hodgkin's Lymphoma

The non-Hodgkin's lymphomas (NHLs) are cancers which originate in lymph node–bearing areas. About 10 percent of all childhood cancers are lymphomas, occurring in fewer than 1 per 100,000 children each year. In the United States, NHL is least common under the age of 5, slightly more common in preadolescents and adolescents, then, the incidence of NHL increases with age. Males are diagnosed with NHL two to three times more frequently than females. In the United States, blacks are diagnosed with NHL less frequently than whites. The incidence of NHL varies significantly by geographic area; for example, in central Africa, a particular form of NHL called Burkitt lymphoma is common, and half of childhood cancers in this area are due to NHL. Burkitt NHL in Africa is associated with Epstein-Barr virus, the virus associated with infectious mononucleosis. In the United States, there is no evidence of this association. The etiology of NHL in most children is unknown; however, because lymphomas are clearly associated with immunodeficiency states, it is projected that a significant increase in childhood NHL may occur because of the increasing number of children with AIDS (Horowitz & Pizzo, 1990).

Because lymph nodes are composed of lymphatic cells whose purpose is to migrate throughout the body as part of the normal immune system, NHL is virtually always a systemic problem, although rare cases are confined to a single nodal area. The most common areas are in the head and neck, the abdomen, or the mediastinum (a space deep in the chest). The usual symptoms of lymphoma include enlarged lymph nodes, difficulty breathing because of enlarged lymph nodes in the chest, an abdominal tumor from enlarged lymph nodes, fevers, weight loss, and lethargy. The most common forms of lymphoma in childhood are rapidly growing, and thus they come to attention early. Lymphomas often metastasize to bone, bone marrow, and the central nervous system. It is not uncommon for a child to come to attention with clinical lymphoma, and bone marrow testing shows significant involvement of the bone marrow. If the bone marrow involvement is greater than 30 percent, or if the blood count shows lymphoma cells are obviously circulating, the child is considered to have leukemia and is treated on leukemia protocols.

Current treatment programs for lymphoma include chemotherapy with multiple medications; medications given directly into the spinal fluid to protect the central nervous system; and, for patients with central nervous system disease at diagnosis or high risk of developing CNS disease, cranial or craniospinal radiation. The intensity of therapy is based on the subtype of lymphoma and the tumor burden at diagnosis. The outlook for children with lymphoma appropriately treated is excellent. A small localized lymphoma may be successfully treated for less than 6 months with a close to 90 percent expectation of cure (Link, Donaldson, Berard, Shuster, & Murphy, 1990). Such children may undergo most of the therapy as outpatients and may be able to attend school and participate in normal activities. An aggressive lymphoma, such as advanced T-cell lymphoma, would be treated far more intensively for about 18 to 24 months with about a 75 percent expectation of cure (Anderson et al., 1983; Muller-Weihrich, Henze, Odenwald & Riehm, 1985). Most of these patients are able to resume normal activities after the most intensive induction phase and, like children with leukemia, are able to attend school. An aggressive rapidly growing lymphoma, such as an advanced Burkitt lymphoma, would be treated very aggressively but only for 4 to 5 months with a good expectation of cure; these patients are hospitalized for most of the short but very intense treatment.

Hodgkin's Lymphoma

Hodgkin's lymphoma is a cancer of the lymph nodes which differs from NHL in that it usually demonstrates a slower onset and an orderly progression, involving contiguous lymph node areas. The incidence of Hodgkin's disease among children in the United States is about 0.5 per 100,000 each year. In industrialized countries the peak ages are late adolescence or early adulthood and middle age. In less industrialized nations, the peak age for children is younger. When Hodgkin's disease is shown to be localized to one or two lymph-bearing areas and the patient is fully grown, radiation therapy alone may be curative. For localized disease in young children, the risk of growth disturbance is great enough to try to avoid radiotherapy or to use decreased radiation dosage. Thus for most children chemotherapy or chemotherapy and radiotherapy combinations are required for cure. Multiple studies show survival rates of 80 to 90 percent for Hodgkin's disease in children (Donaldson and Link, 1987; Maity, Goldwein, Lange, & D'Angio, 1992). As cure rates for Hodgkin's disease, even in advanced stages, are high, and because there is a wide variety of useful chemotherapeutic options, much research in the treatment of Hodgkin's disease is based on developing chemotherapy programs with the least toxic sequelae. Hodgkin's disease patients generally receive most of the therapy as outpatients and are able to continue school and most normal activities.

Wilms' Tumor

Wilms' tumor was the first pediatric solid tumor shown to be responsive to chemotherapy. It is in a sense the quintessential pediatric tumor because it arises from embryonic tissue and virtually never occurs in adults. It is responsive to treatment and increasing success in treatment has come through a series of national studies.

Current cure rates for Wilms' tumor are close to 90 percent (D'Angio et al., 1989). Children with unfavorable histology Wilms' tumor fare less well but about half these children will be cured as well. Wilms' tumor will occur in 1 of 10,000 children. The peak age is between 2 and 3 years, and it is slightly more common in females than males. Wilms' tumor usually is symptom-free; generally a parent notes a lump or mass in a child's abdomen. Most children with Wilms' tumor are free of congenital anomalies, although children with certain anomalies such as hemihypertrophy, congenital absence of the iris, and genitourinary problems such as hypospadias are at high risk of developing Wilms' tumor (Miller, Fraumeni, & Manning, 1964). Rarely, Wilms' tumor occurs in both kidneys, and a proportion of patients with bilateral Wilms' tumor have a heritable form of the tumor. Recent research into the biology of Wilms' tumor demonstrates a consistent chromosomal abnormality in the tumor cells. In a subset of patients, the abnormality also occurs in normal tissues. It is thought that among a subset of patients, Wilms' tumor is a heritable disease. Clinical data to support this contention are still lacking; a survey of 36 Wilms' tumor survivors found 59 healthy offspring, none of whom developed Wilms' tumor (Green, Fine, & Li, 1982).

Wilms' tumor is primarily treated with chemotherapy following surgical resection. Radiation therapy is reserved for patients whose tumors are beyond the kidney at surgery or have disease which has metastasized to the chest at diagnosis. Outpatient treatment is usual. The outlook for children with Wilms' tumor is excellent.

Neuroblastoma

Neuroblastoma is one of the only pediatric neoplasms known to be associated with spontaneous regression in a small subset of patients; the rare patient with the kind of neuroblastoma which may regress is less than 1 year of age, has a small primary tumor, and does not have bone metastases (Evans, Baum, & Chard, 1981). The most common sites for neuroblastoma are the abdomen, the chest, and rarely the neck or pelvis. Early stage neuroblastoma may require nothing more than surgical excision (Matthay, Sather, Seeger, Haase, & Hammond, 1989). Unfortunately, the majority of children with neuroblastoma present with advanced disease and come to attention because the primary tumor is very large, crossing the midline and involving lymph nodes, and/or the disease has metastasized to bone, bone marrow, and, less commonly, distant lymph nodes, skin, and liver. Such children come to attention because of fevers and bone pain; they are quite ill. Children with advanced disease do poorly even with very aggressive chemotherapy and radiation therapy (even including bone marrow transplantation) (Zucker, et al., 1990). Children younger than 1 year have a better outlook than older children, even when they have advanced disease at diagnosis.

The vast difference in the outlook for children with early stage and late stage neuroblastoma has led to intensive investigation of the biology of this tumor. Many investigators feel that despite the apparent similarity of the tumor under the microscope, late and early stages of the disease are biologically separate entities rather than later stages of the same tumors (Woods, Lemieux, & Tuchman, 1992). Neuroblastoma is associated with the excretion of a measurable substance in the urine in the majority of patients. Thus screening programs for early detection of the disease are under way in Japan and Canada. Early results seem to confirm the idea that picking up early stage neuroblastoma does not necessarily lead to a decrease in the advanced tumors and that advanced and early stage neuroblastoma are biologically separate entities. Findings from these screening programs will be very important in advancing understanding of these tumors.

Bone Tumors and Soft Tissue Sarcomas

Osteosarcoma is the most common malignant bone tumor of childhood and is derived of bone tissue. Osteosarcoma occurs in the second decade and is usually associated with rapid growth spurts; on the average, patients with osteosarcoma are taller than their peers. In the past, about 10 to 20 percent of patients with osteosarcoma could be cured with surgery that completely removed the tumor, usually by amputation of the involved bone and soft tissues. The remaining patients eventually would succumb to pulmonary metastases, after apparently successful surgery. Today, with complete resection of the tumor and chemotherapy, over 75 percent of patients with osteosarcoma are cured (Jaffe, 1991). Since osteosarcoma is not very sensitive to radiation, surgery is the primary method of controlling the primary tumor. Surgery may be done immediately, but more commonly chemotherapy is given before and after definitive surgery. Although for some patients amputation is still necessary to eradicate the local tumor, for many patients advances in surgery permit a variety of limb-saving options. Patients who undergo limb-sparing surgery may be subject to a minimally higher risk of local recurrence, and, more important, they still will have functional deficits and cosmetic defects. Repeated surgery is required by many children, particularly those who are not fully grown at the time of initial surgery. The emotional effects of surgery for bone tumors, and the difference in these effects between children undergoing amputation and those undergoing alternative surgical therapies, have not been fully explored. The initial chemotherapy for osteosarcoma usually requires only 2 to 5 days of hospitalization, and ongoing therapy is given in intermittent hospitalizations. Chemotherapy for osteosarcoma is intensive, and many patients with osteosarcoma are unable to manage normal activities such as consistent school attendance during the year of therapy.

Ewing's sarcoma, which is quite rare, is the second most common primary bone tumor. Although Ewing's sarcoma occurs in bone, the cancer itself has its origin in neural tissue. Ewing's sarcoma also occurs most frequently in the second decade. The probability of 5-year relapse-free survival for localized nonpelvic Ewing's sarcoma treated with chemotherapy and effective local control is greater than 60 percent (Burgert et al., 1990). However, for those patients who come to attention because of a primary tumor in the pelvis or with pulmonary metastases, the outlook is less sanguine. For all Ewing's patients, chemotherapy is intensive, lasting for about 1 year. After the initial few courses of chemotherapy, the local tumor is treated. This treatment may be surgery, surgery and radiation therapy, or radiation therapy only, depending on the site, size, and characteristics of the initial tumor. Generally, chemotherapy is given intermittently and, as with osteosarcoma, is intensive enough to significantly interfere with school and normal activities.

Sarcomas are cancers arising in mesenchymal tissue; thus such tumors may develop anywhere in the body. Common sites are the head and neck, the extremities, and the genitourinary tract. The most common soft tissue sarcoma of childhood is rhabdomyosarcoma, accounting for 5 to 8 percent of all childhood cancer. Undifferentiated sarcomas are a rare, somewhat heterogeneous group.

Rhabdomyosarcomas are more common in males than females, and more common in white than black children. The peak incidence is at 2 to 5 years of age; about 70 percent occur before age 10. The prognosis for rhabdomyosarcoma varies significantly depending on the site of origin, the histologic subtype, the size of the primary tumor, the ability to remove the tumor surgically, and the presence or absence of metastases. However, with modern therapy consisting of surgical resection if possible, chemotherapy, and radiation therapy for incompletely removed tumors, overall survival rates of about 70 percent are expected (Mandell, 1993). Current treatment for rhabdomyosarcomas generally requires a year or more of intensive therapy, given in both the outpatient and inpatient setting.

Retinoblastoma

Retinoblastoma is a malignant cancer of the eye. Unlike most other pediatric tumors, it is often congenital. Over 80 percent of cases are recognized before 3 years of age, with a median of less than 2 years of age. It occurs in 1 of about 18,000 live births. Retinoblastoma is diagnosed most often when a child develops squinting or looses the red reflex in the eye, developing a "white pupil." Most often, the disease is localized when recognized. Treatment depends on the extent of the disease, and it may range from cryotherapy, photocoagulation, or laser therapy, which may preserve vision, to enucleation if the tumor is extensive and vision cannot be preserved. Radiation therapy and/or chemotherapy is often indicated for advanced retinoblastoma. Although rare, retinoblastoma is important because much has been learned about the genetic basis of this tumor, which has helped in the understanding of the molecular mechanisms of cancer. About 40 percent of retinoblastomas are hereditary, and in most of these cases the tumor is bilateral. In the hereditary form, each child of an affected parent has a 50 percent risk of developing the tumor. Furthermore, about 10 percent of children cured of bilateral retinoblastoma will develop osteosarcoma later in life. The gene associated with the retinoblastoma tumor is also found in some osteosarcoma tumors, thus providing information which will help us understand the linkage of these tumors (Donaldson & Egbert 1989).

Late Effects

As significant numbers of children survive cancer, the late effects of therapy become more important. In all tumors with significant cure rates, the goal of the pediatric oncologist is to cure without creating long-term disabilities and morbidities. Nonetheless, the current treatment armamentarium results in significant late effects in many patients. As we continue to cure increasing numbers of patients, we will learn more about the incidence of late effects and how to prevent them.

The most feared late effect is a second malignancy. The incidence of second malignancy is estimated at about 8 percent (Mike, Meadows, & D'Angio, 1982). The greatest risk factor for a second tumor is high doses of radiotherapy and/or high doses of the class of chemotherapy medications called alkylating agents. In addition, secondary leukemias have been associated with a class of medications called epipodophylotoxins. The risk of a secondary brain tumor is 2.3 percent in children who received cranial radiation for ALL (Albo, Miller, Leikin, Sather, & Hammond, 1985). Although these risks are far higher than desired, it is necessary to remember that the risk only exists if one survives the first malignancy.

Neuropsychological sequelae are significant late effects in children who receive radiation therapy to the cranium or chemotherapy with significant entry into the CNS. Studies have shown significant sequelae in children with ALL who have received cranial radiation; however, recent work documents important sequelae in children treated for ALL with chemotherapy alone (see Mulhern, Chapter 5, this volume). The patients who are at most risk for neuropsychological sequelae are those treated for brain tumors with high doses of radiation to the CNS. The younger the age at treatment and the higher the dose of radiation, the higher the risk. The neuropsychological sequelae of children treated for extracranial solid tumors have not been carefully investigated. On the surface, cognitive and neurologic function appears normal in these patients. However, further investigations are warranted to determine if this indeed is the case.

Loss of fertility is an important late effect for patients who have received radiation which involves the ovaries or testicles or who have received certain classes of chemotherapy, particularly alkylating agents. Many children treated for leukemia will not have received these agents and will be fertile. However, most children with solid tumors will have received alkylating agents and consequently many will be infertile. Males are more likely to be rendered infertile than females, although it has been noted that women who survive cancer may have an earlier menopause, and thus may have a narrower window for procreation than their peers (Stillman et al., 1981). Although some physicians assure patients who do not receive alkylating agents that they will be fertile, recent reports demonstrate that other drugs may also be associated with infertility (Damewood & Grochow, 1986). Thus care in counseling at diagnosis is important. Many pediatric oncologists fail to give adolescent boys the option of sperm banking before starting therapy and perhaps the feasibility of this option for more patients should be explored. Survivors of cancer who have children generally have healthy children; the risk of most birth defects is not significantly greater compared to healthy individuals in most published series (Blatt, Mulvihill, Ziegler, Young, & Poplack, 1980).

Other treatment-related late effects include growth problems and disturbances in organ function due to specific chemotherapeutic agents. For example, kidney dysfunction and hearing loss may occur as a consequence of treatment with cis-platin, heart failure may occur after prolonged treatment with the class of medications called anthracyclines, and pulmonary problems may occur after treatment with bleomycin. Most patients do not have serious sequelae, but the incidence may be underestimated by inadequate follow-up. Children who survive cancer must be carefully monitored for late effects throughout their life span. Coordinated efforts to understand and to prevent late effects is critical, and many institutions have started "late follow-up" clinics to meet the needs of cancer survivors.

Another significant late effect to be countenanced is the stigma of being a cancer survivor, which may have ramifications in school admissions, admission to national armed service, and employment opportunities. Significant problems obtaining health, life, and disability insurance exist for cancer survivors. These late effects are only now surfacing and must be considered and countered by physicians and patients as well as governing agencies (see Kupst, Chapter 2, this volume). Despite the unfortunate specter of late effects, the fact that about 60 percent of children with cancer survive, and most survive with little functional disability, is a source of satisfaction for all those who care for children with cancer and their families.

References

Albo, V., Miller, D., Leikin, S., Sather, H., & Hammond, D. (1985). Nine brain tumors as a late effect in children "cured" of acute lymphoblastic leukemia from a single protocol study. *Proceedings of the American Society of Clinical Oncology, 4,* 172.

Anderson, J. R., Wilson, J. F., Jenkin, D. T., Meadows, A. T., Kersey, J., Chilcote, R. R., Coccia, P., Exelby, P., Kushner, J., Siegel, S., & Hammond, D. (1983). The results of a randomized trial comparing a 4-drug regimen (COMP) with a 10-drug regimen (LSA2-L2). *New England Journal of Medicine, 308,* 559–565.

Blatt, J., Mulvihill, J. J., Ziegler, J. L., Young, R. C., & Poplack, D. G. (1980). Pregnancy outcome following cancer chemotherapy. *American Journal of Medicine, 69,* 828–832.

Bleyer, W. A. (1990). Acute lymphoblastic leukemia in children, advances and prospectus. *Cancer, 65,* 689–695.

Bleyer, A. W., & Poplack, D. G. (1985). Prophylaxis and treatment of leukemia in the central nervous system and other sanctuaries. *Seminars in Oncology, 12,* 131–148.

Bleyer, W. A. (1988). Central nervous system leukemia. *Pediatric Clinics of North America, 35,* 789–814.

Burgert, O. E., Nesbitt, M. E., Garnsey, L. A., Gehan, E. A., Hermann, J., Vietti, T. A., Cangir, A., Tefft, M., Evans, R., Thomas, P., Aslin, F., Kissane, J. M., Pritchard, D. J., Neff, J., Makley, J. T., & Gilula, L. (1990). Multimodal therapy for the management of nonpelvic, localized Ewing's sarcoma of bone: Intergroup study IESS-II. *Journal of Clinical Oncology, 8,* 1514–1524.

Butterini, A., Rivera, G. K., Bortin, M. M., & Gale, R. P. (1987). Which treatment for childhood acute lymphoblastic leukemia in second remission? *Lancet, 1,* 429–432.

Clavell, L. A., Gelber, R. D., Cohen, H. A., Hitchcock-Bryan, S., Cassady, R. J., Tarbell, N. A., Blattner, S. A., Tantravhi, R., Leavitt, P., & Sallan, S. E. (1986). Four-agent induction and intensive asparaginase therapy for treatment of childhood acute lymphoblastic leukemia. *New England Journal of Medicine, 315,* 657–663.

Cohen, B. H., & Rothner D. A. (1989). Incidence, types, and management of cancer in patients with neurofibromatosis. *Oncology, 3,* 23–38.

Corr, C. A., & Corr, D. M. (1985). Pediatric hospice care. *Pediatrics, 76,* 774–780.

Damewood, M. D., & Grochow, L. B. (1986). Prospects for fertility after chemotherapy or radiation for neoplastic disease. *Fertility and Sterility, 45,* 443–459.

D'Angio, G. J., Breslow, N., Beckwith, B. J., Evans, A. E., Baum, E., Delorimer, A., Fernbach, D., Hrabovsky, E., Jones, B., Kelalis, P., Othersen, H. B., Tefft, M., & Thomas, P. R. M. (1989). Treatment of Wilms' tumor: Results of the third national Wilms' tumor study. *Cancer, 64,* 349–360.

Donaldson, S. S., & Egbert, P. R. (1989). Retinoblastoma. In P. A. Pizzo & D. G. Poplack (Eds.), *Principles and practice of pediatric oncology (pp. 555–568).* Philadelphia: Lippincott.

Donaldson, S. S., & Link, M. P. (1987). Combined modality treatment with low-dose radiation and MOPP chemotherapy for children with Hodgkin's disease. *Journal of Clinical Oncology, 5,* 742–749.

Draper, G. J., Heaf, M. M., & Kennier-Wilson, L. M. (1977). Occurrence of childhood cancers among sibs and estimation of familial risks. *Journal of Medical Genetics, 44,* 81–90.

Duffner, P. K., Cohen M. E., & Freeman, A. A. (1985). Pediatric brain tumors: An overview. *Ca—A Cancer Journal for Clinicians, 35,* 287–301.

Evans, A. E., Baum, E., & Chard, R. (1981). Do infants with stage IV-S neuroblastoma need treatment? *Archives of Disease in Childhood, 56,* 271–274.

Evans, A. W., Gilbert, E. S., & Zandstra, R. (1970). The increasing evidence of central nervous system leukemia in children. *Cancer, 26,* 404–409.

Fletcher, J. C., van Eys, J., & Dorn, L. D. (1989). Ethical considerations in pediatric oncology. In P. A. Pizzo & D. G. Poplack (Eds.), *Principles and practice of pediatric oncology (pp. 309–320).* Philadelphia: Lippincott.

Flores, L. E., Williams, D. L., Bell, B. A., O'Brien, M., & Ragab, A. H. (1986). Delay in diagnosis of pediatric brain tumors. *American Journal of Diseases of Children, 140,* 684–686.

Gaynon, P. S. (1992). Childhood leukemia and lymphoma. *Current Opinion in Pediatrics, 4,* 118–125.

Green, D. M., Fine, N. E., & Li, F. P. (1982). Offspring of patients treated for unilateral Wilms tumor in childhood. *Cancer, 49,* 2285–2288.

Greenberg, R. S., & Shuster, J. L. (1985). Epidemiology of cancer in children. *Epidemiology Reviews, 7,* 22–48.

Harvey, E. B., Boice, J. D., Honbeyman, M., Flannery, J. T. (1985). Prenatal X-ray exposure and childhood cancer in twins. *New England Journal of Medicine, 312,* 541–545.

Horowitz, M. E., & Pizzo, P. A. (1990). Cancer in the child infected with human immunodeficiency virus. *Journal of Pediatrics, 116,* 730–731.

Jaffe, D., Fleisher, G., & Grosflam, G. (1985). Detection of cancer in the pediatric emergency department. *Pediatric Emergency Care,* 1(11), 11–15.

Jaffe, N. (1991). Osteosarcoma. *Pediatric Reviews, 12,* 333–343.

Kaye, S. A., Robison, L. L., Smithson, W. A., Gunderson, P., King, F. L., & Neglia, J. P. (1991). Maternal reproductive history and birth characteristics in childhood acute lymphoblastic leukemia. *Cancer, 68,* 1352–1355.

Kinlen, L. J., Clarke, K., & Hudson, C. (1990). Evidence from population mixing in

British new towns, 1946–1985 of an infective basis for childhood leukemia. *Lancet, 336,* 577–582.

Leikin, S. L. (1985). Beyond proforma consent for childhood cancer research. *Journal of Clinical Oncology, 3,* 420–428.

Lerman, C., Rimer, B. K., & Engstrom, P. F. (1991). Cancer risk notification: Psychosocial and ethical implications. *Journal of Clinical Oncology, 9,* 1275–1282.

Levy, M. H. (1985). Pain management in advanced cancer. *Seminars in Oncology, 12,* 394–410.

Li, F. P., & Fraumeni, J. F., Jr. (1982). Prospective study of a family cancer syndrome. *Journal of the American Medical Association, 247,* 2692–2694.

Link, M. P., Donaldson, S. A., Berard, C. W., Shuster, J. J., & Murphy, S. A. (1990). Results of treatment of childhood localized non-Hodgkin's lymphoma with combination chemotherapy with or without radiotherapy. *New England Journal of Medicine, 322,* 1169–1174.

Macahon, B., & Levy, M. A. (1964). Prenatal origin of childhood leukemia: Evidence from twins. *New England Journal of Medicine, 270,* 1082–1085.

Maity, A., Goldwein, J. W., Lange, B., & D'Angio, G. J. (1992). Comparison of high-dose and low-dose radiation with and without chemotherapy for children with Hodgkin's disease: An analysis of the experience at the Children's Hospital of Philadelphia and the Hospital of the University of Pennsylvania. *Journal of Clinical Oncology, 10,* 929–936.

Malkin, D., Li, F., Strong, L. C., Fraumeni, J. F., Nelson, C. E., Kin, D. H., Kassel, J., Gryker, M. A., Bischof, F. Z., Tainsky, M. A., & Friend, S. A. (1990). Germline p53 mutations in a familial syndrome of breast cancer, sarcomas, and other neoplasms. *Science, 250,* 1233–1238.

Mandell, L. R. (1993). Ongoing progress in the treatment of childhood rhabdomyosarcoma. *Oncology, 7,* 71–90.

Martinson, I. M., Moldow, D. G., Armstrong, G. D., Henry, W. F., Nesbitt, M. E., & Kersey, J. H. (1986). Home care for children dying of cancer. *Research Nursing Health, 9,* 11–16.

Matthay, K. K., Sather, H. N., Seeger, R. C., Haase, G. M., & Hammond, G. D. (1989). Excellent outcome of stage II neuroblastoma is independent of residual disease and radiotherapy. *Journal of Clinical Oncology, 7,* 236–244.

Meadows, A. T., Krejmas, N. L., & Belasco, J. B. (1980). The medical cost of cure: Sequelae in survivors of childhood cancer. In J. van Eys & M. P. Sullivan (Eds.), *Status of the curability of childhood cancers* (pp. 263–268). New York: Raven Press.

Mike, V., Meadows, A. T., & D'Angio, G. J. (1982). Incidence of second malignant neoplasms in children. Results of an international study. *Lancet, 2,* 1326–1331.

Miller, R. W. (1967). Persons with exceptionally high risk of leukemia. *Cancer Research, 27,* 2420–2423.

Miller, R. W. (1970). Neoplasia and Down's syndrome. *Annals of the New York Academy of Science, 171,* 637–644.

Miller, R. W. (1971). Deaths from childhood leukemia and solid tumors among twins and other sibs in the United States, 1960–67. *Journal of the National Cancer Institute, 46,* 203–209.

Miller, R. W., Fraumeni, J. F., Jr., & Manning, M. D. (1964). Association of Wilms' tumor with aniridia, hemihypertrophy, and other congenital malformations. *New England Journal of Medicine, 270,* 922–927.

Miser, A. W., Dothage, J. A., Wesley, R. A., & Miser, J. S. (1987). The prevalence of pain in a pediatric and adult cancer population. *Pain, 29,* 73–83.

Miser, A. W., McCalla, J., Dothage, J. A., Wesley, M., & Miser, J. S. (1987). Pain as a presenting symptom in children and young adults with newly diagnosed malignancy. *Pain, 29,* 85–90.

Müller-Weihrich, S., Henze, G., & Odenwald, E. & Riehm, H. (1985). BFM trials for childhood non-Hodgkin's lymphomas. In F. Cavalli, G. Bonadonna, & M. Rosencweig (Eds.), *Malignant lymphomas and Hodgkin's disease: Experimental and therapeutic advances* (pp. 603–642). Norwell, MA: Martinus Nijhoff.

Mulvihill, J. J. (1989). Clinical genetics of pediatric cancer. In P. A. Pizzo & D. G. Poplack (Eds.), *Principles and practice of pediatric oncology* (pp. 19–37). Philadelphia: Lippincott.

Niemeyer, C. M., Hitchcock-Bryan, S., & Sallan, S. E. (1985). Comparative analysis of treatment programs for childhood acute lymphoblastic leukemia. *Seminars in Oncology, 12,* 122–130.

Nitschke, R., Humphrey B., Sexauer, C. L., Catron, B., Wunder, S., & Jay, S. (1982). Therapeutic choices made by patients with end stage cancer. *Journal of Pediatrics, 101,* 471–476.

Poplack, D. G. (1989). Acute lymphoblastic leukemia. In P. A. Pizzo & D. G. Poplack (Eds.), *Principles and practice of pediatric oncology* (pp. 323–366). Philadelphia: Lippincott.

Rubenstein, A. (1986). Pediatric AIDS. *Current Problems in Pediatics, 16,* 631–409.

Savitz, D. A., & Chen J. (1990). Parental occupation and childhood cancer: Review of epidemiologic studies. *Environmental Health Perspectives, 88,* 325–337.

Savitz, D. A., John, E. M., & Kleckner, R. C. (1990). Magnetic field exposure from electric appliances and childhood cancer. *American Journal of Epidemiology, 131,* 763–775.

Schechter, N. L., Allen, A., & Hanson, K. (1986). Status of pediatric pain control: A comparison of hospital analgesic usage in children and adults. *Pediatrics, 77,* 11–15.

Stillman, R. J., Schinfeld, J. S., Schiff, I., Gelber, R. D., Greenberger, J., Larson, M., Jaffee, N., & Li, F. P. (1981). Ovarian failure in long-term survivors of childhood malignancy. *American Journal of Obstetrics and Gynecology, 139,* 62–66.

Twycross, R. G. (1984). Incidence of pain. *Clinical Oncology, 3,* 5–15.

Vigliani, E. C., & Sarta G. (1964). Benzene and leukemia. *New England Journal of Medicine, 271,* 872–876.

Weinberg, K. I., & Parkman R. B. (1989). Interface between immunodeficiency and pediatric cancer. In P. A. Pizzo & D. G. Poplack (Eds.), *Principles and practice of pediatric oncology.* Philadelphia: Lippincott.

Woods, W. G., Lemieux, B., & Tuchman, M. (1992). Neuroblastoma represents distinct clinical entities: A review and perspective from the Quebec Neuroblastoma Screening Project. *Pediatrics, 89,* 114–118.

Young, J. L., Ries, L. G., Silverberg, E., Horm, J. W., & Miller, R. W. (1986). Cancer incidence, survival and mortality for children younger than 15 years. *Cancer, 58,* 598–602.

Yunis, J. J. (1986). Chromosomal rearrangements, genes, fragile sites in cancer: Clinical and biologic implications. In V. T. De Vita, S. Hellman, & S. Rosenberg (Eds.), *Important advnces in oncology* (pp. 93–128). Philadelphia: Lippincott.

Zucker, J. M., Bernard, J. L., Philip, T., Gentet, J. C., Michon, J., & Bouffet, E. (1990). High dose chemotherapy with BMT as consolidation treatment in neuroblastoma: An unselected group of patients re-visited with a median follow-up of 55 months after BMT. *Proceedings of the American Society of Clinical Oncology, 9,* 294.

2

Coping with Pediatric Cancer: Theoretical and Research Perspectives

MARY JO KUPST

This chapter examines the concept of coping as it pertains to theory and research in pediatric cancer. Over the past 30 years psychosocial functioning in children with pediatric cancer and their families has been the subject of a significant number of studies. Since the 1960s there have been over 200 psychosocial studies of coping, adjustment, or adaptation to pediatric cancer. Most of these have been more concerned with description than with theoretical perspectives or hypothesis testing. Some researchers have used elements of one or more coping theories, but, as in Harper's (1991) review of paradigms in chronic illness, there is a notable lack of theory-driven research in pediatric cancer. Few investigators have explicitly identified a theory or paradigm of coping that guides them in their work, and even fewer have provided a link between theory and research.

It can be argued that the field is still in a descriptive phase and that a theory of how individuals cope with pediatric cancer is premature. However, each study of coping with pediatric cancer proceeds from basic assumptions that affect the choice of research question, methodology employed, and interpretation of results. Even in studies with no explicit theoretical orientation, psychological functioning is defined by the variables selected (e.g., behavior problems, competence), which provide some clues about the investigator's orientation. For example, "adjustment" is the term of choice for those with a traditional child psychiatric perspective, while the term "coping" tends to be used by those who work with nonclinical populations. Those with an intrapsychic orientation may be more interested in personality correlates of coping, and those with a behavioral orientation may be more interested in the reduction of distress behaviors.

Some psychosocial research has gone beyond description and has tested hypotheses about the relationship of adaptation to selected personal and environmental variables. In addition, there are intervention studies that build on previous descriptions and test hypotheses. The problem, then, is less an absence of theory in psychological research in pediatric cancer than a variety of orientations which are frequently fragmented, loosely linked to research, and incomplete.

This chapter considers the primary orientations that have been used in psychological research with pediatric cancer patients and their families. It is not a review of coping paradigms used in clinical work, of coping theory in general, of coping with chronic illness, or of coping in adults who have cancer. A description of these models will help explain the various ways that people in this field view children with cancer and their families and how these orientations affect research and clinical applications.

Basic Assumptions

Several underlying assumptions guide psychological research in pediatric cancer.

1. *Assumptions about the population of children with cancer and their families.* According to a pathology-oriented model, children with cancer are at risk for significant psychological problems. Within this model, then, studies are designed to assess the frequency of psychological problems such as depression, anxiety, and family dysfunction, using common clinical instruments such as personality tests and mental status interviews. Children and families are compared to "normal" (nonclinical) families as well as to test norms.

In a normative-based model, children with cancer and their families are viewed as normal individuals who are facing a series of stressful situations (Kellerman, 1980; Spinetta, 1977). Here the emphasis is on the process of coping with an abnormal situation. Within this model (e.g., Stein & Jessop, 1982), children and families are viewed as a sample of the population of patients with chronic illness and their families. In a more specific approach (Rolland, 1984), cancer patients would be seen as a population to be compared with each other and typical norms would not be relevant or applicable. An even more specific approach would differentiate among types of pediatric cancers, such as children with acute lymphoblastic leukemia, who have different treatment demands and late effects than do children with brain tumors.

2. *Assumptions about subjects.* In early studies, mothers were the primary subjects, but more recently children with cancer, their fathers, siblings, or the entire family have been subjects. Some studies include peers, various comparison groups, the extended family, or members of social networks, depending on the objective.

3. *Assumptions about the situation.* Some studies focus on one particular phase of the experience of pediatric cancer, such as diagnosis, early treatment, long-term survival, dying, or death. Frequently these are cross-sectional studies, although they may include several measurements within that time frame. Some studies narrow the focus even further, for example, to specific treatment procedures like chemotherapy, radiation, or surgery. The choice of situation is an important consideration because it determines the focus of coping within the subjects' experiences of having cancer.

4. *Assumptions about the impact of the situation.* Many studies tacitly assume

equal impact of particular situations across all subjects. Other studies, particularly those that assess predictors of coping, acknowledge the role of individual differences in terms of the subjects' antecedent conditions (personal and environmental variables) and/or their appraisal and interpretation of the situation. Such studies examine the impact of the situation in light of the individual's history, current coping capabilities, or emotional state.

5. *Assumptions about the process of coping.* Retrospective or cross-sectional studies frequently present coping as static and concerned with the occasion at hand. Prospective, longitudinal studies, on the other hand, treat coping as a dynamic process that occurs over time; they are concerned with changes in subjects' coping strategies and adaptation.

6. *Assumptions about the correlates of outcome.* Studies that assess correlates of coping, adaptation, or adjustment generally proceed from assumptions about the importance of these correlates as predictors of coping. Some focus on personal variables such as personality, intelligence, or preferred coping style; others focus on environmental variables such as family functioning, concurrent stresses, or socioeconomic status. Still others focus on the coping strategies used in response to the stressor and the ways that they affect adaptation.

7. *Assumptions about the definition of coping.* Recent reviews (Compas, Worsham, & Ey, 1992; Kupst, 1992) of theories of coping indicate there is no universally accepted definition of coping.

Coping Definitions

In everyday life, coping, adaptation, and adjustment mean the same thing: how well a person deals with some aspect of his or her environment that is particularly challenging to that person's resources. However, as a result of increased interest over the past 30 years in coping theory and research, useful distinctions have been made among these terms. Adjustment is a broad term describing a person's accommodation to or compliance with environmental demands, such as school, work, marriage, peers, or having a serious illness. When used as an outcome variable, adjustment is operationally defined according to various tests and rating scales.

Adaptation, a term derived from biology, means "striving toward acceptable compromise with the environment" (White, 1974, p. 52). According to this definition, adaptation is a more active process than adjustment (Harper, 1991) and implies that the person can act upon the environment as well as merely "fit in." While this definition connotes a dynamic process as one is never fully adapted to an ever-changing environment, it is used in many studies as an outcome or end point, the result of the adaptive strategies one uses. For White (1974), these include defenses, mastery (in which one successfully meets task demands), and coping (which is "an ongoing adaptive process used when the task is difficult," p. 49).

Similarly, Murphy (1974) viewed adaptation as a broad hierarchical concept, with reflexes and instincts at the bottom. Next came coping, which was "all those efforts to deal with the environmental pressures that could not be handled by reflexes or organized skills, but involved struggles, trials, persistent focused energy directed towards a goal'' (p. 71). Mastery, for Murphy, was the result of effective coping efforts, followed by competence, which resulted from cumulative mastery.

The most commonly cited theory of coping was formulated by Lazarus (1991), who defines coping as "cognitive and behavioral efforts to manage specific external or internal demands (and conflicts between them) that are appraised as taxing or exceeding the resources of the person'' (p. 112). Coping is a process that leads to adaptation in three domains: functioning in work and social life, life satisfaction, and physical health.

For these theorists, coping is equivalent to the efforts one makes to deal with situational demands. Thus coping strategy is an intervening variable between stress and adaptation. Although this currently is the most frequent use of the term coping, it also has been defined as a dispositional style or trait (Loevinger, 1976; Vaillant, 1977). The trait definition has been criticized as having low predictive value in terms of actual coping (Lazarus & Folkman 1984); however, it is still used in studies of how people typically cope (repressors, avoiders, information seekers). Still others (e.g., Haan, 1977) define coping as an evaluative function, making coping a more desirable process than defense or fragmentation. In this way, coping can be used as an outcome variable (as in good vs. poor coping) and is frequently equated with adaptation.

How coping is defined determines how it is measured. When coping is defined as a style or a strategy, it is measured in terms of classifications based upon either self-report measures or observations of actual behaviors. When coping is defined as adjustment, it is measured by clinical observations, interviews, standardized psychological tests, or nonreactive measures such as school attendance. When coping is defined as adaptation, it is measured by standardized tests and scales, by scales tailored to more specific situational criteria, or by tasks.

An overview of common paradigmatic models used in coping research with pediatric cancer patients and families follows. These models are not necessarily mutually exclusive, and some researchers may use more than one orientation.

Theoretical Perspectives
Grief and Loss Model

Coping with pediatric cancer has been a topic of considerable research and some theory over the past 30 years, beginning with clinical observation studies (Binger et al., 1969; Bozeman, Orbach, & Sutherland, 1955; Chodoff, Friedman, & Hamburg, 1964; Friedman, Chodoff, Mason, & Hamburg, 1963; Futterman & Hoffman, 1973; Natterson & Knudson, 1960; Townes, Wold & Holmes, 1974). When these studies were conducted, the prognosis for pediatric cancer was poor. For example, there was a less than 10 percent survival rate for acute lymphoblastic leukemia (ALL), the most common form of pediatric cancer. Therefore, most studies at that time employed a grief and loss paradigm (Lindemann, 1944) in which the parents' role was to prepare for the eventual death of their child (anticipatory mourning).

This paradigm focused on the parents' stages of grieving (Chodoff et al., 1964). Parents typically were shocked or stunned to learn of the diagnosis of pediatric cancer. As their child entered treatment, parents began to accept the illness and probability of death intellectually but not emotionally. The most common grief reactions included isolation of affect, denial, flight into activity, and the search for meaning. With time and decline in their child's condition, more acute emotional reactions were displayed, such as anger, blaming, guilt, and somatic distress. Gradually, if these feelings were resolved, parents would be able to participate in the care of their child, maintain emotional equilibrium, come to an affirmation of life rather than a denial of death, and reorganize their lives. Intervention typically was based on Lindemann's crisis-intervention model in which the person is encouraged to do the "work of worrying" in order to resolve his or her grief (Janis, 1958). An optimal period for anticipatory mourning was thought to be at least 4 months prior to the child's death (Natterson & Knudson, 1960). Later, Kaplan, Grobstein, and Smith's (1976) work incorporated this orientation and found that 70 percent of families experienced significant marital, family, health, or functional problems. Koocher & O'Malley's (1981) work with children and adolescents who were long-term survivors of cancer also included some of the basic tenets of anticipatory grief along with other orientations. Most of these investigators did not define explicitly what they meant by coping or adaptation, but Chodoff et al. (1964) used Murphy's earlier (1962) definition: "The sum total of all the strategies employed by an individual to deal with a significant threat to his psychological stability."

In summary, the grief and loss paradigm in terms of a child with cancer and the family included the following assumptions: (1) the diagnosis of pediatric leukemia meant inevitable death for the child and constituted a severe crisis for the family; (2) parents could be expected to go through predictable stages of grief, which, if unresolved, would result in serious dysfunction; (3) with a focus on greater or lesser degrees of pathology, most of the families would exhibit psychosocial problems, and (4) because problems were expected, intensive psychosocial intervention with the family would be necessary to help them work through their grief.

Critique. Although these studies made significant initial contributions to understanding how parents respond during critical phases of their child's cancer, by today's standards they lacked rigor. Later studies called into question the universality of predictable stages of grief or coping (Kupst & Schulman, 1988; Kupst et al., 1984). Despite the positive focus of some (Chodoff et al., 1964; Futterman & Hoffman, 1973), most of these studies treated the diagnosis and treatment of pediatric cancer as uniformly distressing and concluded that many families were left with serious psychosocial sequelae. Given that most of these children died, these observations were perhaps valid for that time. On the other hand, the choice of the grief and loss model led to an expectation of emotional problems and little opportunity to discover healthy forms of coping. The typical methodology in these studies included clinical observations and judgments made by staff, usually without the use of standardized instruments or information from other sources for validation. In addition, the primary subjects of study were not the children with cancer but their parents, usually their mothers.

While the anticipatory grief model is still relevant in cases of relapse and death, it is not comprehensive enough to understand how children and families cope with 2 to 3 years of intensive treatment, the late effects of treatment, and coping with survival. As children and adolescents with cancer began living longer and even being cured, the focus shifted to them as primary subjects. When more clinical knowledge was gained and more systematic studies began to emerge (Kellerman, 1980; Koocher & O'Malley, 1981; Schulman & Kupst, 1980; Spinetta & Deasy-Spinetta, 1981) it became clearer that a pathological orientation did not fit. Instead, these families appeared to be basically normal people who, while they might experience significant stressful situations and losses, did not develop serious psychopathology. Thus studies shifted from focusing on pathology to coping and adaptation.

Stress and Coping Model

This model was developed from the work of Lazarus (1966, 1991; Lazarus & Folkman, 1984). The concept of coping as a process has been emphasized by several investigators (Chodoff et al., 1964; Futterman & Hoffman, 1973; Spinetta, 1977) and has been particularly important in understanding how people experience and exhibit intense emotional reactions and are still able to deal effectively with stresses. Taken in the context of a stressful situation and viewed over time, upsets and suffering are seen as necessary elements of the coping experience. In this model, emphasis is placed on situational characteristics (coping tasks) and what people do to deal with them (coping strategies). Coping is not a state or a disposition; it is what one actually does in a specific situation. It is dynamic and changeable, is separate from adaptation, and can be a mediating variable.

Several theorists have been involved in classifying different types of coping strategies (Lazarus & Folkman, 1984; Moos & Billings, 1982; Weisman & Worden, 1976). For example, problem-focused coping (such as seeking information, seeking social support, planful problem solving) is action-centered and applicable when one sees the possibility of changing a situation. Emotion-focused coping (such as denial, avoidance, minimization, distancing, positive reappraisal) is applicable when one sees no possibility of changing the situation and is designed to change the way one attends to stress or interprets it. The assessment of coping strategies varies from paper and pencil measures, such as the Ways of Coping Scale (Folkman & Lazarus, 1988), the Kidcope (Spirito, Stark, & Williams, 1988), the Coping/Health Inventory for Parents (McCubbin, McCubbin, Nevin, & Cauble, 1981) to ratings based on systematic behavioral observations of children and their families and to self-reports in interviews.

According to Lazarus, coping strategies are not, in themselves, good or bad. Instead, they are appraised in light of the outcome and in relation to adaptation in specific situations. Thus defenses can be adaptive or maladaptive, such as when patients and families "deny" the possibility of death in order to begin treatment. Coping strategies are effective when they help achieve certain tasks. Lazarus's major coping tasks have been adapted by Spinetta (1977) and Koocher & O'Malley (1981) for use with pediatric cancer patients and their families. The child and family must learn (1) to manage distress; (2) to maintain a sense of personal worth; (3) to maintain rewarding interpersonal relationships; and (4) to use available resources to meet the specific situational tasks. Similarly, in Kupst and Schulman's (1988) longitudinal study of family coping with pediatric leukemia, adaptational tasks for family members, as measured by the Family Coping Scale (Hurwitz, Kaplan, & Kaiser, 1962), at each phase were (1) an understanding of the realities and implications of the disease, treatment, and long-term survival; (2) management of emotional reactions; and (3) capability to (a) deal with medical issues, (b) deal with other responsibilities and activities, and (c) use available resources effectively. Coping tasks can also be more specific—for example, to lower the level of procedural distress, or to develop more effective social skills.

There are several basic assumptions to this model. One is that the expected outcome is adaptation rather than psychopathology. While outcome is important, the primary interest is in the efforts of children and their families to cope with the stressors associated with pediatric cancer. Coping is not a trait or a disposition but what one actually does. Coping is not static but a process that is enacted over time. Coping is viewed in the context of the situation and the particular demands it places on individuals. This orientation emphasizes individual differences in appraisal and choice of strategies. The coping strategies used by children and their families are not in themselves good or bad, but they are effective if they lead to a desirable outcome.

Critique. This orientation allows the investigator to study coping in a specific and empirical manner by delineating coping tasks and strategies that can be applied to various situations in the pediatric cancer experience. The nonpathological orientation is more appropriate and is supported in various studies (e.g., Kellerman, Zeltzer, Ellenberg, Dash, & Rigler, 1980; Kupst & Schulman, 1988; Noll, LeRoy, Bukowski, Rogosch, & Kulkarni, 1991; Spinetta & Deasy-Spinetta, 1981; Susman, Hollenbeck, Nannis, & Strope, 1980; Worchel et al., 1988). Much of the research has involved the classification of coping strategies used by children and their parents.

While more descriptive information about coping strategies in certain populations and situations in pediatric cancer is needed, classification alone is not enough. More needs to be done to validate these strategies in terms of their relationships to actual behaviors (e.g., do responses to the Ways of Coping Scale correlate with observable behaviors in the oncology clinic?). In addition, we need to know which strategies actually work, for whom, in what situations, and at what times. For example, one study (Kupst, Mudd, & Schulman, 1990) found that avoidance behaviors in children seen in an oncology clinic were associated with lower evaluative coping scores. This relationship was interpreted to mean that avoidance typically does not work well in procedural distress situations. It is tempting to assume that because studies have found relationships between coping strategies and adaptation, intervention studies can promote these strategies, but some strategies may not be helpful for everyone. For example, if searching for information is used as a strategy by those whose coping style is avoiding, more anxiety may result. In addition, what works at one time may not work later. For example, focusing on procedural details at the beginning of treatment may be helpful, but continued focus during long-term remission may hinder one from getting on with the rest of his or her life. Studies of coping need to address these issues as well as examine individual differences, such as appraisal and personality, in order to advance our understanding of the relationships between coping strategies and adaptation.

Developmental Model

This model, frequently used in combination with other models, acknowledges the necessity of identifying problems and coping strategies and emphasizes that children with cancer are normal people undergoing stress. It recognizes that although a child's developmental course may be altered by the disease, basic normal developmental processes continue in spite of the disease (Spinetta, 1974; Susman, 1980). The basic tenet of this model is that researchers must consider the developmental level of the child and that one must consider the child as more than just a "cancer patient" (Rowland, 1989). Susman, Hollenbeck, Nannis, and Strope (1980) systematically observed specific behaviors in children undergoing long-term hospitalization in a laminar airflow room as a method promoted by this model. The developmental model is also notable in several systematic observational studies of children undergoing aversive medical procedures, such as the work of Kellerman, Katz, and Jay (Jay & Elliott, 1990; Jay, Ozolins, Elliott, & Caldwell, 1983; Katz, Kellerman, & Siegel, 1980). Interventions are aimed at maximizing the development of the child instead of remediating pathology (Susman et al., 1980).

The basic assumptions of this model are (1) that the impact of pediatric cancer must be considered in light of the child's developmental level; (2) in addition to the impact of cancer on the child, the child's normal developmental issues and needs, such as school, peer relationships, and psychosocial development, must be acknowledged; and (3) that a process approach is necessary (Drotar, 1991). In many of these studies, coping per se is not defined except by the behaviors exhibited in response to a stressful situation. A decrease in undesirable behaviors or an increase in desirable behaviors may be assumed to be a positive indicator of adjustment and adaptation.

Critique. This model is valuable for understanding how a child copes with cancer, as there are significant differences based on a child's developmental level. For example, very young children perceive death in different ways than do adolescents (Bluebond-Langer, 1978; Spinetta, 1974); they have different concepts of illness (Bibace & Walsh, 1980); and younger children are often given less disease-related information than older children (Claflin & Barbarin, 1991). Coping strategies may also differ depending upon developmental level (Band, 1990). Some investigators have focused on specific age groups, such as school age (Spinetta & Deasy-Spinetta, 1981; Spirito et al., 1990) or adolescents (Blotcky, Cohen, Conaster, & Klopovich, 1985; Kazak & Meadows, 1989; Kellerman et al., 1980; Zeltzer, 1980). Frequently there are too few subjects in a given institution to stratify them into age groups to conduct comparative analyses. More often children's responses are compared to age norms and given standardized scores that are aggregated in the analysis. There is a need for a greater developmental focus to describe the way different age groups cope with cancer and to provide effective interventions. However, this requires adequate sample sizes that can be attained only if investigators pool their data across institutions.

Cognitive-Behavioral Model

This model is derived from the field of pediatric psychology and is generally espoused by those who are more interested in intervention in pediatric cancer (e.g., Carpenter, 1990; Dahlquist, Gil, Armstrong, Ginsberg, & Jones, 1985; Hilgard & LeBaron, 1982; Jacobsen, Manne, Gorfinkle, & Schorr, 1990; Jay et al., 1983; Katz et al., 1980; Redd, 1989; Zeltzer & LeBaron, 1982). The diagnosis and treatment of pediatric cancer includes conditions such as invasive procedures, negative side effects of treatment, and social changes, to which children and their parents respond in ways that typically avoid or lessen the impact of noxious stimuli. Coping mechanisms that have been effective in other situations often do not work. Thus common problems such as anxiety, distress behavior, pain, nausea and vomiting, anticipatory reactions, and social withdrawal can be understood from this model, and interventions can be designed to alter the inappropriate reinforcement of problem behaviors. Coping in this framework is defined as contingent responses to reduce distress, pain, anxiety, and so on. Armstrong (1992) has expanded this definition to include anticipation of problems. Interventions include systematic desensitization and arousal reduction, including distraction, relaxation, hypnosis, guided imagery, providing information, behavioral rehearsal, and modeling. Some investigators (Jay & Elliott, 1990; Jay et al., 1983) have combined several modalities into a comprehensive package that also might include, as a preventive measure, stress inoculation programs to new patients and their families.

As in the stress and coping model, the assumptions of this model are that children with cancer and their parents are essentially normal people in an abnormal situation (Armstrong, 1992). Studies using this model are concerned not about degree of pathology but instead about how well one meets the criteria for successful coping. Thus for children with cancer success could be pain reduction, lowered anxiety, or acquisition of social skills. Subjects are usually the children with cancer, although parents are sometimes studied as well, for example, to determine whether anxious parents contribute to their child's procedural anxiety. The impact of a given situation (e.g., bone marrow aspirations) is assumed to be similar for all children, but the subjects may vary in the intensity and type of reactions.

Methodology varies from single-subject studies involving traditional behavioral assessment to combining data from groups of subjects. Outcome data are generally in the form of frequencies of behavior, and some well-validated and reliable behavior scales are available (Jay et al., 1983; Katz et al., 1980).

Critique. Concepts such as pain and distress, as well as specific techniques such as relaxation and desensitization, are operationalized and quantifiable. The impact of the intervention, therefore, can be measured and replicated. In addition, this model lends itself to practical applications in pediatric cancer which lessen pain and discomfort and which improve the quality of life for these children. Some have criticized this model for being too molecular and limited in terms of situational specificity and reliance on discrete behaviors. Its narrow focus does not contribute to understanding how children adapt overall to having cancer. Also, the assumption that particular coping strategies are desirable for all subjects or that subjects' preferred modes of coping will be effective is not always valid. The link to coping and adaptation is frequently assumed but not assessed in this model. In addition, while these studies consist of multiple observations, typically they occur at only one phase of treatment, and it is not known whether the coping behavior continues over time.

Social Ecology Model

In recent years this model has gained more adherents, particularly from those with a family systems background. Its basic premise is that the child with cancer must be studied in the context of transactions that occur within social and environmental systems (Kazak, 1992; Michael & Copeland, 1987). This model is derived from Bronfenbrenner's (1979) theory in which development co-occurs within different contexts that constitute a series of concentric rings radiating outward from the child: the microsystem (family), the mesosystem (interactions among family, school, hospital, agencies), the exosystem (social support networks, agencies which indirectly affect the child), and the macrosystem (culture and policy). The child and family members are viewed not as isolated individuals but as they interact with other persons and systems. Issues related to disease and treatment involve siblings, parental employment, medical/nursing staff interactions. These transactions are multidirectional and dynamic. For example, family adaptability may affect the child's coping and vice versa. This orientation emphasizes a developmental, nonpathological perspective that includes the developmental level of the family.

Examples of studies derived from this model include assessments of family configurations as they affect the child (Kazak & Meadows, 1989), assessments of social support systems (Kazak & Meadows, 1989), comparisons of parenting practices in families of children with cancer and with the children's peers (Davies, Noll, DeStefano, Bukowski, & Kulkarni, 1991), assessments of peer relationships and social isolation (Noll et al., 1991), evaluations of the impact of pediatric cancer on parents, siblings, and peers, and comparisons of parental coping styles (Barbarin, Hughes, & Chesler, 1985; Cook, 1984; Sabbeth, 1984), comparisons of parental and adolescent coping styles (Ostroff, Smith, & Lesko, 1990), and evaluations social support networks (Kazak & Meadows, 1989; Morrow, Carpenter, & Hoagland, 1984).

Critique. Although this model reflects a comprehensive approach to understanding that a child's coping is related to his or her social context, few systematic studies have been done beyond the microsystem of the family. Several studies have included family and school influences, but with some exceptions few have studied cultural factors that interact with the child with cancer and his or her family (de Parra, de Cortazar, & Covarrubias-Espinoza, 1983; Pfefferbaum, Adams, & Aceves, 1990; Spinetta, 1984). Even in studies that are limited to the family system, there have been methodological dilemmas (see Kazak & Nachman, 1991). For example, consider the measurement of family coping: Should standard measures for each family member be used so that each could be described individually or should family measures such as the Family Environment Scale (Moos & Moos, 1986) or the Family Adaptability and Cohesion Evaluation Scales (FACES III) (Olson, Portner, & Bell, 1982) be used even though these are not direct measures of coping? Should one use less well-validated but more applicable measures of family coping? According to the social ecology model, intervention studies should go beyond those that target the individual child to include parents, siblings, peers, schools, and medical settings. Because the child does not enter treatment from a vacuum, there is a need to understand how to intervene in the context of the environment to which he or she must return.

Research Overview

Coping research in pediatric cancer can be divided into studies of (1) coping with adjustment as the outcome, (2) coping as a strategy, and (3) correlates of coping and adjustment. This review is limited to studies conducted since 1980, since previous reviews (Michael & Copeland, 1987; Van Dongen-Melman & Sanders-Woudstra, 1984) provide excellent summaries of earlier studies.

Coping with Adjustment as the Outcome

General Adjustment—Children and Adolescents with Cancer

The most comprehensive study of adjustment among cancer survivors is that of Koocher and O'Malley (1981). A heterogeneous group with respect to diagnosis, time since diagnosis, and type of treatment of 117 long-term survivors was given multiple measures of adjustment, including standardized tests and clinical interviews. Their major finding was that nearly half (47 percent) of these survivors were found to experience at least mild psychiatric symptoms based on impressions from clinical interviews. The clinical implication was that a sizable proportion of long-term survivors experienced adjustment problems.

Obetz, Swenson, McCarthy, Gilchrist, and Burgert (1980) studied 18 children who were in remission from leukemia over 4 years. Using standardized tests and interviews (Thematic Apperception Test [TAT], Minnesota Multiphasic Personality Inventory [MMPI], Children's Personality Questionnaire), they found that survivors generally were well-adjusted, while still having some concerns about the permanence of their cure. A study by Powazek, Schyving Payne, Goff, Paulsen, and Stagner (1980) of 35 consecutive admissions of ALL at diagnosis, 6 months, and 1 year postdiagnosis used standardized psychometric instruments, including age-appropriate Catell-designed personality questionnaires and the Piers-Harris Self-Concept Scale. In general, the functioning of children at 1 year was within normal limits, with low levels of anxiety. Chang, Nesbit, Youngren, and Robison (1987) studied 47 survivors of childhood cancer, using the MMPI and Personality Inventory for Children (PIC), and found that one-third of the survivors exhibited moderate to severe maladjustment. However, examination of test profiles revealed that this group was not significantly different from norms. Similarly, a large-scale ($N = 450$) epidemiological study of depression and maladjustment (Teta et al., 1986) found that the prevalence of psychopathology among childhood cancer survivors was not significantly different from that of the general population. A later study (Fritz, Williams, & Amylon, 1989) of 52 long-term survivors found few serious problems and good general adjustment for most survivors. In a study that mixed long-term survivors with children receiving treatment, Sanger, Copeland, & Davidson (1991) compared children with hematological cancers to those with solid tumors. While many children were experiencing somatic concerns, most were found to cope well in general. One-third had difficulties with physical symptoms and academic progress, but there were no significant differences between the two disease groups.

While most of these studies, with the exception of Teta et al. (1986), compared long-term survivors to normative data, few have compared them to controls. In a well-designed study, Greenberg, Kazak, and Meadows (1989) limited the age range (8 to 16 years of age) and the time variable (at least 2 years posttreatment and 5 years postdiagnosis). They compared 138 long-term survivors with controls matched for age, sex, and race who were seen in a walk-in clinic. Using well-validated measures (Piers-Harris Self Concept Scale, Nowicki-Strickland Locus of Control Scale for Children, Children's Depression Inventory (CDI), Family Environment Scale, Derogatis Stress Profile), it was found that, as a group, long-term survivors were well-adjusted and able to adapt posttreatment. Compared to the control group, long-term survivors showed poorer self-concept and more external locus of control, but both groups were within normal limits and were significantly lower in depression. Rates of depression were also low in another study by Worchel, Nolan, Willson, Purser, Copeland, and Pfefferbaum (1988), who compared 76 children undergoing treatment for cancer with 42 children who were psychiatric inpatients and 304 normal schoolchildren. Although parents rated their level of depression as relatively high on the Child Behavior Checklist (CBCL), children with cancer reported lower levels of depression than normal controls based on the CDI. The authors interpreted these results as possible evidence of denial, given the parental ratings and the children's rating of their disease as less severe than physicians. Similar results have been found (Kaplan, Busner, Weinhold, & Lenon, 1987; Tebbi, Bromberg, & Mallon, 1988). Worchel et al. (1988) suggest, as others have (Beisser, 1979; Lazarus, 1981), that denial can serve an adaptive purpose and can be, at times, an appropriate way of coping with the disease and treatment.

Thus assessment of depression alone does not appear to be a particularly useful way to tap coping as reflected by adjustment, given self-report measures alone. As Worchel et al. (1988) recommend, multiple measures should be used to tap this dimension. Also, the distinction should be made between depressive affect and behavior—which are commonly seen and may be appropriate reactions at diagnosis, relapse, or impending death—and clinical depression. This difference is important in terms of intervention decisions.

It is difficult to compare the results of all these studies, since they differ in stage of illness, time since diagnosis, time of assessment, and type of disease. There have been few longitudinal studies that have controlled for these variables. Kupst, Schulman, and colleagues studied the same group of pediatric leukemia patients and their families from the time of diagnosis (Kupst, 1980) through early treatment (Kupst, Schulman, Maurer, Honig, Morgan, & Fochtman, 1983), 1 year (Kupst, Schulman, Honig, Maurer, Morgan, & Fochtman, 1982), 2 years (Kupst, Schulman, Maurer, Morgan, Honig, & Fochtman, 1984), 6 years postdiagnosis (Kupst & Schulman, 1988), and a longer follow-up in progress. Subjects were children who were consecutively admitted with a diagnosis of leukemia over a 3-year period and their families. They were also randomly assigned to two intervention groups or to a no-intervention control group (Kupst, Tylke, Thomas, Mudd, Richardson, & Schulman, 1983) and were compared with a group of children with bacterial meningitis and their families. Results of psychometric tests (Missouri Children's Picture Series, Nowicki-Strickland LOC) and rating scales (Current Adjustment Rating Scale, Family Coping Scale, Mood and Behavior Scale) indicated that, regardless of the type of intervention, most children were coping well at all measurement occasions and even significantly improved at 6 years postdiagnosis.

In a recent meta-analysis (Lavigne & Faier-Routman, 1992) of studies that investigated global adjustment in several pediatric chronic illnesses, cancer was relatively low, ranking 13th of 19 illnesses in terms of risk for adjustment problems. In general, a moderate effect size was found in terms of significant differences from controls or norms, but only seven studies met the criteria for inclusion in the meta-analysis from the many that have been done in this area.

School and Social Adjustment

Since school and peers are a major part of a child's normal development, school adjustment has been viewed as an important indicator of functioning in children with cancer. Because of frequent or long absences due to treatment or illness, these children may miss opportunities to learn as well as to interact with peers. In addition, the location of a tumor may affect learning or memory centers, and treatment may affect cognitive functioning and academic achievement. Several recent studies have found evidence of difficulties in these areas for pediatric cancer patients (Greenberg et al., 1989; Mulhern, Kovnar, Kun, Crisco, & Williams, 1988; Sanger, Copeland, & Davidson, 1991; Sawyer, Toogood, Rice, Haskell, & Baghurst, 1989).

The question remains as to whether these problems in cognitive or academic functioning are related to coping and adjustment. Kupst and Schulman (1988) found that, while one-fourth of the children with leukemia who had been treated with cranial irradiation did indeed have academic problems, most coped well overall with treatment and long-term remission. Children with CNS tumors, however, appear to be more at risk for adjustment problems (see review by Mulhern, Hancock, Fairclough, & Kun, 1992). Given the frequently severe sequelae of CNS cancer and treatment, these results are not particularly surprising. More work needs to be done to determine the relationships among cognitive and academic functioning, school adjustment, and general adjustment in pediatric cancer patients.

With regard to children's social adjustment, social withdrawal was found to be common in long-term survivors (Chang et al., 1987). In a study of 183 long-term survivors ages 7 to 15 seen 5 years postdiagnosis and 2 years posttreatment, Mulhern, Wasserman, Freedman, and Fairclough (1989) found significant deficits on the Social scale of the CBCL. Length of time since treatment was related to increased social problems. Similarly, children with leukemia seen 5 years since diagnosis were found to be lower than norms in Social Competence on the CBCL, with increased aggressiveness and general noncompliance (Sawyer, Crittenden, & Toogood, 1986), but in a follow-up study 2 years later (Sawyer et al., 1989) these problems were not significant. Since children with leukemia who were treated at a young age were seen as being at risk for developing problems, Spirito, Stark, Cobiella, Drigan, Androkites, and Hewett (1990) studied 56 long-term survivors, mostly of ALL, who were treated between 2 and 5 years of age and were compared with a control group of schoolchildren. While survivors reported more feelings of isolation than controls, the groups were not significantly different from one another in terms of social competence and social functioning.

Recently social adjustment, particularly peer adjustment, has been investigated in several studies that involve an improved control group: matched peers from the child's own classroom, controlling for age, sex, socioeconomic status, neighborhood, and school experience. In one such study (Noll, Bukowski, Rogosch, LeRoy, & Kulkarni, 1990) parents, teachers, and older children completed CBCLs and the children with cancer were more socially withdrawn, isolated, and shy than matched peers. However, a later study (Noll et al., 1991) of actual social functioning found few differences between children with cancer and controls. These children with cancer were popular and socially accepted.

Summary. In general, studies that have examined coping in terms of adjustment as a global outcome variable or set of variables have found that the majority of children and adolescents with cancer do not have significant adjustment problems, compared either to test norms or to control or comparison groups. The range of those who do exhibit significant psychosocial problems appears to be from about one-quarter to one-third of these children. Since most of these studies have used groups that are heterogeneous with respect to diagnosis, time, type of treatment, and so on, the role these and other variables play in determining who is at risk for developing adjustment problems remains unclear. It may also be, as some have suggested (Deasy-Spinetta, 1981; Kazak & Meadows, 1989; Perrin, Stein, & Drotar, 1991), that current instrumentation is not sensitive to more subtle issues and concerns, which argues for more specific cancer-related measures of coping.

General Adjustment—Families

As the section on theory indicated, several early clinical studies (Binger et al., 1969; Bozeman et al., 1955; Kaplan, Smith, Grobstein, & Fischman, 1973; Natterson & Knudson, 1960) of anticipatory grief cited a high frequency of emotional disturbances in families, generally parents, of children with cancer, although others (Chodoff et al., 1963; Futterman & Hoffman, 1973; Schulman, 1976; Stehbens & Lascari, 1974) failed to replicate these findings and even noted positive functioning. In one study which was limited to parents in a support group (Morrow, Hoagland, & Carnrike, 1981), however, parents exhibited significant problems based on their ratings in the Psychosocial Adjustment to Illness Scale, especially among those parents whose child had died. While the scores might be significantly different from zero (the best possible score, indicating no problems whatsoever), they were still relatively low, considering the range of possible scores.

Given high levels of stress and distress at diagnosis and during treatment, however, families could still cope adequately (Powazek et al., 1980). Despite high levels of stress, based on the Clinical Analysis Questionnaire, only one parent out of 35 families evidenced serious psychological problems. Similarly, in a longitudinal study of 35 families of cancer survivors, Kazak and Meadows (1989) found that, in general, these families were not significantly different from norms or from a comparison group of friends and neighbors on several standardized measures, including the FACES III, the Langner Symptom Checklist, and the CBCL. A similar cross-sectional comparison (Speechley & Noh, 1992) found no significant differences between parents ($N = 63$ families) of long-term survivors and neighborhood controls ($N = 64$) in anxiety or depression. Low social support, however, tended to be associated with higher anxiety and depression.

The Coping Project, developed by Kupst and colleagues, followed 64 families of children with pediatric leukemia from diagnosis through and after treatment (6 years postdiagnosis, with a 12-year follow-up study in progress). In general, parental coping was normal at all measurement occasions, with significant improvement in staff ratings at 6 years postdiagnosis. Coping was not significantly different in comparing parents of long-term survivors to parents of children who had died. There were no instances of serious psychological dysfunction in these families. In contrast to studies that tallied symptoms or problems, the perspective of this study was to allow for growth as well as for pathology. This did not mean a lack of upsets, anxiety, typical grief reactions to diagnosis and bad news; rather, these were normal reactions given the situation. Despite much distress, most families did remarkably well, and it is hypothesized that similar results will be obtained in the 12-year follow-up study.

How parents behave toward their children can also be an indicator of adjustment. For example, most families in the Coping Project were able to set limits for their children, treating them as normally as possible. Similarly, in a study of child-rearing practices of parents of long-term survivors, Davies, Noll, DeStefano, Bukowski, and Kulkarni (1991) found no significant differences between these parents and parents of matched classroom controls. Despite opinions of professionals surveyed in the study that parents tended to be overinvolved, to have difficulty with discipline, and to worry about their child, the only significant finding was that parents of long-term survivors tended to worry about their child's health and about whether they were too involved in their child's health concerns.

Thus, as with children and adolescents with cancer, parents tend to have few serious adjustment problems overall. As Kazak and Meadows (1989) suggest, perhaps it is time to accept the null hypothesis of no important differences between these families and "normal" families. Rather than continue to focus on finding differences, it is more germane to determine what these children and families do when faced with the diagnosis and treatment of pediatric cancer. Since some children and families do not cope well, it is also more relevant to determine what variables are related to good coping and adjustment to pediatric cancer.

Coping as a Cognitive Style and Strategy

The role of coping style in dealing with disease remains an interest of many clinicians and researchers. Recently, there has been renewed interest in the repression-sensitization dimension of coping style (Byrne, 1964). In a study of mixed-diagnosis chronic illness (Harris, Canning, & Wong, 1991), repressors represented over half of a group of children with mixed chronic illnesses but only one-third of a control group of high school students. The repressive style was associated with a lower self-report of depressive symptoms. However, there were no comparisons with objective measures of depression, no measures of coping with specific situations related to illness, and no attempt to link style to actual coping behaviors. In a review by Field (1992), "repressors," who were more cooperative and stoic, coped more poorly with stressful surgical procedures than did "sensitizers," who were more active and expressive, and the child's coping style was related to that of her or his mother. However, these data were based on the mother's perceptions of the child's style. It was also not clear, in the long run, whether it was more adaptive to be a repressor or a sensitizer. One study (Smith, Ackerson, & Blotcky, 1989) attempted to relate preferred coping style (repressor or sensitizer) based on the Coping Strategy Interview of 28 pediatric cancer patients undergoing painful procedures. Pain rating results were in the opposite direction of what was expected: repressors randomized to distraction conditions had the highest experienced pain ratings, followed by sensitizers provided with sensory information.

There were some problems with the validity of the intervention itself in that the verbal distraction condition seemed vague and open to variation across staff, and the length of time from diagnosis and prior experience with procedures were not controlled. However, the state of knowledge about the role of coping style is still unclear, and repression–sensitization is only one dimension. Fritz, Williams, and Amylon's (1988) study of long-term survivors indicates the wide variability of coping styles and suggests that children with opposing styles can be well-adjusted. The authors conclude that there is no common path to health and no cookbook answers or interventions. Does coping style determine actual behavior in a given situation? Does coping style determine strategy? These questions need to be explored further.

In terms of practical utility, more attention is being focused on the actual coping strategies used by children with chronic illnesses and their parents. In general, studies (e.g., Compas et al., 1992) indicate that problem-focused coping is acquired during the preschool years, while emotion-focused coping develops in later childhood and early adolescence. Worchel, Copeland, and Barker (1987) found that pediatric cancer patients tended to show more cognitive and decisional control strategies than did younger children. Bull and Drotar (1991) conducted a study of stressors and coping strategies in 39 school-age children and adolescents with cancer. This study indicated the need to differentiate coping with cancer from general coping, since coping with general life stressors was not necessarily consistent with cancer-related stressors, such as procedures, side effects, and hospitalization, as measured by a retrospective interview. As had been found in other studies, younger children used more problem-solving strategies, whereas adolescents used more emotional management.

The role of coping strategies and interactions with staff and parents was assessed in a study which utilized audiotapes of actual verbal coping behaviors (Blount, Landolf-Fritsche, Powers, & Sturges, 1991). Twenty-two children undergoing painful procedures in a hematology-oncology clinic were divided into high and low coping groups, depending on the number of coping behaviors noted. Those in the high groups were more likely to use distraction or deep breathing along with coaching by staff or parents. The authors acknowledged the small sample size and the lack of control for previous experience or other subject characteristics. In addition, the definition of high and low coping based on number of behaviors could have been supplemented by other coping indicators. However, this study was an improvement over those that used dispositional measures which assess only how a person coped previously or might cope in a situation.

Coping styles and strategies of families, particularly parents, have been examined in some studies. Kupst and Schulman (1988), using interviews, self-reports and observational data, attempted to determine common strategies used by children and parents and found, as Fritz et al. (1989) did, wide variability among parents. While most children and parents were found to cope well in terms of overall adjustment, sometimes diametrically opposed strategies could be equally effective. Chesler and Barbarin (1987) found that emotion-focused coping strategies (denial, optimism) tended to be more effective in responding to emotional and interpersonal stresses, whereas problem-focused strategies (information seeking, help seeking) were more effective with intellectual and practical stresses of childhood cancer. Mothers tended to seek information more than fathers; fathers tended to use more denial than mothers. Ostroff et al. (1990) compared parents' and adolescent cancer survivors strategies in an attempt to predict the mental health of family members. They found that adolescents' mental health related to strategies of seeking support, mothers' to positive reframing, and fathers' to reliance on positive attitude, which was interpreted as precluding asking for help. In a similar comparison, Kupst, Penati, and Strother (1992), in a study of children with CNS tumors and their families, administered the Ways of Coping Inventory and the Kidcope. Children and parents tended to use multiple coping strategies. The predominant coping strategies of parents and children reflected a primarily cognitive attempt to redefine or refocus: positive reappraisal, cognitive restructuring, wishful thinking, and planful problem solving. However, the action-oriented strategy of seeking social support was also common among family members.

In summary, most of the studies of coping strategies have used paper-and-pencil type measures. It would be helpful to combine these with observational data, as is done in studies of painful procedures, to determine what children and parents actually do in specific situations. A thorough assessment of a child and family's typical coping strategies, as well as observation of current strategies, would be helpful in planning interventions and preventing problems.

Correlates of Coping

Many of the studies that have assessed coping as outcome have also examined the relationship of various disease-related, personal, family, or social and environmental variables. The results of these studies are useful in determining who is at risk for poor coping with cancer and treatment. In terms of disease-related variables, it has been difficult to determine the role of the type of cancer, since most studies that have combined different types have had too few in each diagnostic group to compare. As was suggested previously, children with CNS involvement and their families may be at higher risk for problems in cognitive functioning, and therefore in school adjustment. The differential impact of various cancer diagnoses can be assessed only through intergroup and interinstitutional studies that allow for sufficient sample sizes.

Since there have been few longitudinal studies, stage of disease has not been well studied, but Kupst and Schulman (1988) found that children and adolescents exhibit improved global coping as time from diagnosis increases. Early problems in coping with procedures, however, may not dissipate over time and indeed may worsen with repeated exposures (Armstrong, 1992). Visibility of the disease has been related to problems in adjustment of long-term survivors (O'Malley, Foster, Koocher, Foster, & Slavin, 1979). Severity of late treatment effects also appears to be a correlate of adjustment in long-term survivors (Fritz et al., 1988; Greenberg et al., 1989; Katz, 1980; Lesko, Kern, & Hawkins, 1984). The physical condition of the child is also a correlate of parental coping (Kupst et al., 1982; Morrow et al., 1981; Spinetta & Deasy-Spinetta, 1981).

Other correlates of good coping include a low level of concurrent stresses (Kalnins, Churchill, & Terry, 1980; Kupst & Schulman, 1988); financial security (Fritz et al., 1988; Koocher & O'Malley, 1981; Kupst & Schulman, 1988); family adaptability (Chesler & Barbarin, 1987; Kazak & Meadows, 1989); good family support (Koocher & O'Malley, 1981; Kupst & Schulman, 1988; Morrow et al., 1984); and previously effective coping (Armstrong, in press; Kupst & Schulman, 1988).

Helpful coping strategies have been found to include open communication (Chesler & Barbarin, 1987; Fritz et al., 1988; Koocher & O'Malley, 1981; Kupst & Schulman, 1988; Slavin, O'Malley, Koocher, & Foster, 1982; Spinetta, Swarner, & Sheposh, 1981); use of denial (Beisser, 1979; Chesler & Barbarin, 1987; Koocher & O'Malley, 1981; Zeltzer, 1980); focusing on positive aspects (Chesler & Barbarin, 1987; Koocher & O'Malley, 1981); searching for information (Chesler & Barbarin, 1987); seeking and maintaining social support (Chesler & Barbarin, 1987; Koocher & O'Malley, 1981; Kupst & Schulman, 1988; Morrow et al., 1981); and living "one day at a time" (Chesler & Barbarin, 1987; Kupst & Schulman, 1988). From these findings it can be predicted that those who have more severe physical problems, little support, additional stresses, and few coping resources are at risk for psychological problems. Early assessment of the child and family's status on these risk factors is an important task for the mental health team.

Conclusion

Our theoretical knowledge of coping and the methodologies to study it have improved greatly over the past 30 years. With changes in treatment and prognosis, as well as better instrumentation and design, we continue to reexamine old assumptions and to evolve a clearer picture of the child's and family's experiences of pediatric cancer. Research findings have enabled clinicians to provide more effective interventions, particularly in the area of painful procedures, but also in more general adjustment to the disease.

Despite this positive picture, there is still much to be learned about coping with pediatric cancer, and such knowledge can be achieved only with more theory-driven longitudinal research. Only then can we answer questions about child and family coping over time and determine when problems occur, when they are indicative of serious dysfunction, and when they are temporary regressions as part of a normal coping process. We need to determine not only what the risk factors are but when they are risk factors and what variables provide resistance to these stresses. We also need to determine what strategies work best, when, and for whom. As research continues toward this goal, we will learn more about what people do when faced with the diagnosis and treatment of pediatric cancer, how well they adapt, and how they can be helped to cope with the experience.

References

Armstrong, F. D. (1992). Psychosocial intervention in pediatric cancer: A strategy for prevention of long-term problems. In T. Field, N. Schniederman, & P. McCabe (Eds.), *Stress and coping in infancy and childhood* (pp. 197–218). New York: Lawrence Erlbaum Associates.

Band, E. B. (1990). Children's coping with diabetes: Understanding the role of cognitive development. *Journal of Pediatric Psychology, 15,* 27–42.

Barbarin, O., Hughes, D., & Chesler, M. (1985). Stress, coping, and marital functioning among parents of children with cancer. *Journal of Marriage and the Family, 47,* 473–480.

Beisser, D. (1979). Denial and affirmation in illness and health. *American Journal of Psychiatry, 136,* 1026–1030.

Bibace, R., & Walsh, M. E. (1981). Children's conceptions of illness. In R. Bibace & M. E. Walsh (Eds.), *New directions for child development: Children's conceptions of health, illness, and bodily functions* (pp. 31–48). San Francisco: Jossey-Bass.

Binger, C. M., Ablin, A. R., Feuerstein, R. C., Kushner, J. H., Zoger, S., & Mikkelsen, C. (1969). Childhood leukemia: Emotional impact on patient and family. *New England Journal of Medicine, 280,* 414–418.

Blotcky, A., Cohen, D., Conaster, C., & Klopovich, P. (1985). Psychosocial characteristics of adolescents who refuse cancer treatment. *Journal of Consulting and Clinical Psychology, 53,* 729–731.

Blount, R. L., Landolf-Fritsche, B., Powers, S. W., & Sturges, J. W. (1991). Differences between high and low coping children and between parents and staff behaviors during painful medical procedures. *Journal of Pediatric Psychology, 16,* 795–809.

Bluebond-Langer, M. (1978). *The private worlds of dying children.* Princeton, NJ: Princeton University Press.

Bozeman, M. F., Orbach, C., & Sutherland, M. (1955). Psychological impact of cancer and its treatment: The adaptation of mothers to the threatened loss of their children through leukemia: Part I. *Cancer, 8,* 1–19.

Bronfenbrenner, U. (1979). *The ecology of human development.* Cambridge, MA: Harvard University Press.

Bull, B. A., & Drotar, D. (1991). Coping with cancer in remission: Stressors and strategies reported by children and adolescents. *Journal of Pediatric Psychology, 16,* 767–782.

Byrne, D. (1964). Repression-sensitization as a dimension of personality. In B. A. Maher (Ed.), *Progress in experimental personality research* (Vol. 1, pp. 169–220). New York: Academic Press.

Carpenter, P. J. (1990). New method for measuring young children's self-report of fear and pain. *Journal of Pain and Symptom Management, 5,* 233–240.

Chang, P., Nesbit, M. E., Youngren, N., & Robison, L. L. (1987). Personality characteristics and psychosocial adjustment of long-term survivors of childhood cancer. *Journal of Psychosocial Oncology, 5,* 43–58.

Chesler, M. A. & Barbarin, O. A. (1987). *Childhood cancer and the family.* New York: Brunner/Mazel.

Chodoff, R., Friedman, S. B., & Hamburg, D. A. (1964). Stress, defenses and coping behavior: Observations in parents of children with malignant disease. *American Journal of Psychiatry, 120,* 743–749.

Claflin, C. J., & Barbarin, O. A. (1991). Does "telling" less protect more? Relationships among age, information disclosure, and what children with cancer see and feel. *Journal of Pediatric Psychology, 16,* 169–192.

Compas, B. E., Worsham, N. L., & Ey, S. (1992). Conceptual and developmental issues in children's coping with stress. In A. M. LaGreca, L. J. Siegel, J. L. Wallander, & C. E. Walker (Eds.), *Stress and coping in child health* (pp. 7–24). New York: Guilford Press.

Cook, J. (1984). Influence of gender on the problems of fatally ill children. *Journal of Psychosocial Oncology, 2,* 71–91.

Dahlquist, L., Gil, K. M., Armstrong, F. D., Ginsberg, A., & Jones, B. (1985). Behavioral management of children's distress during chemotherapy. *Journal of Behavior Therapy and Experimental Psychiatry, 16,* 325–329.

Davies, W. H., Noll, R. B., DeStefano, L., Bukowski, W. M., & Kulkarni, R. (1991). Differences in the child-rearing practices of parents of children with cancer and controls: The perspectives of parents and professionals. *Journal of Pediatric Psychology, 16,* 295–306.

de Parra, M., de Cortazar, S., & Covarrubias-Espinoza, G. (1983). The adaptive pattern of families with a leukemic child. *Family Systems Medicine, 1,* 30–35.

Deasy-Spinetta, P. (1981). The school and the child with cancer. In J. J. Spinetta & R. Deasy-Spinetta (Eds.), *Living with childhood cancer* (pp. 153–168). St. Louis: Mosby.

Drotar, D. (1991). Coming of age: Critical challenges to the future development of pediatric psychology. *Journal of Pediatric Psychology, 16,* 1–12.

Field, T. (1992). Infants' and children's responses to invasive procedures. In A. M. LaGreca, L. J. Siegel, J. L. Wallander, & C. E. Walker (Eds.), *Stress and coping in child health* (pp. 123–139). New York: Guilford Press.

Folkman, S., & Lazarus, R. S. (1988). *Manual for the Ways of Coping Questionnaire.* Palo Alto, CA: Consulting Psychologists Press.

Friedman, S. B., Chodoff, P., Mason, J. W., & Hamburg, D. A. (1963). Behavioral observations of parents anticipating the death of a child. *Pediatrics, 32,* 610–625.

Fritz, G. K., Williams, J. R., & Amylon, M. (1988). After treatment ends: Psychosocial sequelae in pediatric cancer survivors. *American Journal of Orthopsychiatry, 58,* 552–561.

Futterman, E. H., & Hoffman, I. (1973). Crisis and adaptation in families of fatally ill children. In E. J. Anthony & C. Koupernik (Eds.), *The child in his family: The impact of disease and death* Vol. 2 (pp. 127–143). New York: Wiley.

Greenberg, H., Kazak, A., & Meadows, A. (1989). Psychological adjustment in 8–16 year old cancer survivors and their parents. *Journal of Pediatrics, 114,* 488–493.

Haan, N. (1977). *Coping and defending: Processes of self-environment organization.* New York: Academic Press.

Harper, D. C. (1991). Paradigms for investigating rehabilitation and adaptation to childhood disability and chronic illness. *Journal of Pediatric Psychology, 16,* 533–542.

Harris, E. S., Canning, R. D., & Wong, J. M. (1991). *Depressive symptoms and adaptive style in chronically ill children.* Paper presented at the Fifth NIMH Research Conference on Classification and Treatment of Mental Disorders in General Medical Settings, Washington, DC.

Hilgard, J. R., & LeBaron, J. R. (1982). Relief of anxiety and pain in children and adolescents with cancer: Quantitative measures and clinical observations. *International Journal of Clinical and Experimental Hypnosis, 30,* 414–442.

Hurwitz, J. I., Kaplan, D. M., & Kaiser, E. (1962). Designing an instrument to assess parental coping mechanisms. *Social Casework, 10,* 527–532.

Jacobsen, P. B., Manne, S. L., Gorfinkle, K., & Schorr, O. (1990) Analysis of child and parent behavior during painful medical procedures. *Health Psychology, 9,* 559–576.

Janis, I. L. (1958). *Psychological stress.* New York: Wiley.

Jay, S. M., & Elliott, C. H. (1990). A stress inoculation program for parents whose children are undergoing painful medical procedures. *Journal of Consulting and Clinical Psychology, 58,* 799–804.

Jay, S. M., Ozolins, M., Elliott, C. H., & Caldwell, S. (1983). Assessment of children's distress during painful medical procedures. *Health Psychology, 2,* 138–149.

Kalnins, I. V., Churchill, M. P., & Terry, G. E. (1980). Concurrent stress in families with a leukemic child. *Journal of Pediatric Psychology, 5,* 81–92.

Kaplan, D. M., Grobstein, R., & Smith, A. (1976). Predicting the impact of severe illness in families. *Health and Social Work, 1,* 71–82.

Kaplan, D. M., Smith, A., Grobstein, R., & Fischman, S. E. (1973). Family mediation of stress. *Social Work, 18,* 60–69.

Kaplan, S. L., Busner, J., Weinhold, C., & Lenon, P. (1987) Depressive symptoms in children and adolescents with cancer: A longitudinal study. *Journal of the American Academy of Child and Adolescent Psychiatry, 26,* 782–787.

Katz, E. R. (1980). Illness impact and social reintegration. In J. Kellerman (Ed.), *Psychological aspects of childhood cancer* (pp. 14–46). Springfield, IL: Charles C Thomas.

Katz, E. R., Kellerman, J., & Siegel, S. E. (1980). Behavioral distress in children with cancer undergoing medical procedures: Developmental considerations. *Journal of Consulting and Clinical Psychology, 48,* 356–365.

Kazak, A. E. (1992) . The social context of coping with childhood chronic illness: Family systems and social support. In A. LaGreca, L. Siegel, J. Wallander, & C. E. Walker (Eds.), *Stress and coping in child health* (pp. 262– 278). New York: Guilford Press.

Kazak, A. E., & Meadows, A. T. (1989). Families of young adolescents who have survived cancer: Social-emotional adjustment, adaptability, and social support. *Journal of Pediatric Psychology, 14,* 175–192.

Kazak, A. E. & Nachman, G. S. (1991). Family research on childhood chronic illness: Pediatric oncology as an example. *Journal of Family Psychology, 4* (4), 462–483.

Kellerman, J. (Ed.) (1980). *Psychological aspects of childhood cancer.* Springfield, IL: Charles C Thomas.

Kellerman, J., Zeltzer, L., Ellenberg, L., Dash, J., & Rigler, D. (1980). Psychological effects of illness in adolescence. *Journal of Pediatrics, 97,* 126–131.

Koocher, G. P., & O'Malley, J. E. (Eds.) (1981). *The Damocles syndrome: Psychological consequences of surviving childhood cancer.* New York: McGraw-Hill.

Kupst, M. J. (1980). Family coping with leukemia in a child: Initial reactions. In J. L. Schulman & M. J. Kupst (Eds.), *The child with cancer* (pp. 111–128). Springfield, IL: Charles C Thomas.

Kupst, M. J. (1992). Long-term family coping with acute lymphoblastic leukemia in childhood. In A. LaGreca, L. Siegel, J. Wallander, & C. E. Walker (Eds.), *Stress and coping in Child Health* (pp. 242–261). New York: Guilford Press.

Kupst, M. J., Mudd, M. E., & Schulman, J. L. (1990). *Predictors of coping and adjustment in long-term pediatric leukemia survivors.* Paper presented at the American Psychological Association Meeting, Boston, MA.

Kupst, M. J., Penati, B., & Strother, D. (1992). *Family coping with pediatric central nervous system tumors.* Paper presented at the American Psychological Association Meeting, Washington, DC.

Kupst, M. J., & Schulman, J. L. (1988). Long-term coping with pediatric leukemia: A six year follow-up study. *Journal of Pediatric Psychology, 13*, 7–22.

Kupst, M. J., Schulman, J. L., Honig, G., Maurer, H., Morgan, E., & Fochtman, D. (1982). Family coping with childhood leukemia: One year after diagnosis. *Journal of Pediatric Psychology, 7*, 157–174.

Kupst, M. J., Schulman, J. L., Maurer, H., Honig, G., Morgan, E., & Fochtman, D. (1983). Family coping with pediatric leukemia: The first six months. *Medical and Pediatric Oncology, 11*, 269–278.

Kupst, M. J., Schulman, J. L., Maurer, H., Morgan, E., Honig, G., & Fochtman, D. (1984). Coping with pediatric leukemia: A two-year follow-up. *Journal of Pediatric Psychology, 9*, 149–163.

Kupst, M. J., Tylke, L., Thomas, L., Mudd, M. E., Richardson, C. C., & Schulman, J. L. (1983). Strategies of intervention with pediatric cancer patients. *Social Work in Health Care, 8*, 31–47.

Lavigne, J. V., & Faier-Routman, J. (1992). Psychological adjustment to pediatric physical disorders: A meta-analytic review. *Journal of Pediatric Psychology, 17*, 133–158.

Lazarus, R. S. (1966). *Psychological stress and the coping process.* New York: McGraw-Hill.

Lazarus, R. S. (1981). The costs and benefits of denial. In J. J . Spinetta and P. Deasy-Spinetta (Eds.), *Living with childhood cancer* (pp. 50–67). St. Louis: Mosby.

Lazarus, R. S. (1991). *Emotion and adaptation.* New York: Oxford University Press.

Lazarus, R. S., Averill, J. R., & Opton, E. M., Jr. (1974). The psychology of coping: Issues of research and assessment. In G. V. Coelho, D. A. Hamburg, & J. E. Adams (Eds.), *Coping and adaptation* (pp. 249–315). New York: Basic Books.

Lazarus, R. S., & Folkman, S. (1984). *Stress, appraisal and coping.* New York: Springer.

Lesko, L. M., Kern, J., & Hawkins, D. R. (1984). Psychological aspects of patients in germ-free isolation: A review of child, adult and patient management literature. *Medical and Pediatric Oncology, 12*, 43–49.

Lindemann, E. (1944). Symptomatology and management of acute grief. *American Journal of Psychiatry, 101*, 141–148.

Loevinger, J. (1976). *Ego development.* San Francisco: Jossey-Bass.

McCubbin, H. I., McCubbin, M. A., Nevin, R. S., & Cauble, E. (1981). *Coping-Health Inventory for Parents.* St. Paul: University of Minnesota Family Social Sciences.

Michael, B. E., & Copeland, D. R. (1987). Psychosocial issues in childhood cancer: An ecological framework for research. *American Journal of Pediatric Hematology/Oncology, 9*, 73–83.

Moos, R. H., & Billings, A. (1982). Conceptualizing and measuring coping resources and processes. In J. Goldberger & S. Breznitz (Eds.), *Handbook of stress: Theoretical and clinical aspects* (pp. 212–230). New York: Macmillan.

Moos, R. H., & Moos, B. S. (1986). *Family Environment Scale manual* (2nd ed.). Palo Alto, CA: Consulting Psychologists Press.

Morrow, G. R., Carpenter, P. J., & Hoagland, A. (1984). The role of social support in parental adjustment to pediatric cancer. *Journal of Pediatric Psychology, 9*, 317–325.

Morrow, G. R., Hoagland, A., & Carnrike, C. L. M. (1981). Social support and parental adjustment to pediatric cancer. *Journal of Consulting and Clinical Psychology, 49*, 763–765.

Mulhern, R. K., Hancock, J., Fairclough, D., & Kun, L. (1992). Neuropsychological status of children treated for brain tumors: A critical review and integrative analysis. *Medical and Pediatric Oncology, 20*, 181–191.

Mulhern, R. K., Kovnar, E. H., Kun, L. E., Crisco, J. J., & Williams, J. M. (1988). Psychologic and neurologic function following treatment for childhood temporal lobe astrocytoma. *Journal of Child Neurology, 3,* 47–52.

Mulhern, R. K., Wasserman, A. L., Friedman, A. G., & Fairclough, D. (1989). Social competence and behavioral adjustment of children who are long-term survivors of cancer. *Pediatrics, 83,* 18–25.

Murphy, L. B. (1962). *The widening world of childhood: Paths toward mastery.* New York: Basic Books.

Murphy, L. B. (1974) Coping, vulnerability and resilience in childhood. In G. V. Coelho, D. A. Hamburg, & J. E. Adams (Eds.), *Coping and adaptation* (pp. 69–100). New York: Basic Books.

Natterson, J. M., & Knudson, A. G. (1960). Observations concerning fear of death in fatally ill children and their mothers. *Psychosomatic Medicine, 22,* 456–465.

Noll, R., Bukowski, W., Rogosch, F., LeRoy, S., & Kulkarni, R. (1990). Social interactions between children and their peers: Teacher ratings. *Journal of Pediatric Psychology, 7,* 75–84.

Noll, R., LeRoy, S., Bukowski, W. M., Rogosch, F. A., & Kulkarni, R. (1991). Peer relationships and adjustment in children with cancer. *Journal of Pediatric Psychology, 16,* 307–326.

Obetz, S. W., Swenson, W. M., McCarthy, C. A., Gilchrist, G. S., & Burgert, E. O. (1980). Children who survive malignant disease: Emotional adaptation of the children and their families. In J. L. Schulman & M. J. Kupst (Eds.), *The child with cancer* (pp. 194–210). Springfield, IL: Charles C Thomas.

Olson, D., Portner, J., & Lavee, Y. (1985). Family Adaptability and Cohesion scales III. In St. Paul: University of Minnesota, Family Social Science.

O'Malley, J. E., Foster, D., Koocher, G., Foster, D., & Slavin, L. (1979). Visible physical impairment and psychological adjustment among pediatric cancer survivors. *American Journal of Psychiatry, 137,* 94–96.

Ostroff, J., Smith, K., & Lesko, L. (1990, August). *Differential effect of family coping on post-cancer treatment adjustment.* Paper presented at the Annual Meeting of the American Psychological Association, Boston, MA.

Perrin, E. C., Stein, R. E. K., & Drotar, D. (1991). Cautions in using the Child Behavior Checklist: Observations based on research about children with a chronic illness. *Journal of Pediatric Psychology, 16,* 411–422.

Pfefferbaum, B., Adams, J., & Aceves, J. , (1990). The influence of culture on pain in Anglo and Hispanic children with cancer. *Journal of the American Academy of Child and Adolescent Psychiatry, 29,* 642–647.

Powazek, M., Schyving Payne, J., Goff, J. R., Paulson, M. A., & Stagner, S. (1980). Psychosocial ramifications of childhood leukemia: One year postdiagnosis. In J. L. Schulman & M. J. Kupst (Eds.), *The child with cancer* (pp. 143–155). Springfield, IL: Charles C Thomas.

Redd, W. (1989). Behavioral interventions to reduce child distress. In J. C. Holland, & J. H. Rowland (Eds.), *Handbook of psychooncology* (pp. 573–584). New York: Oxford University Press.

Rolland, J. (1984). Towards a psychosocial topology of chronic and life threatening illness. *Family Systems Medicine, 2,* 245–262.

Rowland, J. H. (1989). Developmental stage and adaptation: Child and adolescent model. In J. C. Holland & J. H. Rowland (Eds.), *Handbook of Psychooncology* (pp. 519–543). New York: Oxford University Press.

Sabbeth, B. (1984). Understanding the impact of chronic childhood illness on families. *Pediatric Clinics of North America, 31,* 47–58.

Sanger, M. S., Copeland, D. R., & Davidson, E. R. (1991). Psychosocial adjustment among pediatric cancer patients: A multidimensional assessment. *Journal of Pediatric Psychology, 16,* 463–474.

Sawyer, M. G., Crittenden, A., & Toogood, I. (1986). Psychologic adjustment of families of children and adolescents treated for leukemia. *American Journal of Pediatric Hematology/Oncology, 8,* 200–207.

Sawyer, M. G., Toogood, I., Rice, M., Haskell, C., & Baghurst, P. (1989). School performance and psychological adjustment of children treated for leukemia. *American Journal of Pediatric Hematology/Oncology, 11,* 146–152.

Schulman, J. L. (1976). *Coping with tragedy.* Springfield, IL: Charles C Thomas.

Schulman, J. L., & Kupst, M. J. (Eds.) (1980). *The child with cancer.* Springfield, IL: Charles C Thomas.

Slavin, L. A., O'Malley, J. E., Koocher, G. P., & Foster, D. J. (1982). Communication of the cancer diagnosis to pediatric patients: Impact on long-term adjustment. *American Journal of Psychiatry, 139,* 179–183.

Smith, K., Ackerson, J. D., & Blotcky, A. D. (1989). Reducing distress during invasive medical procedures: Relating behavioral interventions to preferred coping style in pediatric cancer patients. *Journal of Pediatric Psychology, 14,* 405–420.

Speechley, K. N., & Noh, S. (1992). Surviving childhood cancer, social support, and parents' psychological adjustment. *Journal of Pediatric Psychology, 17,* 15–32.

Spinetta, J. J. (1974). The dying child's awareness of death. *Psychological Bulletin, 81,* 256–260.

Spinetta, J. J. (1977). Adjustment in children with cancer. *Journal of Pediatric Psychology, 2,* 49–51.

Spinetta, J. J. (1984). Development of psychometric methods by life cycle stages. *Cancer (Supplement), 53,* 2222–2225.

Spinetta, J. J., & Deasy-Spinetta, P. (Eds.) (1981). *Living with childhood cancer.* St. Louis: Mosby.

Spinetta, J. J., Swarner, J. A., & Sheposh, J. P. (1981). Effective parental coping following the death of a child from cancer. *Journal of Pediatric Psychology, 6,* 251–263.

Spirito, A., Stark, L., Cobiella, C., Drigan, R., Androkites, A., & Hewitt, K. (1990). Social adjustment of children successfully treated for cancer. *Journal of Pediatric Psychology, 15,* 359–371.

Spirito, A., Stark, L. J., & Williams, C. (1988). Development of a brief checklist to assess coping in pediatric patients. *Journal of Pediatric Psychology, 13,* 555–574.

Stehbens, J. A., & Lascari, A. D. (1974). Psychological follow-up of families with childhood leukemia. *Journal of Clinical Psychology, 30,* 394–397.

Stein, R., & Jessop, D. (1982). A noncategorical approach to childhood chronic illness. *Public Health Reports, 97,* 354–362.

Susman, E. J., Hollenbeck, A. R., Nannis, E. D., & Strope, B. E. (1980). A developmental perspective on psychosocial aspects of childhood cancer. In J. L. Schulman & M. J. Kupst (Eds.), *The child with cancer* (pp. 128–142). Springfield, IL: Charles C Thomas.

Tebbi, C. K., Bromberg, C., & Mallon, J. (1988). Self-reported depression in adolescent cancer patients. *American Journal of Pediatric Hematology/Oncology, 10,* 185–190.

Teta, M., Po, M., Kasl, S., Meigs, J., Myers, M., & Mulvihill, J. (1986). Psychosocial consequences of childhood and adolescent cancer survival. *Journal of Chronic Diseases, 39,* 751–759.

Townes, B. D., Wold, D. A. & Holmes, T. H. (1974). Parental adjustment to childhood leukemia. *Journal of Psychosomatic Research, 18,* 9–14.

Vaillant, G. E. (1977). *Adaptation to life.* Boston: Little, Brown.

Van Dongen-Melman, J. E. W. M., & Sanders-Woudstra, J. A. R. (1986). Psychosocial aspects of childhood cancer: A review of the literature. *Journal of Child Psychology and Psychiatry, 27,* 145–180.

Weisman, A. D., & Worden, J. W. (1976). The existential plight in cancer. *International Journal of Psychiatry in Medicine, 7,* 1–15.

White, R. W. (1974). Strategies of adaptation. An attempt at systematic description. In G. V. Coelho, D. A. Hamburg, & J. E. Adams (Eds.), *Coping and adaptation* (pp. 47–68). New York: Basic Books.

Worchel, F., Copeland, D., & Barker, D. (1987) Control-related coping strategies in pediatric oncology patients. *Journal of Pediatric Psychology, 12,* 25–38.

Worchel, F., Nolan, B., Willson, V., Purser, J., Copeland, D., & Pfefferbaum, B. (1988). Assessment of depression in children with cancer. *Journal of Pediatric Psychology, 13,* 101–112.

Zeltzer, L. K. (1980). The adolescent with cancer. In J. Kellerman (Ed.), *Psychological aspects of childhood cancer* (pp. 70–99). Springfield, IL: Charles C Thomas.

Zeltzer, L. K., & LeBaron, S. B. (1982). Hypnosis and nonhypnotic techniques for reduction of pain and anxiety during painful procedures in children and adolescents with cancer. *Journal of Pediatrics, 101,* 1032–1035.

3

Pain and Symptom Management

LONNIE ZELTZER

Pain in children with cancer is often unrecognized and is therefore not treated or prevented. Because pain is an experience common to all health-care professionals and specific training in pain evaluation and treatment is a rare commodity, everyone becomes an "expert," a phenomenon resulting in inadequately treated pediatric pain. Often the psychologist or other mental health professional is called upon to treat anticipatory fear after a child has learned that a medical procedure is a highly distressing event. Had this procedure not been so aversive, such referral might not have been necessary, at least for the majority of children. Since there is mounting evidence that undue stress not only may be emotionally toxic but has adverse physiological consequences as well, an integral part of the medical treatment of children with cancer should include reduction of psychologically distressing symptoms.

Why are distressing symptoms, such as pain, not well addressed, despite the now numerous studies that provide supportive evidence for the efficacy of a variety of cognitive-behavioral intervention strategies? The answer may lie in several areas of insufficiency: (1) diminished attention to distressing symptoms until compliance with diagnostic tests or treatment becomes an issue or until parents become vociferous enough to call attention to the problem; (2) inadequate knowledge about pain evaluation and treatment so that there is an assumption that "all is being done that could be done"; and (3) absence of algorithms indicating how to apply research study results to individual patients in the clinical setting.

The intent of this chapter is to provide a rationale for the treatment of pain and other distressing symptoms in children with cancer and to review contemporary symptom management. The goal is to translate research findings into useful information that will find its way into clinical practice. Focusing on acute pain, this chapter builds a framework for understanding variation in symptoms across children undergoing the same procedure or chemotherapy or variation in symptoms for the same child at different points in time. A brief review of the anatomy and physiology of pain transmission and inhibition is included. This information sets the biological stage for the complex psychobiological drama played out in the interactions between the child and his or her environment resulting in the symptom of pain. Medical management of pain is then discussed with the purpose of integrating psychological treatment with appropriate pharmacological approaches to pain management so that individualized care can be provided. Not all children require drugs for symptom control, nor should psychological strategies be used only after all other methods fail.

The goal of optimal symptom treatment is prevention. To accomplish this goal within the realities of a busy pediatric oncology service, the ''stress-vulnerable'' child, who is likely to be at greatest risk for developing pain and other distressing symptoms, must be identified *before* symptoms become a problem. Thus research findings regarding stress vulnerability will be reviewed, especially as they apply to pain in children, and practical algorithms for identifying such children will be offered, as much as study findings permit. Using this same framework, treatment of other symptoms, such as anticipatory anxiety, will be discussed and practical recommendations will be offered. Finally, directions for research will be outlined.

Pain: An Overview

Pain may be viewed as a complex interplay of biological, cognitive-developmental, situational, and affective factors. The adequate evaluation and management of pain in children requires an understanding of how these factors interact for an individual patient. Age, context, and cultural factors moderate the relationship between sensory aspects of the pain experience and the child's emotional response to and behavioral expression of pain. As the child matures and experiences more pain, significant individuals in the environment provide feedback to the child in response to the child's pain behaviors, and this feedback modifies further the child's expressions of personal distress and pain (Zeltzer, Anderson, & Schechter, 1990).

Pain, as defined by the International Association for the Study of Pain (IASP), is ''an unpleasant sensory and emotional experience associated with actual or potential tissue damage, or described in terms of such damage.'' Implicit in the sensation of pain is the process of transmission of signals from the periphery to the central nervous system (CNS). A, B, and C class afferent nerves are the principal types of nerve fibers which carry signals from the periphery to the CNS. Noxious perturbations from thermal, mechanical, or chemical stimuli, which can potentially produce tissue damage if prolonged, typically activate specialized nerve fibers that carry signals to the CNS. This process is termed *nociception*. The receptors on the ends of these specialized nerves are termed *nociceptors*. Nociceptors generate signals that are first transmitted along afferent nerve fibers to the spinal cord through the dorsal root ganglia where their cell bodies reside. Release of compounds such as substance P, histamine, certain protanoids, acetyl-

choline, potassium, bradykinin, and serotonin from damaged tissue increases noci-
ceptor sensitivity and thus enhances the amount of pain experienced.

Small, thinly myelinated A-δ fibers when stimulated produce sharp, rapid,
well-localized pain of short duration. Activation of the unmyelinated C fibers produces a dull, aching, poorly localized pain sensation. In the spinal cord, afferent
A-δ and C pain fibers synapse on a variety of sensory neurons including
nociceptive-specific neurons. The first opportunity for modulation of painful signals occurs at the initial synaptic junctions in the spinal cord. Incoming nociceptive signals are amplified or suppressed by other afferent signals and by descend-
ing signals from higher brain centers. Many neuroactive substances identified
during the past decade modulate afferent and efferent pain signals. Nociceptive
signals are carried to higher centers in the brain such as the thalamus, reticular
formation, the limbic system, and the cerebral cortex through a number of different afferent tracts in the spinal cord.

Multiple areas in the brain appear to be involved in modifying or modulating
afferent pain input (see Zeltzer, Anderson, & Schechter, 1990, for more detail).
Electrical stimulation of discrete areas of the brain can produce analgesia to noxious stimuli. The discovery of the binding of morphine in the periaqueductal/
periventricular gray areas of the midbrain has stimulated the search for endogenous opioid molecules. The first of these opioid peptides to be identified were the
pentapeptides, Leu-enkephalin and Met-enkephalin. Several additional endogenous opioids have been characterized, including dynorphin and β-endorphin.

Considering that the perception of pain is produced by such a dynamic, highly
integrated system, it becomes easy to understand how a child's memory of past
pain experiences, expectations of pain, and affective state (e.g., anxiety), with
fatigue or the presence of other symptoms (e.g., nausea), can combine to influence
the experience of pain. Increased patient attention to the sensory aspect of tissue
damage from a medical procedure might serve to heighten arousal, perhaps enhancing pain perception. Other cognitive and affective factors might serve to increase pain or, conversely, to inhibit pain and thus reduce suffering. There may
also be individual biological differences (perhaps genetic) in the threshold for
noxious stimuli, arousal, and neural integration and self-regulation, as reflected in
differences in recovery following a pain experience (Boyce, Barr, & Zeltzer,
1992).

The concept of individual differences as traits that orient the child's receptivity
and reaction to the environment is not new. Child development theorists have
posited that consistent, inherent predispositions underlie and modulate the expression of activity, reactivity, emotionality, and sociability (Goldsmith et al., 1987).
For example, Rothbart and Posner (1985) suggest that there are relatively stable,
primarily biologically based individual differences in reactivity and self-
regulation. Others (Goldsmith & Campos, 1982) suggest that these individual differences are manifest in the probability of experiencing and expressing the primary
emotions and arousal. The link between behavioral styles and biological reactivity
under stress has been demonstrated in the studies of Kagan and colleagues (Kagan,
Reznick, & Snidman, 1987, 1988; Kagan, Reznick, Clarke, Snidman, & Garcia-
Coll, 1987), who documented a characteristic pattern of biological reactivity in

children who are behaviorally inhibited (e.g., elevated heart rates and increases in plasma cortisol). Suomi (1988) found similar rises in heart rates, sympathetic adrenomedullary activation, and increases in plasma cortisol in behaviorally inhibited monkeys. Type A personality in children has also been associated with heightened cardiovascular and adrenergic responses to threat or challenge (Krantz & Manuck, 1984; Manuck, Kaplan, & Matthews, 1986). Thus individual differences in pain and anxiety associated with the same medical procedures may relate, at least in part, to inherent biological characteristics of the child. However, it is important to emphasize that the structure of the CNS is such that there is extensive flexibility in psychological response to a pain experience. Thus psychological interventions can activate the pain inhibitory system and can be as powerful an influence on pain as pharmacological interventions.

The Problem of Pain in Pediatric Oncology

Cancer treatment and evaluation, especially for leukemia and non-Hodgkin's lymphoma, often necessitate repeated bone marrow aspirations (BMAs) and lumbar punctures (LPs). A BMA is the insertion of a needle at the anterior or posterior hip site through the skin and periosteum into the bone in order to withdraw a sample of marrow at the center of the bone. If the skin and periosteum are not anesthetized, acute pain may be experienced because of the many afferent nociceptive nerve fibers in this region. Often intense pressure is experienced as the needle pierces the bone. However, most children report that the most severe pain is elicited by the withdrawal of marrow as a vacuum is created within the bone. Local anesthetics cannot reduce the nociception activated by this event. Unlike a BMA performed on the anterior hip bone, an LP cannot be witnessed by the child because it involves the insertion of a needle between two lumbar vertebrae of the back into the spinal canal to withdraw spinal fluid and also, in some cases, inject chemotherapeutic agents. If this procedure is performed rapidly and with skill, it may involve minimal discomfort for most children, although they may still have significant anxiety. For the LP to be technically efficient, the child must be curled tightly into a "ball" and not move. Not uncommonly, the child may squirm and there may be several attempts at needle insertion. If the child is not in the proper position, the needle may land on the vertebral bone rather than entering the space between the bones, which can elicit much pain. All children with cancer, regardless of diagnosis, will also undergo numerous venipunctures for blood tests and for administration of chemotherapy.

Acute medical procedure pain and distress for children with cancer can be so extreme that some children refuse further therapy, thus compromising their survival (Dolgin, Katz, Doctors, & Siegel, 1986; Jay, Ozolins, Elliott, & Caldwell, 1983; Kellerman, & Siegel, 1980; LeBaron & Zeltzer, 1984; Smith, Rosen, Trueworthy, & Lowman, 1979). Medical procedure distress, once established, may become difficult to treat. Thus early identification and preventive treatment could reduce intervention personnel time, medical treatment delays due to child distress, and noncompliance. Chronic pain related to intensive treatment or treatment failure (i.e., relapse or tumor progression) can also become problematic. Pain in children with cancer is generally underestimated by health-care personnel and consequently undertreated (Miser, Dothage, Wesley, & Miser, 1987; Miser, McCalla, Dothage, Wesley, & Miser, 1987).

Children with cancer may undergo surgery for diagnostic purposes (e.g., tumor biopsy) or for treatment (i.e., tumor excision). Hospitalized children typically experience a multitude of acute pain stressors, in addition to surgery-related pain. For example, during the postoperative period, children are expected to cope with acute procedural pain related to dressing changes, suture and drain removals, and wound probing, besides the usual venipunctures. Children who are hospitalized for nonsurgical reasons may have disease-related pain which is also insufficiently managed. These children may have to undergo other painful perturbations in the course of their diagnostic evaluation and/or medical treatment. The child whose current level of pain has not been adequately addressed may have reduced tolerance to cope with new perturbations and thus respond with what may seem like inappropriately severe distress and lack of self-control. Once children have one or more negative painful experiences (e.g., with invasive medical procedures), the memory of that pain experience may contribute to the development of anxiety reactions in anticipation of future procedures (Anderson, Fanurik, & Zeltzer, in press-a; Zeltzer, Jay, & Fisher, 1989). Anticipatory fear with expectations of pain can then contribute to the overall aversiveness of the pain experience. A cascade of different manifestations of stress can ensue, including behavioral withdrawal or irritability, difficulty sleeping, and physiological signs of arousal such as elevated adrenal cortical and medullary stress hormones and metabolic sequelae based on the actions of these hormones (Anand, Carr, & Hickey, 1987; Anand, Hansen, & Hickey, 1990; Anand & Hickey, 1987, 1992; Anand Sippell, & Aynsley-Green, 1987; Anand et al., 1985).

Children with cancer may not only suffer emotionally from undertreated pain, but there may also be medical risks inherent in persistent or recurrent acute pain in children who are already medically unstable or vulnerable. Recent findings in an animal model have shown that pain reduced natural killer (NK) cell levels and, without adequate analgesics, an implanted NK-sensitive tumor metastasized to the lungs. In contrast, no metastases and normal NK levels were found when morphine was administered for postoperative pain control (Page, Ben-Eliyahu, Yirmiya, & Liebeskind, in press). Thus attention to pain, especially in ill and immunocompromised children, is a clinically relevant issue of major importance.

Symptom Evaluation

The undertreatment of pain in children highlights the issue of definition and measurement of any symptom that is a personal experience. By traditional definition, pain is defined at the level of the individual. That is, to understand an individual's personal suffering, the individual must be asked to describe that experience. The nature of human development complicates the presumably simple task of learning if a child is experiencing pain, without considering the added task of quantifying the magnitude of the pain. Pain descriptors used by children, depending on their cognitive stage and previous pain experiences, may have different meanings than those of the querying adult. Similarly, a child may be afraid to express to others his or her personal suffering, as illustrated by a child whose postoperative analgesic orders are written for intramuscular injections to be given when the child complains of pain. Fearing the "shot," the child might suppress behavioral expression of personal suffering.

If pain can be determined only by asking children for self-reports of this experience, then how is pain defined and measured in preverbal children and infants? This issue is similar to the problem of defining and measuring stress in young children. Just because there is difficulty in measurement, phenomena such as pain and other stress experiences cannot be said to not exist. Rather, "proxy variables" are used to imply pain. In infants, the term nociception is used to indicate the infant's observable behavior or physiological reactions in response to a presumably noxious (painful) perturbation, which can be an acute event (e.g., bone marrow aspiration) or a continued aversive experience (e.g., metastatic disease). However, other, nonnociceptive stressors (e.g., having an X-ray taken) might also produce these same responses. For some children, especially very young children and infants, the only way to learn if pain is present is to observe *changes* in the child's behavioral and physiological responses following treatment directed to alleviate pain (Zeltzer & Zeltzer, 1989). If the child can then become engaged in play and can eat and sleep better than before treatment, it can be assumed that the child was in pain prior to treatment.

The problem of evaluating pain and other symptoms in children is compounded by individual and contextual differences in children's verbal and nonverbal expressions of pain. For example, in clinical settings such as the hospital, children differ in their expression of pain. A quiet, withdrawn child who does not complain may be assumed to be comfortable, while an irritable, whiny child may be assumed to be anxious. Both children, in fact, may be experiencing severe pain and both may exhibit concurrent physiological proxy indicators of nociception (e.g., hypertension, tachycardia, tachypnea).

The context may also exert an influence on pain-related behaviors. A boy who injures his arm during a baseball game may not complain about pain until the game is over and he is alone with his parents with no friends to observe his behavior. Yet that same child in the pediatric oncology clinic when experiencing the same amount of tissue injury related to a medical procedure may exhibit a multitude of distress behaviors. As shown by Shaw and Routh (1982), children undergoing bone marrow aspirations display more "distress behaviors" when mothers are present in the treatment room than when they are excluded. In the case of medical procedures, pain behaviors form part of the child's communication repertoire in seeking the parent's aid and comfort. Thus overt behavior is only one potential indicator of pain and is not, in itself, a direct measure of nociception, just as there are many reasons for crying besides pain.

As noted by LeBaron and Zeltzer (1984), an understanding of the extent of a child's pain or other symptoms involves asking the child, observing the child's behavior, and, based on clinical experience, forming an overall impression of the extent of pain. There are a variety of instruments available to assess these dimensions of pain. For further discussion of these instruments, readers are referred to McGrath (1990). In general, useful self-reports can be obtained in children as young as 3 to 5 years of age. Beyer and Wells (1989) found that children 7 years or younger provide more reliable ratings with a vertical rather than horizontal visual analogue scale (e.g., a 10-centimeter line anchored with happy and sad faces). While there are several behavioral checklists (McGrath, 1990; McGrath & Unruh, 1987; Zeltzer & LeBaron, 1986a), LeBaron and Zeltzer (1984) pointed out the importance of using measures that are not age-biased, since older children and adolescents tend to exhibit more controlled behaviors (e.g., flinching, muscle tension) than younger children when in pain. If these behaviors, for example, are not included on the checklist, it might be erroneously assumed that adolescents have less pain than younger children. The accuracy of inferences of pain by observations of the child's distress or suffering depends on the clinical experience of the observer as well as knowledge of the child.

Planning Pain Treatment

A problem with a variety of available pain measurement tools is that they do not capture sufficient information to plan treatment. Psychological intervention is usually not routinely incorporated into pediatric care, and intervention is sought typically only for those children who have demonstrated significant distress. Generally, psychosocial staff time and availability are the rate-limiting steps for such preventive intervention. While all children can benefit from some type of support or intervention during painful medical procedures, there are some children who are at higher risk than others for developing pain problems. Guidelines derived from research findings and clinical experience that can be used to plan treatment for children who exhibit procedure-related distress will be summarized shortly. There are also recent preliminary findings related to identification of the "pain-vulnerable child" that can aid in targeting children for psychological referral in advance of the development of significant pain and anxiety.

A careful assessment must be undertaken at the time of referral, in order to learn about the child, his or her family, and the factors that may influence how the pain or distress is experienced. The efficacy of specific interventions will depend on a number of factors including the extent of the pain or distress experienced by the child, cognitive-developmental level, individual characteristics such as coping style and perceived self-efficacy (perceived ability to cope), and environmental influences which enhance or interfere with the child's ability to cope successfully. The child and parents should be interviewed to obtain information concerning the child's previous experience with the specific or similar medical procedures, pain in other situations, the child's social support system, and characteristics of the child.

A quantitative and qualitative assessment of the child's pain and anxiety should be undertaken both prior to and following intervention. As noted in the previous section, the assessment should not be limited to behavioral observation.

Pain behaviors can be deceiving and the importance of interviewing the child regarding pain should not be underestimated, especially to learn about the child's coping strategies. For example, older children and adolescents exhibit less behavioral distress and develop more cognitive strategies to cope with painful events (LeBaron & Zeltzer, 1984). Therefore, anticipatory anxiety and procedure-related pain may be well hidden in some adolescents, although these patients may subjectively suffer as much as younger children who scream and behaviorally resist procedures. Children's difficulties in coping with procedural pain may be overlooked if the children are cooperative because they are not specifically asked about their experience and extent of suffering.

A child's previous experience with the same or a related pain situation can have both positive and negative consequences. For example, previous pain situations experienced as distressing may create anticipatory anxiety for future procedures. Unsuccessful coping attempts may result in decreased self-confidence, a poor perception of coping abilities, and negative expectations for handling future procedures. Conversely, the successful use of coping skills during a pain situation can contribute to feelings of mastery and confidence regarding abilities to cope with future procedures. Therefore, it is crucial to ask the child to describe in detail those aspects of prior medical procedures that were most or least distressing, coping strategies used, including those that were most helpful, and those factors that interfered with adaptive coping.

Environmental or situational factors that can increase or decrease the amount of pain and anxiety a child experiences during an invasive procedure include the behavior and comments of people present, expectations the child holds based on what she or he has been told in advance of the procedure, and the meaning attached to the procedure (i.e., diagnostic or therapeutic). Parents and others present may make inadvertent comments that do not promote adaptive coping, such as "catastrophizing" statements regarding the procedure or expectations of pain (e.g., "If you don't hold still it will hurt more"). Frustrated parents, in efforts to make their child cooperate, can use punishment or threats (e.g., "Stop screaming or the doctor will give you two shots"). Such efforts to control their child's behavior may increase the child's arousal and affect the relationship with the parents.

Often parents' anxiety and distress result from lack of knowledge about how to help their child cope. Intervention for these children should be directed toward helping the parents learn how to help their child. In cases where there is overwhelming distress, parents may need to be referred to an appropriate professional for dealing with issues surrounding their child's treatment and illness. Expectations of the child about the procedure can affect how well he or she is prepared to cope and how the procedure is experienced. For example, anticipation of pain beyond the child's perceptions of her or his abilities to cope can enhance anticipatory anxiety. Thus children who have developed anticipatory fears can benefit from preparation by discussion of the mechanical and sensory aspects of the procedure and from practice in coping (Zeltzer, Jay, & Fisher, 1989).

Planning treatment also involves assessment of level and type of parental support of the child. Parents or other close relatives are usually the child's primary source of support during medical procedures. However, as mentioned previously, parents may not always be able or know how to provide the kind of support their child needs. Parental anxiety and children's distress during bone marrow aspirations have been found to be positively related (Jay et al., 1983). Several studies have suggested that children are more likely to inhibit behavioral expression of their distress if they are not accompanied by a parent during the procedure (Shaw & Routh, 1982). However, Ross and Ross (1984) found that 99 percent of 720 children (aged 9 to 12 years) interviewed reported that the "thing that helped most," regardless of the type of pain experience, was to have one's parent present.

These observations suggest the need for concurrent parent-child intervention, although only few reports have described interventions for parents. These have consisted of preparation and cognitive-behavioral interventions for parents and children about to undergo surgery (Wolfer & Visintainer, 1979), catheterization (Campbell, Clark, & Kirkpatrick, 1986), and BMAs and LPs (Jay & Elliott, 1990). Older children and adolescents should be asked whether they want a parent (and which parent) to be present while they are undergoing a medical procedure. Intervention planning should include consideration of parent involvement, if needed.

In developing effective interventions, the child's perceptions and experiences of different phases of a procedure must be considered. Peterson, Harbeck, Chaney, Farmer, and Thomas (1990) describe two aspects of coping, anticipatory and encounter; the child's experience of both aspects of a medical procedure must be considered in planning intervention. Evaluation and treatment of anticipatory distress will be reviewed in more detail later in this chapter.

The child's cognitive-developmental level will also play a major role in determining his or her understanding of the pain experience, as well as his or her abilities to utilize or respond to specific intervention techniques. Behavioral strategies for the management of pain in preverbal and very young children (infancy through 2 years) should not be overlooked. Behavioral approaches for pain control in infants include rocking, soothing talk, stroking, and nonnutritive sucking (Berman, Duncan, & Zeltzer, 1992). Whether the demonstrated efficacy of these techniques results from distraction away from the painful stimulus, increased neural organization and self-regulation of the infant, stimulation of larger afferent fibers which might interfere with pain transmission, or effects of vestibular stimulation is unknown. Pacifiers decrease irritability and crying associated with heel sticks and circumcisions (Gunnar, 1992). Restraint of infant movement may also have some benefits. Swaddling, like a pacifier, may reduce arousal and thus help the infant become more self-regulated. However, formal research within this age range has been limited.

Young children (aged 2 to 7) will likely have difficulty understanding the reasons for medical procedures. A procedure may often be perceived as punishment. Young children frequently blame their parents for allowing the painful procedure to occur. Attempts to reason with very young children will not likely be helpful. Rather, young children may benefit more by desensitization techniques or play therapy in advance of procedures, by reinforcing the child's positive behaviors during the procedure, and by simple distraction techniques. The child 8 years and older will usually have the capacity to understand the reasons for medical procedures and can respond to psychological interventions commonly used with older children and adolescents. Younger children, those with less self-control, and those with developmental delays will benefit more from behavioral techniques which require less cognitive effort on their part, such as mutual storytelling, visual distraction, counting, or breathing.

Adolescents may regress when they become acutely anxious and may require help in controlling their fear and in utilizing effective coping mechanisms. Often a discussion of the procedure with plans for coping and practice of coping techniques can be quite useful. How best to help an individual child or adolescent will depend on the child's own natural styles of coping and other factors to be discussed shortly.

The natural coping skills that a child brings to a painful situation can mediate his or her experience and expression of pain and influence the effectiveness of pain management intervention. It is generally accepted that with increasing age and cognitive maturity, a broader array of strategies to control pain and anxiety are developed, replacing behavioral strategies with cognitive methods of alleviating or controlling pain and anxiety (Anderson et al., in press-a). Increasing attention has now been directed toward characterizing children's individual styles of coping in order to develop more effective, individualized methods of pain intervention. Siegel and Smith (1989) and Peterson et al. (1990), among others, have described children's coping styles in response to medical events on a continuum from active (information-seeking) to avoidant (information-avoiding). The information-seeking–information-avoiding continuum appears to have the most relevance for coping in anticipation of medical events and for learning how best to prepare a child for procedures.

A number of studies (Hubert, Jay, Saltoun, & Hayes, 1988; Peterson & Toler, 1986; Smith, Ackerson, & Blotcky, 1989) have indicated that children using more active coping strategies generally appear to have more beneficial responses during pain situations. Thus children who ask more questions, who look at and want to touch and play with hospital preparatory materials, and who show increased physiological arousal while watching a preparation film are more likely to be cooperative during medical procedures and to report medical procedures or surgery as more tolerable than are children who are "avoiders." However, children's methods of coping *during* medical procedures can be very different from coping in *anticipation* of an upcoming procedure. For example, in another study (Fanurik et al., 1991), "attenders" during a painful event had less pain tolerance than did "distractors" (children who kept their attention on something other than the pain). Thus it is important to evaluate children's coping styles *before* an expected pain event as well as *during* the painful experience.

Clinical observation during medical procedures suggests that some interventions are more effective for certain children than others. For example, some children are observed to resist attempts at distraction and appear to become more distressed when they are unable to watch or monitor the steps of a procedure. Unfortunately, little exists in the pediatric literature concerning how to select the most effective techniques to implement with children during painful procedures, although methods of individualizing intervention to maximize successful outcome are beginning to receive empirical attention (Smith et al., 1989).

Fanurik, Zeltzer, Roberts, and Blount (in press) have examined styles of coping with a laboratory pain paradigm, the cold pressor procedure (prolonged arm immersion in cold water). Based on children's behavioral pain tolerance, they classified children into "attenders," those who primarily direct their focus of attention toward the cold pressor–induced sensations, or "distractors," those who divert their attention away from the cold pressor sensations. Over a 2-week period, high within-child stability has been demonstrated in choice of coping strategy. Distractors, as a group, were found to have the highest pain tolerance.

To determine whether coping style is a salient variable in determining selection of an intervention strategy, they designed an experiment in which children were taught pain control strategies that were either "matched" or "mismatched" to their preferred coping style. Children were randomized to three groups (control, matched, and mismatched interventions), with each group balanced for coping style (attenders, distractors). A significant interaction was found between coping style and intervention, with the greatest increase in pain tolerance found for the distractors who were taught self-hypnosis (matched intervention) and greatest *decrease* in tolerance found for the distractors provided with sensory monitoring (mismatched intervention). The attenders did not significantly change their pain tolerance with either intervention strategy. One explanation of this lack of effect is that attenders may comprise a heterogeneous population whose subgroups are yet to be identified. Some of these children may not benefit from any psychological strategy and may require pharmacological intervention to prevent the development of anticipatory distress.

In addition to coping style, perceived source of control in anticipation of a procedure may be an important factor predicting the child's likely effectiveness in maintaining behavioral cooperativeness during the procedure. Carpenter (1990) has found that children who believed that no one could help them cope with an impending phlebotomy were significantly more likely to delay or extend the procedure than were children who perceived some source of control (self, parent, or mutual). Neither age nor gender was related to perceived source of control.

Current practice continues to rely on clinical judgment for intervention to help children cope with painful procedures. Until the emergence of more research in this area, current findings suggest that children's perceived sources of control in anticipation of a procedure and coping skills during the procedure should be assessed through interviews with both the child and the parent, and appropriate individualized intervention should then be initiated. Children can be asked in advance of a procedure how well they believe they will be able to cope with the procedure and who, if anyone, will help them do this. They can also be asked what they have found to be most effective (as well as ineffective) for coping with previous procedures, in addition to what they believe would be helpful for the upcoming procedure. Interventions based on the information provided might include parent-child strategies aimed at enhancing the child's expectations of effective coping or trust in the parent to help her or him cope.

Peterson et al. (1990) called attention to the importance of anticipatory coping. Training the child and parent in effective strategies for coping with the actual procedure ("encounter coping") should be based on the child's level of anxiety, perceived self-effectiveness, prior experience, and coping style. However, continual assessment of the effectiveness of these strategies from the child's perspective, as well as observation, will be needed to modify any strategies that appear ineffective or counterproductive to children's own efforts at coping. Children who are unable to divert their attention away from the aversive aspects of the procedure and cannot reframe these aspects to reduce their aversiveness may need pharmacological intervention, such as conscious sedation, at least until they can develop enhanced abilities to cope. The ultimate goal of psychological intervention is to maximize children's own coping abilities and to increase feelings of self-efficacy and mastery.

Pharmacological Management of Acute Pain

General guidelines regarding pharmacological management of medical procedure pain and anxiety have been outlined previously (Zeltzer, Jay, & Fisher, 1989). For example, optimal pharmacological treatment of the initial diagnostic procedures (e.g., bone marrow aspiration, lumbar puncture) can reduce fear of subsequent procedures and permit time for evaluation of the child and family in order to plan and carry out psychological intervention. Medical procedures should be performed only by medical personnel who are or will be performing them often on a regular basis (e.g., oncology fellows rather than pediatric house staff) to ensure optimal technical skill. If analgesia and sedation with intravenous short-acting opiates and benzodiazepines (e.g., fentanyl, midazolam) are to be used, there should be appropriate monitoring and resuscitation equipment and personnel available. Drugs should be used in appropriate doses and the patient should be evaluated to determine pharmacological efficacy and need for changes in doses or types of drugs used. Thus the determining factor in dosing should be efficacy in controlling pain rather than expected results based on drug pharmacokinetics.

Decisions regarding the use of pharmacological agents for treating procedure-related pain should be individualized and based on the invasiveness and duration of the procedure, anxiety level of the child, coping abilities and distress of the child during past procedures, and context. A child who requires medication for a procedure at one point in time may cope well without drugs after psychological intervention for a subsequent procedure. Pharmacological and psychological interventions are not mutually exclusive and can be used successfully in combination for many children. Readers are referred to Zeltzer, Jay, and Fisher (1989), Zeltzer, Anderson, and Schechter (1990), Anderson, Fanurik, and Zeltzer (in press-a), Anderson and Zeltzer (in press), and Anderson, Fanurik, and Zeltzer (in press-b) for more details regarding pharmacological treatment of pain and anxiety among children with cancer.

Psychological Treatment of Acute Pain and Anxiety

There are a number of specific psychological interventions that can be helpful in reducing children's procedure-related pain and distress. The selection of one or more techniques should be based on assessment of the child and family and consideration of other factors discussed previously. As noted by Carpenter (1991), studies of psychological interventions have been based primarily on strategy testing rather than model building. Thus a variety of approaches have been compared in terms of efficacy (e.g., hypnosis versus nonimagery support). Generally speaking, psychological intervention is better than no intervention; especially useful are intervention "packages" that include a smorgasbord of strategies (Jay, 1988; Jay, Elliott, Katz, & Siegel, 1987; Jay, Elliott, Ozolins, Olson, & Pruitt, 1985). What these studies have typically *not* provided are algorithms permitting optimal intervention for an individual child. As will be discussed under research directions, there are current investigative moves in this direction that should enhance the likelihood of effective intervention. The most commonly studied interventions will be described next.

Preparation

Preparation is perhaps the most widely used psychological intervention to help children cope with anxiety related to anticipation of a painful event. The central core of preparation is the provision of information, including sensory (what it may feel like) and mechanical (what will be done) aspects of the procedure. Sensory information might include being told that the cleansing of the body part upon which the procedure will be performed might feel "cool" and perhaps pleasantly "tingly" while the local anesthetic might feel like a "pinch" or a "prick," allowing the "skin and nerves to go to sleep and feel numb." Mechanical information involves the steps of the procedure. A combination of sensory and mechanical information appears to be most effective (Zeltzer, Jay, & Fisher, 1989).

The rationale underlying preparatory interventions is that unexpected stress is more anxiety provoking and more difficult to cope with than anticipated or predictable stress (Siegel, 1976). Preparation is often best provided by nursing staff or child life specialists who know the child well, because the amount of information provided will depend on the child's level of anxiety, perceived control over the anticipated procedure, and coping styles (anticipatory and encounter). For example, provision of procedural information both before and during the procedure for a child with an "avoidant" anticipatory style and a "distractor" encounter style might be counterproductive, especially if the child's natural coping abilities are already effective.

Desensitization

For children who have anticipatory distress or severe fears of medical procedures, desensitization can be an effective intervention. This behavioral technique involves gradually exposing the child to the stimuli associated with the medical procedure in hierarchical steps, perhaps beginning with practice imagining the procedure, advancing to the child performing the procedure on a doll, and eventually concluding with practice in coping effectively with a "mock" procedure in the actual treatment room if this is possible (Poster & Betz, 1983). This technique should be combined with training in effective coping skills to permit mastery in coping with procedure-related pain and anxiety.

Positive Self-Statements and Thought-Stopping

The use of positive self-statements involves teaching a number of simple statements that the child can repeat to himself or herself during times of fear, for example, when a child receives a venipuncture (IV stick). These statements would relate to appraisal of the situation (e.g., "This is an IV stick. I've had this before."), self-efficacy (e.g., "I know what to do during an IV stick."), and positive expectations ("I know that the IV stick will go quickly and it won't bother me.").

Positive self-statements are often coupled with thought-stopping (Ross, 1984). In this strategy, the child is told that whenever he starts thinking about the feared procedure (e.g., an IV stick), he should stop whatever he is doing and say "stop!" These techniques are most effective for dealing with anticipatory distress, but they can be used during the actual procedure as well.

Positive Reinforcement

Positive reinforcement is a relatively simple intervention that involves encouragement with positive statements about the child and tangible rewards (e.g., stickers, badges, prizes) immediately following the procedure. A child should be rewarded for any positive behavior or even for just coping with the procedure. On the other hand, uncooperative behaviors should *not* be punished and the child should never be threatened or made to feel ashamed if he or she is unable to cooperate. Reward contingencies should not be set up in advance for behavior that the child is unlikely to control such as crying. Positive reinforcement will likely be most effective if the child is also taught coping strategies to use during the procedure.

Distraction Techniques

Distraction techniques help children reduce pain and distress during the actual procedure. The goal of distraction is to focus children's attention away from the painful aspects of the procedure. While there are a variety of ways of distracting children's attention away from aversive stimuli (e.g., counting, blowing bubbles, using noisemakers or roll-out objects, looking at pop-up books, concentrating on another body part), hypnosis, emphasizing imaginative involvement, often can be an effective way to maintain continued attention and interest and reframe sensory experiences (Zeltzer & LeBaron, 1986b). For example, the child might imagine burying her hand in snow until it is numb in preparation for an IV stick or pouring a magic liquid on it to make it "go to sleep." Knowledge of the child's interests, hobbies, favorite television programs and movies, friends, and desires can make the imaginative experience absorbing and meaningful to the child. Maintenance of the imaginative involvement can be accomplished often with the help of therapist- or parent-initiated pleasant surprises along the way to pique the child's curiosity and to engage the child in the development of the fantasy. Young children (3 to 6 years) may need props to help them in fantasy play, and children who are highly anxious or who have difficulty maintaining focused attention for other reasons may need to shift their attention back and forth between the medical procedure and the fantasy. These children often require information about the progress of the procedure and benefit from frequent reassurance throughout the procedure that all is progressing well. Children whose natural coping style is to focus their attention on the pain may not benefit at all from hypnosis and should be considered for other types of treatment. For further discussion of hypnotherapy, readers are referred to Zeltzer and LeBaron (1986b), Hilgard and LeBaron (1984), and Olness and Gardner (1989). For further information on distraction techniques for younger children, see Kuttner, Bowman, and Teasdale (1988) and McGrath (1990).

Distraction strategies, including hypnosis, may be associated with and facilitate relaxation. Deep breathing and progressive relaxation of muscle groups (with or without preceding selective muscle tension) are other methods for achieving a relaxed state. Not uncommonly a child can be engaged in an active imaginative experience, such as playing football, that is highly effective in controlling procedural distress without being "relaxed."

Modeling and Rehearsal

Methods of teaching and reinforcing coping techniques for use prior to or during medical procedures include modeling and rehearsal. Modeling involves some type of actual demonstration that displays positive coping behavior. For example, as in the studies of Jay (1988; Jay et al., 1985, 1987), the child views a videotape of another child undergoing the same medical procedure, where positive coping behaviors can be observed. Another effective use of modeling is to teach parents coping behaviors that they can demonstrate to their child.

After the child is taught specific coping strategies that best suit the needs and characteristics of the child, it is beneficial to provide the child with opportunities to practice these techniques. Such rehearsal not only reinforces these positive behaviors but also gives the child reassurance about his or her own abilities to cope effectively.

Management of Chronic Pain and Other Distressing Symptoms

Evaluation and treatment of persistent pain and other symptoms that might last longer than acute, procedure-related pain and anxiety, such as chemotherapy-related nausea and vomiting, involve the same principles already discussed. These include evaluation of the symptom through child self-report with ratings and interview-obtained descriptors of the experience, behavioral observation, and physiological indicators. Even for symptoms such as nausea and vomiting, children as young as 5 years of age can provide reliable self-reports through the use a rating scale (Zeltzer, LeBaron, Richie, & Reed, 1988). Important information for planning treatment includes assessment of coping style, perceived control over the symptom, parental support style, and the child's past history of similar symptoms. Many of the same psychological and pharmacological interventions can be used for either acute or chronic symptoms.

Studies of psychological interventions such as hypnosis and other distraction techniques are effective for reduction of nausea and vomiting, symptoms that tend to get worse over time with no intervention (Zeltzer, Dolgin, LeBaron, & LeBaron, 1991). As with acute pain, there is great variability in chemotherapy-related distress, usually measured by nausea, vomiting, and subjective "bother," even for the same chemotherapeutic agents (LeBaron, Zeltzer, LeBaron, Scott, & Zeltzer, 1988; Zeltzer, LeBaron, & Zeltzer, 1984b). Thus there are many factors besides the direct drug effects that appear to be strong moderators of symptom production such as anxiety level, prior chemotherapy experience, medical status (e.g., presence of other symptoms such as fatigue), and expectations. There may also be differences in vulnerability to these potential moderators, resulting in large variance in symptoms within a disease category or treatment protocol. The direction of research needs to be the identification of the environmental moderators and child characteristics that result in individual differences in cancer-related distress so that more individualized treatments can be developed.

Despite similarities in evaluation and treatment of a variety of symptoms, there are some unique considerations related to persistent symptoms that will be reviewed here. For recurrent symptoms, such as those associated with chemotherapy, aversiveness of initial experiences (unconditioned stimuli) may come to elicit anticipatory symptoms through association with stimuli that have been repeatedly associated with the chemotherapy (conditioned stimuli; Burish & Lyles, 1981; Morrow, 1982; Redd, Andreson, & Minagawa, 1982). One example is the child who becomes nauseated every time he sees the chemotherapy nurse in his neighborhood supermarket. More commonly, children often vomit when an antiemetic drug is administered intravenously, although the chemical action of the drug should prevent emesis. Beliefs and expectations can play powerful roles in symptom production, as indicated by one study (Zeltzer et al., 1984b) that found significantly more nausea and vomiting in the same children for chemotherapy courses with preventive antiemetics than when no antiemetics were administered for the same type of chemotherapy. The findings of this study dispel the myth that antiemetics are always better than no antiemetics and signify the importance of the child's expectations in symptom production. While advances in the development of antiemetics, such as ordansetron, have reduced the broad-spectrum need for psychological intervention for chemotherapy-related nausea and vomiting, there are still many children who develop these symptoms despite the use of these agents. In some ways, the drug advances have helped identify the vulnerable subpopulation of children that previous psychological intervention studies ignored, focusing instead on modal effects rather than the outliers in psychological treatment trials. Characterizing these children and identifying factors that exacerbate or mitigate their symptoms should be the direction of future psychobiological studies, since these are not being examined in antiemetic drug trials.

There are many factors that influence a child's experience and tolerance of pain and other persistent symptoms. For hospitalized children, the benefit of distractors during the day are evident when pain becomes intolerable only at night. The role of anxiety and fear in the pain experience is highlighted when potentially bad news related to disease or diagnostic testing is the only new event associated with an increase in pain and reduced pain tolerance. The impact of feelings of helplessness on the pain experience and on total analgesic requirements is evident in improved comfort and reduced drug needs when children can administer their own opiates through patient-controlled analgesia (PCA) delivery systems.

PCA involves the use of a computerized method of drug administration to the patient in which the child pushes a button located on the end of a cord at bedside to self-administer analgesic medication when she or he feels the need to do so. The physician programs the computer to provide a certain dose of medication, such as morphine or dilaudid®, when the patient pushes the button. A "lockout period," say, 6 or 8 minutes, is also programmed as a safety factor to prevent overdosage. Thus the child might press the button 40 times in an hour but only receive a maximum of 10 doses if the lockout period were set at 6 minutes. The other safety factor is that the child will become too sedated to press the button further if she or he is receiving too much medication. This is a safety factor only if no one but the child pushes the button. Thus parents and nurses must be instructed that the button is for the child's use exclusively.

Every time the button is pushed, most PCA machines provide a "ding" or other such sound to indicate that the button has been pushed. This sound occurs whether or not an actual dose of drug has been delivered. The rationale for the sound is that it reinforces the patient's belief that pain medication has been received. As noted previously, the child's beliefs about his or her pain are powerful moderators of the pain experience. The computer records the number of attempts and actual doses of drug delivered each hour, so that a profile of the patient's use of the machine can be obtained. For children with persistent severe pain, or perhaps during the first day after surgery, a "basal rate" can be programmed so that the child will receive a continuous infusion of opiate. The child can then push the button to self-administer additional medication as needed.

The concept behind PCA is that enhanced self-control over pain will reduce attentional focus on the pain, enhance feelings of self-efficacy, and reduce worry about the pain getting worse and becoming intolerable. Additionally, in comparison to periodic nurse-administered analgesia at specific time intervals in response to the child's pain complaints or behaviors, self-administration of frequent minidoses of drug, with or without continuous infusion of opiate, allows ongoing comfort, rather than the typical cycles of "peaks and valleys" of pain–drug administration–comfort–toxicity, and pain again when the drug effects wear off. This latter pattern often leads to clock watching with a focus on symptoms in order to ensure that there is sufficient time to call the nurse, have the nurse respond and get the medicine, receive the drug, and allow time for it to work. Through these mechanisms involved in self-administered analgesia, the total analgesic drug doses received are less than for nurse-administered analgesia (Rodgers, Webb, Stergios, & Newman, 1988). Contrary to popular belief, even adolescents titrate a balance between comfort and opiate side effects rather than pushing the button to a point of stupor (Tyler, 1990). We and others have used PCAs in children as young as 4 years of age, if they have the cognitive capacity to understand pushing a button "when it hurts."

Another factor in a child's ability to cope with chronic pain that is often overlooked, especially in hospitalized children, is the frequency with which the child is exposed to acute pain and nonpainful stressors. For example, a hospitalized child (e.g., during the postoperative period following bone marrow transplantation) typically has multiple phlebotomies, dressing changes, mouth care, and other repeated aversive events with which he or she is expected to cope. Even children who coped well with medical procedure pain as outpatients may lose their effectiveness in coping during intensive or prolonged hospitalization as fatigue, depression, anxiety, and feelings of loss of control set in. As the child continues to experience the repeated stressors of acute pain, abilities to cope with chronic pain may break down, a condition resulting in withdrawal, increased irritability and complaining, or oppositional behavior.

Future Directions

Most research in symptom management for children with cancer is directed toward (1) refined assessment, including identification of pain-vulnerable children; (2) improved methods of individualizing intervention; (3) more effective pharmacological treatment of pain and methods of drug delivery; and (4) determination of the impact of stress, and pain in particular, on immunocompetence, medical sequelae of pain-related immune dysfunction, and tumor growth and spread.

With regard to the first objective, studies from the laboratory of Zeltzer and Fanurik have shown that the cold pressor pain paradigm is a feasible and useful model in which to study individual differences in pain responsivity (LeBaron, Zeltzer, & Fanurik, 1989; Zeltzer, Fanurik & LeBaron, 1989). They found that children's responses were stable over a 2-week period (Fanurik et al., in press) and that laboratory pain responsivity predicted lumbar puncture pain responses (Mizell, Fanurik, & Zeltzer, 1992) in children with cancer and a variety of symptoms and health outcomes in healthy children (Shin, Fanurik, Ifekwunigwe, Le-Gagnous, & Zeltzer, 1992). In this school-based study of cold pressor responses in healthy children, high laboratory pain ratings were associated with more somatic complaints (vague pains, stomach aches, headaches, feeling "unwell" or other vague symptoms), higher symptom intensity, more school nurse visits for acute illnesses (upper respiratory symptoms or other observable signs of illness), and more school absences. These findings suggest that individual characteristics that lead to "pain vulnerability" may be the same or similar to child characteristics that render a child "stress vulnerable" as well.

Such laboratory studies of pain remove the "background noise" inherent in the clinical setting in order to help characterize child factors that lead to pain vulnerability. Conversely, the laboratory also removes important potential moderators of pain and other symptoms that aggregate to enhance the likelihood of the development of clinical pain problems. Thus pain and other symptoms must be studied both in the laboratory and in clinical settings in order to develop and test models that will aid in identifying pain- or symptom-vulnerable children and permit evaluation of targeted individualized intervention.

Studies are also needed to assist physicians in optimal pharmacological management of pain, preferably to reduce suffering and to mitigate the likelihood of the development of anticipatory pain and coping breakdown. Such studies might include evaluation of presurgery nociceptive inhibition through epidural analgesia of intravenous opiates, including the development of self-administered drug delivery systems for epidural and transdermal analgesia and anesthesia. Finally, likely the most powerful way to change medical treatment of pain and incorporate pain and symptom management as an integral part of cancer treatment is to document the impact of these aversive symptoms on disease course, including evaluation of mechanisms of action, such as immune effects of pain or changes in neural growth related to pain. Animal studies are a beginning in this avenue of research and careful clinical and laboratory child studies are also now indicated.

Acknowledgment

Preparation of this chapter was supported, in part, by the William T. Grant Foundation Research consortium, "The Developmental Psychobiology of Stress."

References

Anand, K. J. S., Brown, M. J., Causon, R. C., Christofides, N. D., Bloom, S. R., & Aynsley-Green, A. (1985). Can the human neonate mount an endocrine and metabolic response to surgery? *Journal of Pediatric Surgery, 20,* 41–48.

Anand, K. J. S., Carr, D. B., & Hickey, P. R. (1987). Randomized trial of high-dose sufentanil anesthesia in neonates undergoing cardiac surgery: Hormonal and hemodynamic stress responses. *Anesthesiology, 67,* A502.

Anand, K. J. S., Hansen, D. D., & Hickey, P. R. (1990). Hormonal-metabolic stress responses in neonates undergoing cardiac surgery. *Anesthesiology, 73,* 661–670.

Anand, K. J. S., & Hickey, P. R. (1987). Pain and its effects in the human neonate and fetus. *New England Journal of Medicine, 317,* 1321–1347.

Anand, K. J. S., & Hickey, P. R. (1992). Halothane-morphine compared with high-dose sufentanil for anesthesia and postoperative analgesia in neonatal cardiac surgery. *New England Journal of Medicine, 326,* 1–9.

Anand, K. J. S., Sippell, W. G., & Aynsley-Green, A. (1987). Randomised trial of fentanyl anesthesia in preterm babies undergoing surgery: Effects on the stress response. *Lancet, 1,* 243–248.

Anderson, C. T. M., Fanurik, D., & Zeltzer, L. K. (in press-a). The management of procedure-related pain. In N. L. Schechter, C. Berde, & M. Yaster (Eds.), *Pain management in children and adolescents.* Baltimore: Williams & Wilkins.

Anderson, C. T. M., Fanurik, D., & Zeltzer, L. K. (in press-b). Pain in adolescence. In E. McAnarnery, R. E. Kriepe, D. P. Orr, & G. D. Comerci (Eds.), *Textbook of adolescent medicine.* Philadelphia: Saunders.

Anderson, C. T. M., & Zeltzer, L. K. (in press). Pain mechanisms and pain control in children. In C. Pochedly (Ed.), *Neoplastic diseases of childhood.* New York: Harwood Academic Publishers (Gordon and Breach).

Barr, R. G., Boyce, T., & Zeltzer, L. K. (in press). The stress and illness connection in children: A perspective from the biobehavioral interface. In N. Garmezy & M. Rutter (Eds.), *Risk and resilience in children* (3rd ed.). New York: Cambridge University Press.

Berman, D., Duncan, A. M., & Zeltzer, L. K. (1992). The evaluation and management of pain in the infant and young child with cancer. *British Journal of Cancer, 66,* S84–S91.

Beyer, J., & Wells, N. (1989). Assessment of pain in children. *Pediatric Clinics of North America, 36,* 837–854.

Boyce, T., Barr, R. G. & Zeltzer, L. K. (1992). Temperment and the psychobiology of childhood stress. *Pediatrics, 90,* 483–486.

Burish, T. G., & Lyles, J. N. (1981). Effectiveness of relaxation training in reducing adverse reactions to cancer chemotherapy. *Journal of Behavioral Medicine, 4,* 65–78.

Campbell, L., Clark, M., & Kirkpatrick, S. E. (1986). Stress management training for parents and their children undergoing cardiac catheterization. *American Journal of Orthopsychiatry, 56,* 234–243.

Carpenter, P. J. (1990). New method for measuring young children's self-report of fear and pain. *Journal of Pain and Symptom Management, 5*(4), 233–240.

Carpenter, P. J. (1991). Scientific inquiry in childhood cancer psychosocial research: Theoretical, conceptual, and methodologic issues in the investigation and behavioral treatment of procedure-related distress. *Cancer* (Supplement), *67*(3), 833–838.

Dolgin, M. J., Katz, E. R., Doctors, S. R., & Siegel, S. E. (1986). Caregivers' perception of medical compliance in adolescents with cancer. *Journal of Adolescent Health Care, 7,* 22–27.

Fanurik, D., Mizell, T., & Zeltzer, L. K. (1991). Individual differences in children's responses to cold-pressor pain. *Journal of Pain and Symptom Management, 6,* 180 (abstract).

Fanurik, D., Zeltzer, L., Roberts, M. C., & Blount, R. L. (in press). The relationship between children's coping styles and psychological interventions for cold pressor pain. *Pain.*

Goldsmith, H., Buss, A., Plomin, R., Rothbart, M., Thomas, A., Chess, S., Hinde, R., & McCall, R. (1987). Roundtable: What is temperament? Four approaches. *Child Development, 58,* 505–529.

Goldsmith, H., & Campos, J. (1982). Toward a theory of infant temperament. In R. Emde & R. Harmon (Eds.), *The development of attachment and affiliative systems* (pp. 51–103). Hillsdale, NJ: Lawrence Erlbaum Associates.

Gunnar, M. (1992). Stress hormones: Biologic markers of vulnerability in infants and children. *Pediatrics, 90,* 491–497.

Hilgard, J. H., & LeBaron, S. (1984). *Hypnotherapy of pain in children with cancer.* Los Altos, CA: William Kaufmann.

Hubert, N. C., Jay, S. M., Saltoun, M. S., & Hayes, M. H. (1988). Approach-avoidance and distress in children undergoing preparation for painful medical procedures. *Journal of Clinical Child Psychology, 17,* 194–202.

Jay, S. M. (1988). Invasive medical procedures: Psychological intervention and assessment. In D. K. Routh (Ed.), *Handbook of pediatric psychology* (pp. 401–425). New York: Guilford Press.

Jay, S. M., & Elliott, C. H. (1990). A stress inoculation program for parents whose children are undergoing painful medical procedures. *Journal of Consulting and Clinical Psychology, 58,* 799–804.

Jay, S. M., Elliott, C. H., Katz, E. R., & Siegel, S. E. (1987). Cognitive behavioral interventions and pharmacologic interventions for children undergoing painful medical procedures. *Journal of Consulting and Clinical Psychology, 55,* 860–865.

Jay, S., Elliott, C., Ozolins, M., Olson, R., & Pruitt, S. (1985). Behavioral management of children's distress during painful medical procedures. *Behaviour Research and Therapy, 5,* 513–520.

Jay, S. M., Ozolins, M., Elliott, C., & Caldwell, S. (1983). Assessment of children's distress during painful medical procedures. *Journal of Health Psychology, 2,* 133–147.

Kagan, J., Reznick, J., Clarke, C., Snidman, N., & Garcia-Coll, C. (1987). Behavioral inhibition to the unfamiliar. *Child Development, 58,* 1459–1473.

Kagan, J., Reznick, J., & Snidman, N. (1987). The physiology and psychology of behavioral inhibition in young children. *Child Development, 58,* 1459–1473.

Kagan, J., Reznick, J., & Snidman, N. (1988). Biological bases of childhood shyness. *Science, 240,* 167–171.

Katz, E. R., Kellerman, J., & Siegel, S. E. (1980). Behavioral distress in children with cancer undergoing medical procedures: Developmental considerations. *Journal of Consulting and Clinical Psychology, 48,* 356–365.

Krantz, D., & Manuck, S. (1984). Acute psychophysiological reactivity and risk of cardiovascular disease: A review and methodologic critique. *Psychological Bulletin, 96,* 435–464.

Kuttner, L., Bowman, M., & Teasdale, M. (1988). Psychological treatment of distress, pain and anxiety for young children with cancer. *Developmental and Behavioral Pediatrics, 9,* 374–381.

LeBaron, S., & Zeltzer, L. (1984). Assessment of acute pain and anxiety in children and adolescents by self-reports, observer reports, and a behavior checklist. *Journal of Consulting and Clinical Psychology, 55,* 729–738.

LeBaron, S., Zeltzer, L., & Fanurik, D. (1989). An investigation of cold pressor pain in children: Part I. *Pain, 37,* 161–171.

LeBaron, S., Zeltzer, L. K., LeBaron, C., Scott, S. E., & Zeltzer, P. (1988). Chemotherapy side effects in pediatric oncology patients: Drugs, age, and sex as risk factors. *Medical and Pediatric Oncology, 16,* 263–268.

Manuck, S., Kaplan, J., & Matthews, K. (1986). Behavioral antecedents of coronary heart disease and atherosclerosis. *Arteriosclerosis, 26,* 2–14.

McGrath, P. A. (1990). *Pain in children.* New York: Guilford Press.

McGrath, P. J., & Unruh, A. (1987). *Pain in children and adolescents.* Amsterdam: Elsevier.

Miser, A. W., Dothage, J. A., Wesley, R. A., & Miser, J. S. (1987). The prevalence of pain in a pediatric and young adult cancer population. *Pain, 29,* 73–83.

Miser, A. W., McCalla, J., Dothage, J. A., Wesley, M., & Miser, J. S. (1987). Pain as a presenting symptom in children and young adults with newly diagnosed malignancy. *Pain, 29,* 85–90.

Mizell, T., Fanurik, D., & Zeltzer, L. K. (1992). Development of a laboratory model to predict pain in children with cancer. *Clinical Research,* 117A. (From Western Society for Pediatric Research Abstracts.)

Morrow, G. R. (1982). Prevalence and correlates of anticipatory nausea and vomiting in chemotherapy patients. *Journal of the National Cancer Institute, 68,* 585–588.

Olness, K., & Gardner, G. G. (1989). *Hypnosis and hypnotherapy in children* (2nd ed.). New York: Grune & Stratton.

Page, G. G., Ben-Eliyahu, S., Yirmiya, R., & Liebeskind, J. C. (in press). Surgical stress promotes the metastatic growth and suppresses killer cell function in rats. *Journal of Pain and Symptom Management.*

Peterson, L., Harbeck, C., Chaney, J., Farmer, J., & Thomas, A. M. (1990). Children's coping with medical procedures: A conceptual overview and integration. *Behavioral Assessment, 12,* 197–212.

Peterson, L., & Toler, S. M. (1986). An information seeking disposition in child surgery patients. *Health Psychology, 5,* 343–358.

Poster, E. C., & Betz, C. L. (1983). Allaying the anxiety of hospitalized children using stress immunization techniques. *Issues in Comprehensive Pediatric Nursing, 6,* 227–233.

Redd, W., Andresen, G. V., & Minagawa, R. Y. (1982). Hypnotic control of anticipatory emesis in patients receiving cancer chemotherapy. *Journal of Consulting and Clinical Psychology, 50,* 14–19.

Rodgers, B. M., Webb, C. J., Stergios, D., & Newman, B. M. (1988). Patient controlled analgesia in pediatric surgery. *Journal of Pediatric Surgery, 23,* 259–262.

Ross, D. M. (1984). Thought-stopping: A coping strategy for impending feared events. *Issues in Comprehensive Pediatric Nursing, 7,* 83–89.

Ross, D. M., & Ross, S. A. (1984). The importance of type of question, psychological climate and subject set in interviewing children about pain. *Pain, 19,* 71–79.

Rothbart, M., & Posner, M. (1985). Temperament and the development of self-regulation. In I. Hartlage & C. Teizrow (Eds.), *The neuropsychology of individual differences: A developmental perspective* (pp. 93–123). New York: Plenum.

Shaw, E. G., & Routh, D. K. (1982). Effect of mother presence on children's reaction to aversive procedures. *Journal of Pediatric Psychology, 7,* 33–42.

Shin, D., Fanurik, D., Ifekwunigwe, M., LeGagnoux, G., & Zeltzer, L. K. (1992). The relationship between children's laboratory pain responses and their health behaviors. *Clinical Research,* 117A. (From Western Society for Pediatric Research Abstracts.)

Siegel, L. J. (1976). Preparation of children for hospitalization: A selected review of the research literature. *Journal of Pediatric Psychology, 1,* 26–30.

Siegel, L. J., & Smith, K. E. (1989). Children's strategies for coping with pain. *Pediatrician, 16,* 110–118.

Smith, K., Ackerson, J. D., & Blotcky, A. D. (1989). Reducing distress during invasive medical procedures. Relating behavioral interventions to preferred coping style in pediatric cancer patients. *Journal of Pediatric Psychology, 14,* 405–419.

Smith, S. D., Rosen, D., Trueworthy, R. C., & Lowman, J. T. (1979). A reliable method for evaluating drug compliance in children with cancer. *Cancer, 43,* 169–173.

Suomi, S. (1988). Genetic and maternal contributions to individual differences in Rhesus monkey biobehavioral development. In N. Krasnagor (Ed.), *Psychobiological aspects of behavioral development.* New York: Academic Press.

Tyler, D. C. (1990). Patient-controlled analgesia in adolescents. *Journal of Adolescent Health Care, 11,* 154–158.

Wolfer, J. A., & Visintainer, M. A. (1979). Prehospital psychological preparation for tonsillectomy patients: Effects on children's and parents' adjustment. *Pediatrics, 64,* 646–655.

Zeltzer, L. K., Anderson, C. T. M., & Schechter, N. L. (1990). Pediatric pain: Current status and new directions. In J. Lockhart (Ed.), *Current problems in pediatrics.* St. Louis: Mosby-Year Book.

Zeltzer, L. K., Dolgin, M. J., LeBaron, S., & LeBaron, C. (1991). A randomized, controlled study of behavioral intervention for chemotherapy distress in children with cancer. *Pediatrics, 88* (1), 34–42.

Zeltzer, L. K., Fanurik, D., & LeBaron, S. (1989). The cold pressor pain paradigm in children: Feasibility of an intervention model: Part II. *Pain, 37,* 305–313.

Zeltzer, L. K., Jay, S. M., & Fisher, D. M. (1989). The management of pain associated with pediatric procedures. *Pediatric Clinics of North America, 36,* 1–24.

Zeltzer, L., & LeBaron, S. (1986a). Assessment of acute pain and anxiety and chemotherapy related nausea and vomiting in children and adolescents with cancer. In D. M. Dush, B. Cassileth, & D. Turk (Eds.), *Psychosocial assessment in terminal care.* New York: Haworth Press.

Zeltzer, L., & LeBaron, S. (1986b). The hypnotic treatment of children in pain. *Advances in Developmental and Behavioral Pediatrics, 7,* 197–234.

Zeltzer, L. K., LeBaron, S., Richie, M. D., & Reed, D. (1988). Can children understand and use a rating scale to quantify somatic symptoms? Assessment of nausea and vomiting as a model. *Journal of Consulting and Clinical Psychology, 56,* 567–572.

Zeltzer, L., LeBaron, S., & Zeltzer, P. M. (1984a). Paradoxical effects of prophylactic phenothiazine antiemetics in children receiving chemotherapy. *Journal of Clinical Oncology, 2,* 930–936.

Zeltzer, L. K., LeBaron, S., & Zeltzer, P. M. (1984b). A prospective assessment of chemotherapy related nausea and vomiting in children with cancer. *American Journal of Pediatric Hematology and Oncology, 6,* 5–16.

Zeltzer, L. K., & Zeltzer, P. M. (1989). Clinical assessment and pharmacologic treatment of pain in children: Cancer as a model for the management of chronic or persistent pain. *Pediatrician* (Special edition) 64–70.

4

Medication Compliance in Pediatric Oncology

DAVID J. BEARISON

The successful medical treatment of children depends not only on adequate pre-scribed treatment but also on patients' compliance with treatment. Therefore, it is crucial that health-care providers ensure that patients receive maximal benefit from prescribed treatment programs so that their therapeutic outcomes will depend on the biologic responsiveness of the disease rather than on their compliance with accepting appropriate treatment (Festa, Tamaroff, Chasalow, & Lanzkowsky, 1992). This chapter reviews findings in medical compliance in pediatric oncology within the broader context of medical compliance in pediatrics. It considers com-pliance research in terms of how compliance is measured, how it is influenced by corollary variables, and how it can lead to effective interventions to increase levels of compliance.

Studies of medical compliance in the treatment of various diseases among children and adolescents has increased dramatically in the past 20 years. Noncom-pliance in the treatment of diabetes ranks first in the number of studies followed by asthma and epilepsy (Dunbar, Dunning, & Dwyer, 1992). Other chronic pediatric diseases in which noncompliance has been recognized as a problem include cystic fibrosis, renal dialysis, otitis media (inner ear infection), recurrent urinary tract infections, and juvenile rheumatoid arthritis. There are few studies of children and adolescents' compliance with short-term medication regimens.

Studies typically have found an overall rate of compliance for self-administration (parent administration in the case of young children) of medication in pediatrics to be about 50 percent. This rate is comparable to that found among adults (Dunbar, 1983; Dunbar et al., 1992). Although it might be expected that patients with more severe or life-threatening illness would be at lower risk for noncompliance, there is no consistent evidence to support this conclusion. In some cases but not in others, compliance rates for children with less pernicious illnesses have been reported to be lower. For example, one study in a private practice setting reported rates as low as 18 percent for compliance on the ninth day of a 10-day penicillin regimen (Bergman & Werner, 1963), but another study (Charney et al., 1967) found 56 percent compliance on the ninth day for penicillin therapy. In general and contrary to common wisdom, studies of disease severity or severity of symptoms generally have not correlated with compliance rates (Haynes, 1979). Furthermore, the various adverse side effects of medication do not typically appear to have an important effect on medication compliance, although they do affect the likelihood of patients keeping their clinic appointments (Richardson, Marks, & Levine, 1988; Richardson, Shelton, Krailo, & Levine, 1990). An exception to this finding is a study of adolescent females with renal transplants who cited the cosmetic side effects (i.e., cushingoid features) of steroid medication as a reason for medication noncompliance (Korsch, Fine, & Negrete, 1978). Also, such variables as the age and gender of the pediatric patient, the duration of symptoms, and the educational level of the parents do not generally distinguish compliers from noncompliers. The failure to find relationships between compliance rates and the severity of different disease states, medication side effects, or common patient demographic variables substantiates the complexity of this phenomenon in medical practice and the challenge it poses to investigators to formulate empirical studies that would enhance compliance.

Studies of noncompliance have considered several different kinds of behaviors including refusal, to varying extent, of a procedure or treatment, failure to keep appointments, delays (usually defined as a lapse of more than 3 months) or "lag-time" between the appearance of symptoms and seeking medical consultation, and failure to reliably self-administer prescribed amounts of oral medication at the specified times. These different kinds of compliance behaviors have been found to be intercorrelated in some studies (Dolgin, Katz, Doctors, & Siegel, 1986) but not in others (Inui, Carter, Pecorato, Pearlman, & Dohan, 1980; Taylor, Lichtman, & Wood, 1984).

Although compliance typically is reported in terms of the proportion of patients who either are or are not compliant, there is not a common marker or threshold among investigators to indicate noncompliance. Similarly, in cases where compliance refers to medication and is measured according to biological assay procedures, there is not a common threshold of the amount of medication consumed to indicate noncompliance.

In this chapter noncompliance is considered primarily as the failure to reliably self-administer prescribed amounts of oral medication. Adherence to medication regimens is the most reliable form in which noncompliance has been studied in pediatric oncology, and it reflects its most direct and pernicious effects. Specific procedures used in studies to measure medication compliance are discussed later in this chapter.

Compliance in Pediatric Oncology

Among pediatric cancer patients, medication compliance is becoming an increasingly important area of study consistent with the dramatic improvements in the past few decades in the treatment of childhood malignancies. Although it was assumed at one time that the severity of cancer and its life-threatening condition would ensure compliance among patients, there is to date sufficient evidence to indicate, especially among adolescents with cancer, that medication compliance cannot be assumed for any patient at any time during treatment. Adolescents who have cancer are significantly more likely than younger patients to be noncompliant. In the most frequently referenced study on medication noncompliance among pediatric cancer patients, Smith, Rosen, Trueworthy, and Lowman (1979) found that 59 percent of adolescents with acute leukemia were noncompliant based on random urine levels of oral prednisone, a commonly used and self-administered drug with potentially unpleasant side effects such as weight gain and skin changes. The rate of noncompliance among children under 13 years in the study was 33 percent.

These findings have been replicated by Lansky, Smith, Cairns, and Cairns (1983), Dolgin et al. (1986), Tebbi et al. (1986), and Festa et al. (1992). Compliance is better among children than adolescents because of direct parental administration of oral medication for children. Among adolescents with cancer, compliance issues are exacerbated because of problems that often arise in the parent-child relationship around issues regarding the transfer of responsibilities for self-care at a time when they normally are assuming greater autonomy and independence, as well as ambiguous and evasive patterns of communicating illness-related issues between parents and adolescents (Mulhern, Crisco, & Camitta, 1981; Spinetta & Maloney, 1978). In addition, noncompliance among adolescents may reflect their denial of illness and its life-threatening consequences (Zeltzer, 1980). Despite the difference in compliance rates between children and adolescents, noncompliance even among young children is high enough to consider it a significant risk factor in the clinical management of all patients in pediatric oncology.

Noncompliance with oral prednisone has been found during initial induction and in late remission (Klopovich & Trueworthy, 1985). Compliance has generally been found to decline over the course of therapy (Dolgin et al., 1986; Haynes, 1979; Tebbi et al., 1986). For example, using validated self-reports, Tebbi et al. (1986) found a decline from 81 percent compliance at 2 weeks from diagnosis to 61 percent compliance at 20 weeks.

Among adult oncology patients, it has been found that self-administration of one medication (e.g., prednisone) correlated significantly with the self-administration of another medication (e.g., allopurinol), suggesting that medications routinely are either taken or not taken as a group (Richardson et al., 1990). This, in turn, suggests consistency of patient behavior that might reflect a kind of personality trait.

Compliance and Cure

It is apparent from these findings that noncompliance with oral therapy is a significant problem for fully half of all adolescents and one-third of all children with cancer. These rates of medication noncompliance can potentially confound experimental treatment effects (Feinstein, 1979; Goldsmith, 1979). They could explain, in part, why children with the same kinds of cancer and receiving the same drug regimens show such wide variations in response (i.e., induction rates and remission lengths; Smith et al., 1979). For example, according to some, the differential compliance rates between children and adolescents with acute lymphoblastic leukemia (ALL) might contribute to the poorer outcomes for adolescents compared to younger children (Lansky, List, & Ritter-Sterr, 1989; Sather, 1986). Also, it has been suggested that difficulties in replicating treatment effects across institutions using the same protocols might be attributed to poor patient compliance rates (Smith et al., 1979). Furthermore, differential rates of compliance occurring in different arms of an experimental treatment protocol could bias findings (Bonadonna & Valaquessa, 1981). Consequently, studies of experimental treatment effects must consider the influence of protocol compliance on the efficacy of the treatment protocols being tested.

Although compliance would be expected to have a causal influence on therapeutic response rates, a few studies, including a study of prophylactic antibiotic therapy to prevent infection from chemotherapy-induced granulocytopenia in patients with cancer (Pizzo et al., 1983), found that treatment outcome was independent of whether the patient was administered the actual drug or a placebo. Patients with less than total compliance showed no significant decrease in infection incidence while patients with excellent compliance had a significant decrease regardless of whether they had been randomly selected to receive the drug or a placebo. Such a finding implies that patient compliance can function as a significant independent variable when assessing treatment outcomes.

The logical test for the effect of compliance on treatment efficacy calls for a two-by-two factorial design in which patients are randomly assigned to a drug or placebo condition and retrospectively assigned to compliant or noncompliant groups. Statistical analyses of the results from such a study would provide a test of the efficacy of the experimental drug as a main effect on treatment outcome, compliance as a main effect on treatment outcome, and an interaction effect between drug and compliance on outcome (Epstein, 1984). However, in pediatric oncology, this kind of factorial design of an experimental protocol typically would be precluded because it would be inappropriate to use placebo-controlled chemotherapy trials. Instead, new drugs typically are compared to conventional standards of known efficacy. However, the finding by Pizzo et al. (1983) suggests that medication compliance reflects a broader range of behaviors and attitudes (hygiene, diet, etc.) that can potentially influence outcomes in ways that are not yet understood.

Causal Relationship

Compliance with prescribed medication regimens is not typically measured in clinical trials. However, there is some evidence of a direct causal relationship between compliance and prognosis. Richardson et al. (1990) found a causal relationship between medication compliance with allopurinol and survival rates among adult cancer patients. Allopurinol is a supportive drug in cancer treatment and although it would not be expected to directly affect survival rates, it served as a marker for the self-administration of other medications that would have direct affects. True-worthy (1982) found a causal relationship between noncompliance with prednisone treatment in children and the occurrence of relapses. Among 17 children with ALL, 12 had urine assays consistent with taking prednisone and had no relapses. Among the 5 patients who did not have urine values consistent with taking predni-sone, 4 relapsed. The relationship between compliance and relapses was indepen-dent of the initial prognostic conditions of the patients (Klopovich & Trueworthy, 1985). Another study of prednisone adherence among adolescent ALL patients (Festa et al., 1992) found that 5 of 11 noncompliers had relapses compared to 1 of 10 compliers. Although further studies using larger samples of patients are warranted, these initial findings mark the critical consequences of medication non-compliance among pediatric oncology patients and establish noncompliance as a significant risk factor for survival in pediatric oncology.

Measures of Medication Compliance

There are several *indirect* methods that have been used to measure compliance with self-administration of oral medications in pediatric oncology. These include patients' and/or parents' self-reports, physician estimates, pill counts, prescription renewals, the occurrence of predictable side effects, and indexes of therapeutic outcome. These kinds of indirect methods, however, have been found to overesti-mate rates of compliance (Evans & Spellman, 1983; Ruth, Caron, & Bartholo-mew, 1970; Wilson & Endres, 1986). For example, in medical contexts other than pediatric oncology, physician estimates, surprisingly, have been found to be one of the least accurate methods (Brody, 1980; Roth & Casen, 1978). A more valid and *direct* method of assessing compliance is using biological assays that measure levels of drugs in urine, serum, or saliva. In pediatric oncology, the prototype for biological measures of compliance, developed by Smith et al. (1979), has been urine assays for the absorption of oral prednisone. Other reliable methods of as-sessing oral prednisone adherence include measuring serum levels of dehydroepi-androsterone sulfate (DHEA-S), an adrenal androgenic steroid which is suppressed by prednisone administration (Festa et al., 1992), and high-pressure liquid chro-matography (Fry, Fry, & Benet, 1979). Serum assays for 6-mercaptopurine (6-MP) and methotrexate also have been developed. Consequently, there are today methods to assess compliance with the three oral drugs most commonly used in the treatment of children with ALL (Klopovich & Trueworthy, 1985; Lennard, 1987). Although biological indexes of compliance of the kind described constitute the most objective method of measuring compliance, they are expensive and gen-erally not available in most community laboratories. In addition, altered or differ-ential rates of metabolism between patients for some medications can compromise the validity of these techniques.

     To provide a reliable measure of medication compliance without the need to resort to the expense and effort of biological assay procedures, a new kind of tablet bottle has been developed, which, unknown to the patient, is electronically sensitive to light entering the part containing the pills and thus provides a continuous record of times of bottle opening (Lee, Nicholson, Souhami, & Deshmukh, 1992). Because the time as well as the number of bottle openings is recorded, investigators can determine whether the pattern of bottle openings for a given patient represents a regular or irregular regimen of self-medication. However, this method obviously cannot account for deliberate subversion by a patient, such as opening and taking the medication out of the bottle on time but then discarding it.

Factors Associated with Noncompliance
Demographic Correlates of Noncompliance

There appears to be no reliable pattern of demographic variables that predicts compliance. Surprisingly, noncompliance has *not* been found to be associated with such demographic variables as patient's age, gender, ethnicity, or socioeconomic status among adult cancer patients (Richardson et al., 1988), adolescent patients in general (Litt & Cuskey, 1980), and adolescent cancer patients (Tamaroff, Festa, Adesman, & Walco, 1992; Tebbi et al., 1986). Although one study found that female adolescents with renal transplants were poorer compliers than males (Korsch et al., 1978), gender differences in compliance rates have not been found in other studies. Treatment variables such as the presence of medical complications and the number of infections among children and adolescents with leukemia have not been found to be related to compliance levels (Tebbi et al., 1986). Although parental marital status did not correlate with compliance among adolescent cancer patients, one study found that patients who had fewer siblings were more compliant (Tebbi et al., 1986). The effects of drug toxicity such as hair loss, nausea, loss of appetite, fever, weakness, pain, and bleeding also have not been correlated with compliance levels in pediatric oncology (Richardson et al., 1988, 1990; Tebbi et al., 1986), with the exception of a study by Dolgin et al. (1986) that relied only on physicians' reports as the measure of compliance.

Knowledge of Illness and Patient Education

Despite the high incidence of medication noncompliance in pediatric oncology, studies to date have been unable to explain why patients are noncompliant or to reliably predict which patients are at risk for noncompliance. Patients' knowledge of their illness and medication procedures would seem to be an obvious prerequisite for compliance and, consequently, it has been the principal variable in most compliance studies. However, findings regarding a relationship between compliance and knowledge of patients' disease states in general and their medication in particular have been equivocal in both correlational and experimental intervention studies among adolescents and adults. For example, studies with pediatric patients with renal transplants (Beck et al., 1980), juvenile diabetes (Etzwiler & Robb,

1972), hematologic malignancies (Richardson et al., 1987), and adults with diabetes (Graber, Christman, Alonga, & Davidson, 1977) found that intervention programs that increased patients' medication knowledge did not increase their medication compliance. Richardson et al., (1987) concluded that "knowledge did not affect any aspect of compliance" (p. 184), Graber et al. (1977) concluded that "correlations of test scores (knowledge) with the patients' compliance . . . have shown no consistent trends" (p. 62), and Beck et al. (1980) that "there was no association between compliance and the patient's initial, final, or improvement in medication knowledge" (p. 1096).

Tamaroff et al. (1992) found no differences between compliers and noncompliers among adolescent cancer patients in their knowledge of their illness and their understanding of treatment; however, they reported that compliers had greater insight about the causality of their illness and issues related to its prognosis. However, it is not clear from their report how patients were questioned about the causality and prognosis of their cancer, particularly when there are no known causes for the kinds of cancer their patients had. Tebbi et al. (1986) found that adolescent cancer patients' knowledge of their illness and belief in the effectiveness of their medication was not correlated with compliance; moreover, compliant adolescents were no more likely than noncompliant ones to actively seek information about their cancer and its treatment from their physician or anyone else. They did find, however, that compliers reported being better informed than noncompliers about instructions concerning how to self-administer their medications, but such an association between reported knowledge of medication instructions and compliance is more likely to be a consequence of compliance than a causal factor.

In general, attempts to enhance adolescents' understanding of disease processes has not yielded greater adherence to treatment regimens (Cromer & Tarnowski, 1989). In the few cases where interventions that were aimed specifically at improving patients' medication knowledge have been shown to enhance compliance, the effects were not long lasting (Litt & Cuskey, 1980). Haynes (1976) conducted a "methodologic analysis" of 185 compliance studies and found that "the problem of noncompliance is rarely one of lack of knowledge" (p. 81). Similarly, Shope (1981) in an extensive review of studies of pediatric medication compliance concluded that "knowledge about the disease being treated has rarely had any relationship to compliance behavior" (p. 19) and that "the provision of information alone without assistance in changing or adapting behavior is not likely to achieve the desired results of better medication compliance" (p. 16). Despite repeated failures to confirm a causal or even correlational association between medication compliance and patients' knowledge of their illness, treatment, and medical instructions, most intervention programs designed to enhance medication compliance among adolescent cancer patients continue to focus on educational efforts.

The failure to find associations between compliance and patient education should not belie the importance of educating cancer patients, even when they are very young children, about their condition and complex treatment regimens. Also, in the reported studies on knowledge and compliance, it must be assumed that all patients were advised about their treatment and its effects, as is the practice at all medical centers, at least in this country. Thus in considering patients' knowledge as a correlate of their compliance or some aspect of medical education as an intervention to enhance compliance, the base rate is not ignorance but varying extent of knowledge as it is acquired within the overall context of communication between patient or family and staff.

Psychological Variables

Patients' emotional demeanor, personality traits, modes of coping with stress, and sense of control of the clinical outcome of their illness all influence how they come to understand and make sense of their medical condition and, accordingly, these kinds of psychosocial variables would be expected to affect their adherence to medical procedures. Thus if patients' knowledge of cancer, treatment, and medical instructions has not been found to correlate with compliance, how patients adjust to having cancer might mediate the relationship between having cancer and adhering to treatment procedures. This approach to the problem is more consistent with advances in cognitive-developmental psychology than simply considering compliance in terms of whether the patient knows what to do and understands the need to do it. According to a cognitive-developmental perspective, there is a dynamic and reciprocal relationship between how individuals come to understand and organize their experiences and how they emotionally adjust to them (Bearison & Zimiles, 1986). Because of the continuing uncertainties associated with the treatment of cancer in children, it is expected that they will experience emotional stress and adjustment problems. Thus issues of compliance in pediatric oncology can be reconceptualized from being a focal problem in patient management to an integral aspect of the psychological changes that the patient and family members undergo in the face of cancer. Accordingly, compliance might then be studied as one aspect of their psychological adjustment and coping mechanisms and, as such, it would be expected to correlate with other signs of patients' adjustment reactions.

In support of such an approach, the only variables that have been found to be consistently associated with levels of compliance in studies of chronically ill adults and adolescents with diagnoses other than cancer as well as with adults with cancer have been those associated with different aspects of psychosocial adjustment. In general, findings have shown that noncompliant patients have significantly greater adjustment problems than compliant patients, although it usually is not clear whether these are preexisting or reactive. For example, scores on anxiety (Kleiger & Dirks, 1979), depression, and locus of control measures (Blackwell, 1973; Duke & Cohen, 1975; Kirscht, 1972) have been associated with compliance among adults with chronic illness. Richardson et al. (1987) reported that among adult cancer patients perceived satisfaction with their overall medical care, but not their knowledge, was correlated with compliance in terms of keeping appointments. They further found that patients' level of depression about their illness was inversely related to their perceived satisfaction and thus served to mediate overall compliance rates. Increasing levels of depression also correlated with poorer compliance for prednisone self-administration. Among adolescent patients, Korsch et al. (1978) found that noncompliance with immunosuppressive therapy following renal transplants was associated with poor self-esteem and socialization as well as psychological problems prior to the onset of illness. In a study of adolescents with juvenile rheumatoid arthritis, noncompliers had significantly poorer self-esteem and felt that they had less autonomy than did compliers (Litt, Cuskey, & Rosenberg, 1982). Self-esteem (and parent reports of children's social functioning) also was found to correlate with compliance among children and adolescents with diabetes mellitus (Jacobson et al., 1987).

There are only a few systematic studies of the relationship between psychosocial adjustment and medication compliance among pediatric cancer patients. Jamison, Lewis, and Burish (1986) found that overall treatment compliance, based on nurse's ratings including but not limited to medication compliance, was inversely correlated with adolescents' poor self-image and a sense of external locus of control. When adolescents with cancer were compared to their healthy peers, the patients had significantly lower internal and higher external locus of control scores about health-related issues, which was interpreted as a sign of an increased sense of helplessness among these cancer patients (Jamison, Lewis, Burish, 1986; Kellerman, Zeltzer, Ellenberg, Dash, & Rigler, 1980).

The construct of locus of control has received considerable attention in studies of how individuals adjust to illness. It supposedly reflects the degree to which individuals perceive that they have the ability to control factors affecting their lives. It generally has been reported that individuals who have an internal locus of control adjust better to illness than those with an external locus of control, the latter reflecting a relative inability to control health-related events. However, the locus of control construct, as it pertains to children and adolescents with cancer, is particularly problematic because (1) patients can't be expected to assume responsibility for the cause of their cancer given the unknown etiologies of childhood cancers, and (2) there is relatively little that they can do for themselves in the treatment of cancer, particularly during the initial critical periods and during relapses. By comparison, a disease such as insulin-dependent diabetes mellitus (DDM) allows patients greater control over their treatment in terms of diet, exercise, insulin intake, and rotation of injection sites; consequently, there is a strong positive association between medication compliance and an internal locus of control (Brown, Kaslow, Sansbury, Meacham, & Culler 1991).

In pediatric oncology, however, the relationship between locus of control and compliance among adolescents with cancer has been equivocal (Cromer & Tarnowski, 1989). Despite findings reported by Jamison, Lewis, and Burish (1986) of a relationship between compliance and an external locus of control, Tamaroff et al. (1992) and Tebbi et al. (1986) found no relationship among adolescent cancer patients between health locus of control and medication compliance. Tamaroff et al. (1992) did find, however, that noncompliers used denial as a defense in the context of health-related issues significantly more than compliers.

Parents and Compliance

Because parents are inextricably involved in their children's treatment, correlates of noncompliance include parental factors as well as patient characteristics. In one of the few studies that systematically considered personality traits of both parents and their children, it was found that compliance with oral prednisone was related more to the parents' personality (as measured by the MMPI scales) than that of their children (Lansky et al., 1983). Although the rates of compliance were equal for boys and girls, psychological traits associated with compliance were different for boys and girls as well as for their mothers and fathers. Several personality traits among the parents which usually are considered maladaptive were found to correlate positively with compliance among boys. Mothers of compliant boys were compulsive, anxious, and high in self-control whereas fathers of compliant boys were hostile and aggressive. Mothers of compliant girls, on the other hand, were calm instead of anxious and their fathers tended to avoid facing problems. The compliant girls themselves were more anxious than boys and noncompliant girls. The authors interpreted their findings as reflecting different expectations about compliance that parents have for their sons compared to their daughters; they expected their sons to be more vulnerable and in need of supervision and their daughters to be more responsible. While there is a compelling need for more studies of the psychological correlates of compliance behaviors among children and adolescents with cancer, the Lansky et al. (1983) study illustrates the value of including measures of parents' (and also siblings') reactions to having a child with cancer in the family and statistically testing for interaction effects between patient and family variables.

Refusal of Treatment

Although the focus of this chapter has been on medication noncompliance, the blatant refusal of treatment among adolescents with cancer is a remarkable, albeit infrequent, form of noncompliance. Blotcky, Cohen, Conatser, and Klopovich (1985) compared 10 adolescents (8 of whom had ALL and 5, progressive disease) who refused cancer treatment for a mean of 6.6 months and their mothers with 10 control patients and their mothers. The controls were carefully matched on a number of demographic and illness-related variables. They found that adolescent cancer patients who refused treatment scored lower than consenting adolescents on measures of immediate (i.e., "state") anxiety and subjective distress but scored higher on characterologic (i.e., "trait") anxiety, religiosity, and external locus of control. The mothers of adolescent refusers also scored higher than the consenting group mothers on measures of religiosity and trait anxiety. No significant differences were found on measures of family satisfaction, hopelessness, satisfaction with physician, mother's coping, and mother's state anxiety. In interpreting their findings Blotcky et al. (1985) suggested that the adolescent refusers' tendency to be threatened by stressful situations (i.e., high trait anxiety) exacerbated their high degree of religiosity and external locus of control (i.e., believing that their lives are controlled by luck, fate, or God) and that these factors defended them from having severe immediate anxiety and contributed to their belief that their illness was beyond the realm of control (either their own or their physicians'). Accordingly, the investigators recommended interventions that lessened anxiety and fostered a greater sense of self-mastery (i.e., internal locus of control) in coping with cancer. The use of confrontational or aversive kinds of interventions (e.g., scare tactics) with these kinds of patients would heighten their defensiveness and rigidify their focus on treatment refusal.

At other times, adolescents refuse treatment because they sense that their parents or others are making all the major treatment decisions and, consequently, their refusal is a means for them to assert control in a frightening situation. In other cases, the life-threatening nature of their condition might not be fully grasped, so that the prolonged distress and discomforts of treatment do not seem justified.

A patient's decision to resort to unproven methods of treatment or faith healing is, from the medical team's perspective, another form of treatment refusal, even though it generally is not seen this way by the patient. Refusal of treatment can occur as an initial reaction to learning of the diagnosis of cancer or at any point during treatment, particularly at stressful times, such as a relapse or an invasive medical procedure.

How to respond to situations in which a minor refuses treatment (with the parent's consent) depends on the patient's prognosis. In cases where it is not urgent that treatment be immediately initiated, appropriate counseling can be provided. However, when the prognosis is good and there is evidence that the patient's condition will respond to immediate medical procedures, legal interventions should be obtained. When initiating or continuing treatment is not likely to yield cure, the patient's decision to refuse treatment or seek alternative nonconventional treatment may be honored (Lansky, Vats, & Cairns, 1979).

Future Directions

Despite increasing interest and research on compliance issues, our understanding of the multivariate causes of noncompliance is very limited. Most research efforts in pediatric oncology have been aimed at either documenting the extent of the problem or deriving correlates of the problem. At this stage, there is sufficient evidence documenting the extent of the problem, although more research is needed to establish the pattern of causal relationships between noncompliance and clinical outcomes. If documentation is an appropriate initial phase in compliance research programs, then finding correlates of compliance might be seen as the next phase, which ultimately could support the third and primary purpose of research in this area—the implementation of effective interventions to ameliorate the risk of noncompliance among children and adolescents with cancer. To date, however, there have been very few systematic and controlled studies to test interventions in the broad area of general patient compliance and even fewer in the specific area of pediatric oncology.

As evident in the present review of findings, the demographic and psychological correlates of poor compliance have not been clearly identified, findings have been equivocal, and, consequently, it is difficult to identify prospectively which patients will present a compliance risk. There presently is not a sufficient knowledge base on which to design or implement successful intervention procedures. Nevertheless, given the climate of psychological research in other areas of pediatric oncology, it is time to move beyond the search for correlates and predictors and to design studies around intervention procedures. Properly designed experimental studies of intervention, employing appropriate control and experimental conditions along with pre- and postintervention measures of both compliance and its correlative variables, would yield findings relevant to all three phases of compliance research: documentation, correlation, and intervention.

Previous findings make it clear that simple interventions designed around educational issues, while providing a direct and univariate approach to the problem of compliance, do not address the problem in a meaningful way. Instead, the focus of compliance research in pediatric oncology should shift from concerns about patients' knowledge of cancer, treatment, and medical instructions to issues concerning the adjustment to having cancer. The best predictors of compliance are likely to be other indices of "good coping." Also, it is likely that children with premorbid adjustment problems who are part of dysfunctional families will cope poorly and will be poor compliers. Interventions designed to enhance compliance, therefore, should be aimed at enhancing both patients' and their families' adjustment to the uncertainties, frustrations, anger, and fears about having cancer and test how these kinds of adjustment variables mediate compliance.

When considering the range and nature of the various kinds of adjustment variables worth including in proposed intervention studies, investigators should be guided by general findings indicating that it is the patient's and family's uncertainty regarding the duration of treatment and its ultimate outcome which remain the greatest psychological stressors in the treatment of cancer (Koocher, 1986; Kupst, Chapter 2, this volume). Until we have better means of predicting which children from which families will have compliance problems, and given the findings documenting the extent of noncompliance, all children should be considered at risk for medication noncompliance and should be monitored for medication compliance as part of their standard therapeutic regimen.

References

Bearison, D. J., & Zimiles, H. (Eds.) (1986). *Thought and emotion: Developmental perspectives.* Hillsdale, NJ: Lawrence Erlbaum Associates.

Beck, D. E., Fennel, R. S., Yost, R. L., Robinson, J. D., Geary, M. B., & Richards, G. A. (1980). Evaluation of an education program on compliance with medication regimens in pediatric patients with renal transplants. *Journal of Pediatrics, 96,* 1094–1097.

Bergman, A., & Werner, R. (1963). Failure of children to receive penicillin by mouth. *New England Journal of Medicine, 268,* 1334–1338.

Blackwell, B. (1973). Patient compliance. *New England Journal of Medicine, 289,* 249–252.

Blotcky, A. D., Cohen, D. G., Conatser, C., & Klopovich, P. (1985). Psychosocial characteristics of adolescents who refuse cancer treatment. *Journal of Consulting and Clinical Psychology, 53,* 729–731.

Bonadonna, G., & Valaquessa, P. (1981). Dose-response effect of adjuvant chemotherapy in breast cancer. *New England Journal of Medicine, 43,* 169.

Brody, D. S. (1980). Physician recognition of behavioral, psychological and social aspects of medical care. *Archives of Internal Medicine, 140,* 1286–1289.

Brown, R. T., Kaslow, N. J., Sansbury, L., Meacham, L., & Culler, F. L. (1991). Internalizing and externalizing symptoms and attributional style in youth with diabetes. *American Academy of Child and Adolescent Psychiatry, 30,* 921–925.

Charney, E., Bynum, R., Eldredge, D., Frank, D., MacWhinney, J. B., McNabb, N., Scheiner, A., Sumpter, E. A., & Iker, H. (1967). How well do patients take oral penicillin? A collaborative study in private practice. *Pediatrics, 40,* 188–195.

Cromer, B. A., & Tarnowski, K. J. (1989). Noncompliance in adolescents: A review. *Journal of Developmental Behavioral Pediatrics, 10,* 207–215.

Dolgin, M. J., Katz, E. R., Doctors, S. R., & Siegel, S. E. (1986). Caregivers' perceptions of medical compliance in adolescents with cancer. *Journal of Adolescent Health Care, 7,* 22–27.

Duke, M., & Cohen, B. (1975). Locus of control as an indicator of patient cooperation. *Journal of the American College of Dentistry, 42,* 174–178.

Dunbar, J. (1983). Compliance in pediatrics populations. A review. In P. J. McGrath & P. Fireston (Eds.), *Pediatric and adolescent medicine: Issues in treatment.* New York: Springer.

Dunbar, J., Dunning, E. J., & Dwyer, K. (1992). The development of compliance research in pediatric and adolescent populations: Two decades of research. In N. Krasnegor, S. Johnson, I. Epstein, & S. Jaffe (Eds.), *Developmental aspects of health compliance behavior.* Hillsdale, NJ: Lawrence Erlbaum Associates.

Epstein, L. H. (1984). The direct effects of compliance on health outcome. *Health Psychology, 3,* 385–393.

Etzwiler, D. D., & Robb, J. R. (1972). Evaluation of programmed education among juvenile diabetics and their families. *Diabetes, 21,* 967–971.

Evans, L., & Spelman, M. (1983). The problem of non-compliance with drug therapy. *Drugs, 25,* 63–76.

Feinstein, A. R. (1979). Compliance bias and the interpretation of therapeutic trials. In R. B. Haynes, D. W. Taylor, & D. L. Sackett (Eds.), *Compliance in health care.* Baltimore: Johns Hopkins University Press.

Festa, R., Tamaroff, M. H., Chasalow, F., & Lanzkowsky, P. (1992). Therapeutic adherence to oral medication regimens by adolescents with cancer: I. Laboratory assessment. *Journal of Pediatrics, 120,* 807–811.

Fry, J., Frey, B. M., & Benet, L. (1979). Liquid chromatographic measurement of endogenous and exogenous glucocorticoids in plasma. *Clinical Chemistry, 25,* 1944–1947.

Goldsmith, C. H. (1979). The effect of compliance distributions on therapeutic trials. In R. B. Haynes, D. W. Taylor, & D. L. Sackett (Eds.), *Compliance in health care.* Baltimore: Johns Hopkins University Press.

Graber, A., Christman, B., Alonga, M., & Davidson, J. K. (1977). Evaluation of diabetes patient education programs. *Diabetes, 26,* 61–64.

Haynes, R. B. (1976). Strategies for improving compliance: A methodological analysis and review. In D. L. Sackett & R. B. Haynes (Eds.), *Compliance with therapeutic regimens*. Baltimore: Johns Hopkins University Press.

Haynes, R. B. (1979). Determinants of compliance: The disease and the mechanics of treatment. In R. B. Haynes, D. W. Taylor, & D. L. Sackett (Eds.), *Compliance in health care*. Baltimore: Johns Hopkins University Press.

Inui, T. S., Carter, W. B., Pecorato, R. E., Pearlman, R. A., & Dohan, J. J. (1980). Variation in patient compliance with common long term drugs. *Medical Care, 18*, 986–993.

Jacobson, A. M., Hauser, S. T., Wolfsdorf, J. I., Houlihan, J., Milley, J. E., Herskowitz, R. D., Wertlief, D., & Watt, E. (1987). Psychologic predictors of compliance in children with recent onset of diabetes mellitus. *Journal of Pediatrics, 110*, 805–811.

Jamison, R. N., Lewis, S., & Burish, T. G. (1986). Cooperation with treatment in adolescent cancer patients. *Journal of Adolescent Health Care, 7*, 162–167.

Jamison, R. N., Lewis, S., Burish, T. G. (1986). Psychological impact of cancer on adolescents: Self-image, locus of control, perception of illness and knowledge of cancer. *Journal of Chronic Diseases, 39*, 609–617.

Kellerman, J., Zeltzer, L., Ellenberg, L., Dash, J., & Rigler, D. (1980). Psychological effects of illness in adolescence: Anxiety, self-esteem and perception of control. *Journal of Pediatrics, 97*, 126–131.

Kirscht, J. P. (1972). Perceptions of control and health beliefs. *Canadian Journal of Behavioral Sciences, 4*, 225–237.

Kleiger, J. H., & Dirks, J. F. (1979). Medication compliance in chronic asthmatic patients. *Journal of Asthma Research, 16*, 95–96.

Klopovich, P. M., & Trueworthy, R. C. (1985). Adherence to chemotherapy regimens among children with cancer. *Topics in Clinical Nursing, 7*, 19–25.

Koocher, G. P. (1986). Psychosocial issues during the acute treatment of pediatric cancer. *Cancer, 58*, 468–472.

Korsch, B. M., Fine, R. N., & Negrete, V. F. (1978). Noncompliance in adolescents with renal transplants. *Pediatrics, 61*, 872–876.

Lansky, S. B., List, M. A., & Ritter-Sterr, C. (1989). Psychiatric and psychological support of the child and adolescent with cancer. In P. A. Pizzo & D. G. Poplack (Eds.), *Principles and practice of pediatric oncology*. Philadelphia: Lippincott.

Lansky, S. B., Smith, S. D., Cairns, N. U., & Cairns, G. F. (1983). Psychological correlates of compliance. *American Journal of Pediatric Hematology/Oncology, 5*, 87–92.

Lansky, S. B., Vats, T., & Cairns, N. U. (1979). Refusal of treatment. *American Journal of Pediatric Hematology/Oncology, 1*, 277–282.

Lee, C. R., Nicholson, P. W., Souhami, R. L., & Deshmukh, A. A. (1992). Patient compliance with oral chemotherapy as assessed by a novel electronic technique. *Journal of Clinical Oncology, 10*, 1007–1013.

Lennard, L. (1987). Assay of 6-thioinosinic acid and 6-thioguanine nucleotides, active metabolites of 6-mercaptopurine in human red blood cells. *Journal of Chromatography, 423*, 169–178.

Litt, I. F., & Cuskey, W. R. (1980). Compliance with medical regimens during adolescence. *Pediatric Clinics of North America, 27*, 3–15.

Litt, I. F., Cuskey, W. R., & Rosenberg, A. (1982). Role of self-esteem and autonomy in determining medical compliance among adolescents with juvenile rheumatoid arthritis. *Pediatrics, 69*, 15–17.

Mulhern, R. K., Crisco, J. J., & Camitta, B. M. (1981). Patterns of communication among pediatric patients with leukemia, parents and physicians: Prognostic disagreements and misunderstandings. *Journal of Pediatrics, 99*, 480–483.

Pizzo, P. A., Robichaud, K. J., Edwards, B. K., Schumaker, C., Kramer, B. S., & Johnson, S. (1983). Oral antibiotic prophylaxis in patients with cancer: A double-blind randomized placebo-controlled trial. *Journal of Pediatrics, 102*, 125–133.

Richardson, J. L., Marks, G., Johnson, C., Graham, J. W., Chan, K. K., Sesler, J. N., Kishbaugh, C., Barranday, Y., & Levine, A. M. (1987). Path model of multidimensional compliance with cancer therapy. *Health Psychology, 6*, 183–207.

Richardson, J. L., Marks, G., & Levine, A. (1988). The influence of symptoms of disease and side effects of treatment on compliance with cancer therapy. *Journal of Clinical Oncology, 6*, 1746–1752.

Richardson, J., Shelton, D. R., Krailo, M., & Levine, M. (1990). The effect of compliance with treatment on survival among patients with hematologic malignancies. *Journal of Clinical Oncology, 8*, 356–364.

Roth, H., & Casen, H. D. (1978). Accuracy of doctors' estimates and patients' statements on adherence in a drug regimen. *Clinical Pharmacological Therapy, 23*, 361–370.

Ruth, H. P., Caron, H. S., & Bartholomew, P. H. (1970). Measuring intake of prescribed medication: A bottle count and a tracer technique compared. *Clinical Pharmacology Therapy, 11*, 228–237.

Sather, H. N. (1986). Age at diagnosis of childhood acute lymphoblastic leukemia. *Medical and Pediatric Oncology, 14*, 166–172.

Shope, J. T. (1981). Medication compliance. *Pediatric Clinics of North America, 28*, 5–21.

Smith, S. D., Rosen, D., Trueworthy, R. C., & Lowman, J. T. (1979). A reliable method for evaluating drug compliance in children with cancer. *Cancer, 43*, 169–173.

Spinetta, J. J., & Maloney, L. J. (1978). The child with cancer. Patterns of communication and denial. *Journal of Consulting and Clinical Psychology, 46*, 1540–1541.

Tamaroff, M. H., Festa, R. S., Adesman, A. R., & Walco, G. A. (1992). Therapeutic adherence to oral medication regimens by adolescents with cancer: II. Clinical and psychologic correlates. *Journal of Pediatrics, 120*, 812–817.

Taylor, S. E., Lichtman, R. R., & Wood, J. V. (1984). Compliance with chemotherapy among breast cancer patients. *Health Psychology, 3*, 553–562.

Tebbi, C. K., Cummings, K. M., Zevon, M. A., Smith, L., Richards, M., & Mallon, J. (1986). Compliance of pediatric and adolescent cancer patients. *Cancer, 58*, 1179–1184.

Trueworthy, R. C. (1982, April 11). *A new prognostic factor for childhood acute lymphoblastic leukemia: Drug absorption and compliance.* Proceedings of the Fourth Annual Pediatric Hematology/Oncology Symposium at University of Kansas Medical Center. Kansas City, KN.

Wilson, D. P., & Endres, R. K. (1986). Compliance with blood glucose monitoring in children with type 1 diabetes mellitus. *Journal of Pediatrics, 108*, 1022–1024.

Zeltzer, L. K. (1980). The adolescent with cancer. In J. Kellerman (Ed.), *Psychological aspects of childhood cancer.* Springfield, IL: Charles C Thomas.

5

Neuropsychological Late Effects

RAYMOND K. MULHERN

The study of late effects of cancer among children presupposes that the children are long-term survivors, if not permanently cured, of their disease. Late effects are temporally defined as occurring after the successful completion of medical therapy, usually 2 or more years from the time of diagnosis. It is generally assumed that late effects are chronic, if not progressive, in their course. This definition separates late effects from those effects of disease and treatment which are acute and time-limited such as chemotherapy-induced nausea and vomiting.

Research interest in psychological late effects, as well as medical late effects, has shown an increase commensurate with improvements in effective therapy for childhood cancer. For example, 30 years ago, when few children were cured of cancer, questions relating to the school performance of long-term survivors were trivial compared to the need for improved therapy. In contrast today, more than 60 percent of children diagnosed with cancer can be cured (e.g., Neglia & Robison, 1988) and issues relating to their quality of life as long-term survivors now receive increased emphasis.

Neuropsychological late effects, as a subset of psychological late effects, are defined by a special emphasis on pathological changes in the child's central nervous system (CNS) secondary to cancer or its treatment that are manifested by stable changes in the child's behavior. The most frequently studied behavioral correlates include intellectual and cognitive as well as academic performance. At best, research designs are quasi-experimental because of limitations in controlling essential features of the child's disease and medical therapy. For example, in contrast to traditional manipulations of independent variables in psychological research, one cannot control which children will be diagnosed with cancer, when they will be diagnosed, what type of cancer they will develop, what type of CNS therapy they will receive, or how they will respond to their therapy. Although some of these factors may be controlled with appropriate comparison groups or statistical analyses, one generally cannot expect the same level of rigor as possible in samples of children without life-threatening disease. Clearly the most troublesome issue resulting from this lack of experimental control is the representativeness of patient samples for valid generalization of results to other children.

This chapter discusses the evidence for neuropsychological deficits associated with pediatric acute lymphoblastic leukemia (ALL) and brain tumors, the two most prevalent forms of childhood malignancy. Both ALL and brain tumors are fatal if untreated. It is worth noting that medical treatments previously used for the children who are now participating in late-effects studies have undergone major changes for today's newly diagnosed patient. One must therefore select information from late-effects studies which is pertinent to the clinical question currently being asked about treatment-related toxicity.

Epidemiology

Acute Lymphoblastic Leukemia

ALL is the single most common form of childhood cancer and accounts for almost 30 percent of all newly diagnosed patients. Approximately 6000 new cases will be diagnosed annually with an overall incidence of 126 per million children under the age of 15 years. The peak incidence of ALL is between the ages of 3 and 5 years. The causes are unknown, although previous exposure to ionizing irradiation has been implicated (Neglia & Robison, 1988).

The disease is characterized by an uncontrolled proliferation of malignant white blood cells (lymphoblasts) within the bone marrow, which causes a pathological reduction of normal blood cells and their corresponding functions. Symptoms include fatigue, bruising, and fever, which vary in duration from days to weeks preceding diagnosis (Poplack & Reaman, 1988).

Brain Tumors

The etiology of primary pediatric brain tumors is also unknown. Brain tumors account for approximately 20 percent of all childhood malignancies, second only to the leukemias in terms of incidence. Annually, between 1200 and 1500 children below the age of 16 will be newly diagnosed. The approximate incidence is 0.24 per million in the general population of similarly aged children (Duffner, Cohen, & Freeman, 1985; Leviton, 1984). The diagnosis of brain tumors peaks between the ages of 3 and 9 years with a slightly greater risk in males than females (1.2:1). Brain tumors are quite heterogeneous in terms of site and histology; pediatric patterns do not reflect those found in adult patients. Overall, only 15 to 25 percent of all pediatric brain tumors originate in the cerebral hemispheres.

There are no pathognomonic signs for brain tumors. The presenting signs and symptoms depend on tumor location but are also found in other neurologic and nonneurologic diseases. Among the most common nonspecific signs are those secondary to increased intracranial pressure (hydrocephalus), most often because of tumor obstruction of the flow of cerebral spinal fluid within the ventricles of the brain (Cohen & Duffner, 1984). Irritability, lethargy, diplopia, vomiting, headache, and unexplained changes in behavior and personality may occur. Longstanding hydrocephalus may result in optic atrophy with permanent visual loss as well as mental retardation. Because of the frequent presenting features of headache and vomiting, many children with brain tumors are initially treated as if they have a flulike illness.

Treatment Methods and Survival
Acute Lymphoblastic Leukemia

Approximately 70 percent of children diagnosed with ALL today can be cured with chemotherapy alone. Usually, a three-drug combination is used to induce remission of the leukemia over a 4- to 6-week interval. Following this, 30 months of combination chemotherapy with additional drugs is required. In today's treating institutions, the trend is to provide an increasing proportion of the therapy in an outpatient setting and to encourage resumption of normal activities as soon as possible.

Specific therapy directed at the CNS is also required with the purpose of eradicating leukemia in the brain and spine. Effective CNS therapy, including chemotherapy with or without cranial radiation therapy (CRT), reduces the likelihood of disease relapse and mortality but carries an increased risk of late neurotoxicities. Approximately 10 percent of children treated for ALL will nevertheless experience an isolated CNS relapse requiring even more aggressive treatment with chemotherapy and irradiation of the brain and spine.

Brain Tumors

Primary medical treatment of pediatric brain tumors involves surgery, radiation therapy, and more recently chemotherapy. Although some low-grade tumors may be successfully cured with surgery alone, most tumors will require a multimodal approach to therapy. In addition to the insult to the CNS caused by the tumor and associated pathology such as hydrocephalus, each therapeutic modality is associated with recognized risks of sensory, motor, and cognitive deficits.

Until the 1970s, the operative morbidity and mortality for pediatric brain tumors was extremely high, at least partially because of aggressive attempts to obtain maximal tumor resection in the absence of any other potentially curative therapy. The more recent use of stereoscopic microsurgery, bipolar coagulation forceps, and especially lasers has allowed for decreased patient morbidity and greater precision of tumor resection. Despite these technical advances, neurosurgery provides curative therapy for only a minority of patients with malignant brain tumors.

Ionizing irradiation will be necessary, in some form, for most children with malignant brain tumors. Delivered in one or more fractions per day, fields may encompass the tumor region only, a wide local field may be used, or for highly malignant tumors irradiation is given to the entire neuraxis with a "boost" to the tumor location (Kun, 1984).

Chemotherapy is the most recent addition to the armamentarium of those treating pediatric brain tumors. As with other pediatric malignancies, multiple agents are usually used in combination or sequentially in order to maximize tumor cell kill. Short-term complications (e.g., nausea and vomiting) are common. Some active agents, such as cisplatin, also have significant long-term toxicities in interaction with CRT such as progressive hearing loss and diffuse encephalopathy (Duffner et al., 1985).

With contemporary treatment approaches that combine the therapeutic modalities of chemotherapy, CRT, and surgery, survival remains variable and depends largely upon tumor histology and, secondarily, tumor location. For less aggressive tumors such as low-grade astrocytomas, craniopharyngiomas, or optic and hypothalamic gliomas, the 5-year survival rates generally exceed 70 percent. On the other hand, cerebellar medulloblastoma, the single most common tumor of childhood, can be cured in only 30 to 60 percent of the cases, depending on presenting features such as metastasis at diagnosis. At the most discouraging end of the survival spectrum are high-grade gliomas, such as glioblastoma multiforme, and tumors of the brain stem, which are rarely cured (Kun, 1984).

Pathophysiology of Late Effects in the Central Nervous System

Relevant sources of neuropathology include chemotherapy and CRT for both children with ALL and those with brain tumors. Unique threats to the CNS associated with treatment for ALL and brain tumors are also discussed.

Cranial Radiation Therapy

The goal of CRT is the selective destruction of malignant cells. Irradiation produces intracellular ionization, which causes DNA damage and cell death within the first or second attempt at division. Cells of more rapidly growing normal organ systems are therefore most vulnerable to the adverse side effects of radiation therapy (Kun, 1984). CRT is given in daily fractions to maximize the ratio of tumor to normal cell kill to a total dose of 18 to 24 grays (Gy) for ALL and up to 54 Gy for brain tumors. The gray is a unit that measures the amount of radiation absorbed by tissue.

Irradiation-induced encephalopathies are a major interest area for neuropsychologists. Although acute and subacute irradiation side effects such as anorexia, confusion, and somnolence (a temporary condition of decreased concentration and lethargy) are reversible within weeks of stopping treatment, late CNS effects may

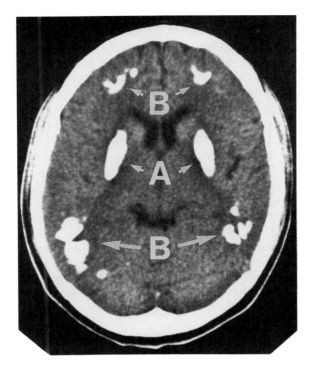

Figure 5.1. Computed tomography of the brain demonstrating bilateral calcification of the basal ganglia (A) and anterior and posterior gray-white matter junctions (B) following treatment for ALL with cranial radiation therapy.

be irreversible if not progressive. Radiation damage to the normal tissues of the central nervous system may manifest as cortical atrophy, vascular damage (mineralizing microangiopathy), or white matter destruction (leukoencephalopathy), as illustrated in Figure 5.1 (Price & Birdwell, 1978). Areas of involvement and severity are associated with the volume of brain irradiated, dose of irradiation per fraction, and total dose of irradiation received (Kun, 1984). However, correlation of these abnormalities as detected on neuroimaging studies such as computed tomography (CT) or magnetic resonance imaging (MRI) with neuropsychological function is not consistently high, except in selected series of patients (Brouwers, Riccardi, Fedio, & Poplack, 1985). At least some recent evidence indicates that calcification of the basal ganglia and/or gray or white matter junctions predicts poor intellectual and memory functioning (Mulhern et al., 1992).

Chemotherapy

Various forms of chemotherapy, administered intravenously or intrathecally (injected into the spinal canal), have been used for CNS treatment of leukemia in combination with CRT. Recent efforts to eliminate the need for CRT have prompted the use of more intensive CNS chemotherapy, most often with methotrexate, in the hopes of avoiding the neurophysiological and neuropsychological adverse effects of irradiation. However, the potential neurotoxicity of methotrexate has been documented for at least the past 10 years and is especially problematic following CRT, supposedly because of changes in the blood-brain barrier following irradiation (Bleyer, 1981). Meadows and Evans (1976) reported that of 13 patients previously treated for ALL, 10 demonstrated neurological and psychological deficits. Of the 10 children with neurotoxicity 4 had been treated with methotrexate but without CRT.

Reduction of CRT-induced brain damage has also been used to justify the administration of chemotherapy to children, especially very young children, with malignant brain tumors. The neurotoxicity of chemotherapy in this clinical setting is less well described, although the drug cisplatin causes dose-related sensorineural hearing loss, which is irreversible. Hearing loss extending into the speech frequencies can limit normal cognitive development and academic progress. In one study of infants and very young children treated for brain tumors with preirradiation chemotherapy, physical and psychological growth was abnormal in the majority of children and showed no "catch-up" effect during the time that CRT was delayed (Mulhern et al., 1989).

Other Sources of Central Nervous System Insult

Conditions that antedate the diagnosis of cancer may also influence the neuropsychological status of survivors. For example, children with Down's syndrome are at greater risk for ALL and children with neurofibromatosis, a genetically transmitted disease involving abnormal proliferation of Schwann cells, are at greater risk for brain tumors than normal children.

Neurological conditions which are secondary to the progression of brain tumors, such as obstructive hydrocephalus and seizures, also have independent importance in determining the neuropsychological functioning of these children. For example, in children without brain tumors poorly controlled seizures are associated with inadequate intellectual and academic development (e.g., Bourgeouis, Prensky, Palkes, Talent, & Busch, 1983).

The normal areas of the CNS of the child with a brain tumor are also at risk for damage secondary to medical treatment of the tumor. Surveys have found that 25 to 30 percent of surviving patients have clinically significant visual (optic atrophy, hemianopia), auditory, and motor disabilities (hemiparesis, ataxia) or seizures which grossly affect their performance of age-appropriate activities of daily living such as self-care and socialization (e.g., Mulhern, Crisco, & Kun, 1983). Short stature, due to irradiation of the spine, or growth hormone deficiency, due to irradiation of the hypothalamic-pituitary axis, are not uncommon problems in long-term survivors (Kun, 1984). Perhaps more than most other clinical populations, close attention should be focused upon these somatic toxicities in the interpretation of neuropsychological test performance, especially with older children who have learned to mask sensory and motor deficiencies through behavioral compensation. Unexpected changes in intracranial pressure, toxic reactions to multiple seizure medications, and the acute but reversible effects of chemotherapy and irradiation make otherwise reliable assessments more difficult.

Age and Time Variables

The various sources of potential brain damage discussed thus far undoubtedly interact with the child's age at the time of exposure and the amount of time elapsed since exposure. Very young children treated for cancer, especially those below age 4 years, receive exposure to neurotoxic agents during a time of accelerated neuroanatomic as well as psychological development. Some of these neurotoxic events may be focal in nature, such as a tumor, and others may have a diffuse impact, such as radiation therapy. In general, the prevailing opinion is that children exposed to diffuse insults at a young age are at greater risk than those exposed to focal insults because of their diminished capacity to use normal brain to adopt functions originally devoted to impaired areas. This hypothesis has received no formal validation with respect to treatment of children with cancer; however, studies of children with brain tumors may eventually provide an answer.

The timing of evaluations which form the basis for conclusions about the late neuropsychological effects of cancer and its treatment is also critical because of the lag between events such as CRT and detectable changes on psychometric testing or neuroimaging. Unless otherwise specified, the following discussion is limited to studies which have assessed children who are long-term survivors of their disease, defined by living 2 or more years following completion of their therapy.

Neuropsychological Deficits Associated with Acute Lymphoblastic Leukemia and Its Treatment

The most commonly used psychological index of neurotoxicity has been the IQ score or pattern of IQ subtest scores displayed by long-term survivors. Following discussion of the effects of CRT, young age at treatment, time since treatment, and gender as factors placing children at high risk for neuropsychological deficits, a discussion of alternative neuropsychological outcome measures is presented. Results of studies using IQs as the primary outcome are summarized in Table 5.1.

Treatment with Cranial Radiation Therapy

Retrospective studies that have demonstrated significantly lower IQ in irradiated compared to nonirradiated patients include Moss, Nannis, and Poplack (98.6 vs. 102.8; 1981), Schlieper, Esseltine, and Tarshis (95.1 vs. 102.1; 1989), Copeland et al. (91.2 vs. 105.6; 1985), and Rowland, Glidewell, and Sibley (91.6 vs.

Table 5.1. Late Effects of Treatment for ALL on Intellectual Development

Factor	Adverse Effects on IQ	
	Yes	No
CRT	Moss et al. (1981)	Longeway et al. (1990)
	Rowland et al. (1984)	Ivnik et al. (1984)
	Copeland et al. (1985)	Whitt et al. (1984)
	Moore et al. (1991)	Mulhern et al. (1991)
	Schlieper et al. (1989)	Jannoun and Chessells (1987)
	Mulhern et al. (1992)	
	Meadows et al. (1981)	
	Waber et al. (1990)	
	Rubenstein et al. (1990)	
Younger age	Moss et al. (1981)	Ivnik et al. (1981)
	Jannoun and Chessells (1987)	Whitt et al. (1984)
	Mulhern (1992)	Rowland et al. (1984)
	Meadows et al. (1981)	Schlieper et al. (1989)
	Waber et al. (1990)	Copeland et al. (1985)
	Robison et al. (1984)	Mulhern et al. (1991)
	Said et al. (1989)	Longeway et al. (1990)
		Rubenstein et al. (1990)
Increased time	Moore et al. (1991)	Schlieper et al. (1989)
	Mulhern et al. (1992)	Said et al. (1989)
	Rubenstein et al. (1990)	
	Mulhern et al. (1991)	
CNS relapse	Ochs et al. (1985)	
	Kun et al. (1984)	
	Mulhern et al. (1987)	
	Longeway et al. (1990)	

106.2; 1984), whereas studies by Ivnik et al. (100.1 vs. 108.9; 1984) and Whitt, Wells, Lauria, Wilhelm, & McMillan (94.6 vs. 96.3; 1984) failed to find an effect. In a recent study of survivors of ALL treated in infancy, discussed in detail later in the chapter, Mulhern et al. (1992) found that nonirradiated infants had nearly normal intellectual development in contrast to those irradiated with 18, 20, or 24 Gy, who generally fell in the low average range of intellectual development. Few studies have been able to establish the relationship between CRT dose and neuropsychological toxicity. However, Moore, Kramer, Wara, Halberg, and Ablin (1991) found that children receiving 18 Gy had mean IQ scores approximately 9 points higher than those children receiving 24 Gy (103.5 vs. 94.6). Waber et al. (1990) reported mean deficits of 14 to 21 IQ points between children with ALL treated with 24 Gy CRT and age- and gender-matched cancer controls.

Among longitudinal studies, Meadows et al. (89.0 vs. 109.0; 1981) and Rubenstein, Varni, and Katz (102.0 vs. 108.7; 1990) have documented significant declines in IQ from first to last observations among long-term survivors receiving CRT, whereas Jannoun and Chessells (1987) and Longeway et al. (1990) did not report a decline with time. In the Meadows et al. (1981) and Rubenstein et al.

(1990) studies, no correction was made for the use of different IQ tests as children became older. When this correction was made in the study by Mulhern, Fairclough, and Ochs (1991), initially significant declines in IQ became nonsignificant.

Younger Age at Treatment

The effects of the child's age at the time of CNS treatment remain ambiguous. Moss et al. (1981), Meadows et al. (1981), Robison et al. (1984), Said, Waters, Cousens, and Stevens (1989), and Jannoun and Chessells (1987) reported increased risk of lowered IQ among children treated at a younger age, whereas Rubenstein et al. (1990), Ivnik et al. (1981), Whitt et al. (1984), Schlieper et al. (1989), Longeway et al. (1990), Copeland et al. (1985), Rowland et al. (1984), and Mulhern et al. (1991) failed to find age-related effects. Waber et al. (1990) found that a younger age at treatment placed females, but not males, at greater risk. As discussed in Mulhern et al. (1991), even among similarly irradiated children, differences in the amount and type of chemotherapy given may help explain these discrepancies.

Because the prognosis for survival among infants with ALL is less favorable than that for older children, little is known about this subgroup of children, although they should be at greatest risk for neuropsychological impairment. With the expectation of clarifying discrepancies in the literature as to the importance of age at diagnosis, Mulhern et al. (1992) compared the functional and neuropsychological status of 26 long-term survivors of ALL diagnosed in the first 24 months of life to 26 children previously treated for Wilms tumor. Of the children with ALL, CNS prophylaxis included no CRT in six, 18 Gy CRT in five, 20 Gy CRT in seven, and 24 Gy CRT in five. Three additional children experienced CNS relapse and received total CRT doses of 24, 40, and 44 Gy. As a group, the children treated for ALL did not differ significantly from those treated for Wilms tumor on objective measures of global functional status (ability to engage in age-appropriate activities). However, children treated for ALL had significantly lower mean IQ (87 vs. 96), poorer performance on four of six measures of visual and auditory memory, lower achievement with regard to arithmetic skills, and a greater frequency of special educational interventions than those treated for Wilms tumor. IQ performance in the ALL group was inversely correlated with total CRT dose: those not receiving CRT had the highest IQs, those receiving 18, 20, and 24 Gy CRT performed less well, and those receiving 40 to 44 Gy displayed the greatest deficits. Similar CRT dose–toxicity relationships were observed with regard to auditory memory function and neurological and neuroimaging abnormalities. These results support the contemporary practice of omitting prophylactic CRT in very young children, except those who are at risk for CNS relapse. For infants and very young children requiring CRT, there was a significant positive correlation between age at CRT and IQ, providing support for delaying CRT until the child is older.

Increasing Time since Treatment

The deleterious biological effects of CNS therapy for ALL are not immediately apparent on radiographic studies, oftentimes taking 2 or more years to materialize on CT or MRI results. Likewise, neuropsychological deficits are usually delayed in those children who will manifest chronic adverse reactions, but this relationship has not always been easy to demonstrate. In a retrospective study, one would attempt to correlate time elapsed from CNS therapy with IQ outcome. A significant negative correlation would suggest IQ decline with increasing time since treatment. In a prospective study, one would attempt to document intra-individual decline with multiple evaluations over time. For both methods, other potentially confounding variables must be ruled out. For example, in retrospective studies, age and time variables are usually highly correlated, making it difficult to separate their effects. In prospective studies, investigators frequently must switch IQ test versions as the children become older during the course of the study (e.g., WPPSI-R to WISC III). This presents a difficult problem, especially because such transitions in the general population are known to result in small changes in IQ scores when different groups of children are used for test standardization.

There have been contradictory findings regarding the relationship between time since treatment and IQ changes. Schlieper, Esseltine, and Tarshis (1989) and Said et al. (1989) failed to find a significant correlation between time elapsed from treatment and IQ levels in their retrospective studies of children surviving ALL, although Schlieper et al. (1989) detected effects of CRT relative to controls. In another retrospective study, Moore et al. (1991) evaluated 35 long-term survivors of ALL, all of whom had received CRT and reported that Verbal IQ but not other IQ measures was inversely correlated with time elapsed from CRT. Mulhern et al. (1992) also found a significant inverse correlation between the IQ levels of children treated for ALL in infancy and time elapsed from therapy. This relationship was not noted in a group of children treated for cancer without CNS therapy.

At least two prospective studies have reported declines in intellectual function over time. Rubenstein et al. (1990) evaluated 24 children with ALL prior to CRT, 1 year later, and 4 to 5 years later. The age-appropriate Wechsler scales were used (WPPSI, WISC-R, WAIS-R). Statistically significant declines of approximately 6 to 7 points were observed with respect to Verbal, Performance, and Full-Scale IQ. Mulhern et al. (1991) presented two alternative methods of analysis of longitudinal IQ data from long-term survivors of ALL that either did or did not make statistical adjustments for changes in IQ test version throughout the study. When no adjustment was made, there was a significant negative correlation between time since treatment and IQ scores of about the same magnitude reported by Rubenstein et al. (1990). When adjustments for test change were incorporated into the design, an otherwise significant time effect was eliminated, suggesting that the size of the experimental effect approximated the size of error introduced by changing IQ tests.

Central Nervous System Relapse

Approximately 5 to 10 percent of children will experience a CNS relapse of their leukemia and 25 percent of these children will become long-term survivors (Kun et al., 1984). Because of the increased aggressiveness of CNS therapies necessitated by their relapse, these children are at increased risk for neuropsychological problems. Kun et al. (1984) reported an average 10-point drop in full-scale IQ approximately 1 year following the second course of CRT in children having CNS relapse. Ochs et al. (1985) compared long-term survivors of ALL who had or had not experienced a CNS relapse. Survivors following CNS relapse had a mean IQ 16 points lower than the comparison group, which had a high incidence of seizure disorders and intracerebral calcification apparent on CT scan. Subsequently, Mulhern et al. (1987) used multiple regression analyses to establish the association between abnormalities seen on CT scan, seizures, and a second course of CRT with lower IQ in this population.

Only one longitudinal controlled study has been reported. Longeway et al. (1990) prospectively assessed 24 children who had received identical CNS therapy, including CRT, early in their treatment: 16 remained in remission and 8 experienced a CNS relapse requiring additional CRT. No change in IQ scores was observed in the group that remained in remission at 5 years posttreatment. In the CNS relapse group, the average IQ decline was a dramatic 25 points.

Gender

Recent interest has developed in the differential vulnerability of male and female children to the effects of CNS treatment for ALL. Although the mechanisms are not yet clear, at least some evidence suggests that girls are more likely to suffer deleterious effects than boys.

Robison et al. (1984), using multiple regression analyses of 50 long-term survivors, identified female gender as a risk factor accounting for mean Verbal and Full-Scale IQ differences of almost 10 points compared to males. Schlieper, Esseltine, and Tarshis (1989) compared the intellectual performance of male and female long-term survivors of ALL who had received CNS treatment with CRT or chemotherapy alone. Few differences were seen between the males and females who had received chemotherapy only. Among the children receiving CRT, however, females consistently scored significantly lower than males on Performance and Full-Scale IQ.

Waber et al. (1990) compared the neuropsychological performance of 27 females and 24 males who were long-term survivors of ALL treated with chemotherapy and 24 Gy CRT. Male and female patients were closely matched for age at diagnosis and relevant treatment features. Results of intellectual testing indicated significantly lower scores on the Arithmetic and Digit Span subtests of the WISC-R and the Arithmetic subtest of the WRAT-R for females. Although females had a mean IQ 8.5 points lower than that of males, this difference failed to reach statistical significance. Interestingly, the proportion of females who were short and overweight for age was also significantly greater than that of males, implying that females are more vulnerable to neuroendocrine as well as cognitive impairment secondary to treatment of the CNS.

In a prospective evaluation of children treated for ALL covering a period of almost 10 years, Mulhern et al. (1991) used regression analysis to identify factors associated with IQ declines from pre-CNS treatment levels. Female gender accounted for a significant amount of variance in Verbal IQ decline; this effect was most pronounced among children in the group given a higher CRT dose (24 Gy).

Specific Neuropsychological Impairments

Several investigators have moved beyond characterizing deficits merely in terms of patterns of IQ scores toward evaluation of more specific neuropsychological functions. Memory functions have been among the more frequently investigated deficits in this context. Copeland et al. (1985) compared long-term survivors of ALL who did or did not have CRT to a cancer control group who did not have any CNS therapy. The Verbal Selective Reminding Test and the Nonverbal Selective Reminding Test were included in the battery to assess memory functioning. Nonirradiated patients with ALL and controls did not differ on these measures but the irradiated patients with ALL exhibited lower nonverbal memory scores than the other two groups. Because the irradiated patients also had significantly lower IQs, it is possible that this difference was secondary to a generalized cognitive impairment.

Mulhern, Wasserman, Fairclough, & Ochs (1988) observed significant deficits in (1) long-term recall of visually and aurally presented verbal material (Learning Efficiency Test) and (2) recall and reproduction of geometric patterns (Target Test) relative to test norms for children treated for ALL with high-dose chemotherapy without CRT or low-dose chemotherapy with CRT. These deficits remained significant after adjusting scores for IQ. There were no differences between treatment groups.

Summary

The sometimes contradictory findings regarding the neuropsychological toxicity of treatment for ALL have most often been attributed to methodological factors such as small sample sizes in some studies, which limited statistical power to detect differences, variance with regard to length of follow-up and measures used, and differences with regard to chemotherapy beyond the inclusion or exclusion of CRT (Fletcher & Copeland, 1988; Mulhern et al., 1991; Williams & Davis, 1986). One might expect that a statistical interaction between the intensity of CNS treatment, age of the child at the time of treatment, and time elapsed from the completion of treatment would explain at least some of these discrepancies. However, we are unaware of any such analysis to date. It is unlikely that a study large enough for this type of analysis could be completed in other than an interinstitutional collaborative setting.

Table 5.2. Late Effects of Treatment of Brain Tumors
on Intellectual Development

Factor	Adverse Effects on IQ	
	Yes	No
CRT	Kun et al. (1983) Ellenberg et al. (1987) Duffner et al. (1988)	
Younger age	Danoff et al. (1982) Kun (1983) Mulhern and Kun (1985) Ellenberg et al. (1987) Packer et al. (1989)	
Increasing time	Ellenberg et al. (1987) Packer et al. (1989) Kun and Mulhern (1983) Cavazutti et al. (1980) Mulhern and Kun (1985)	
Tumor location	Kun et al. (1983) Ellenberg et al. (1987) Hirsch et al. (1989) Mulhern & Kun (1985) Danoff et al. (1982)	
Hydrocephalus	Ellenberg et al. (1987)	Danoff et al. (1982) Kun et al. (1983) Mulhern & Kun (1985)

For children who receive CRT at the age of 2 years or younger and for those who experience a CNS relapse, especially those who will receive a second course of CRT, all available evidence points to an increased risk of chronic and pervasive neurological and neuropsychological deficits. For older children who receive CRT and remain in remission, the risk of clinically significant intellectual or neuropsychological decline is equivocal. Independent of IQ changes, memory functions may be differentially affected. The contribution of other risk factors, such as female gender, are less well documented but are potentially important areas for future research.

Neuropsychological Deficits Associated with Brain Tumors and Their Treatment

Factors which appear to place children at risk for IQ deficits following treatment for pediatric brain tumors are now discussed in detail. Findings are summarized in Table 5.2. Following this, evidence is presented which associates more specific neuropsychological deficits with tumor and treatment variables.

Treatment with Cranial Radiation Therapy

The deleterious effects of CRT for brain tumors in children have been demonstrated using a variety of designs, primarily comparing the presence versus absence of brain irradiation or comparing brain areas irradiated. No studies relating irradiation dose to IQ toxicity were noted. Longitudinal studies of irradiated patients (e.g., Duffner, Cohen, & Parker, 1988) as well as comparisons between irradiated and nonirradiated patients and between irradiated patients and normal controls have all concluded that radiation therapy has adverse effects on intellectual development. Two studies have also demonstrated greater decrements among children receiving whole brain (cranial) irradiation compared to those receiving only a localized field of treatment (Ellenberg, McComb, Siegel, & Stowe, 1987; Kun, Mulhern, & Crisco, 1983).

Younger Age at Treatment

The association between age at treatment and neuropsychological impairment has been difficult to specify because of variations in the definition of "younger." Investigators have defined young children as those below 3, 6, 7, 7.5, and 8 years. Danoff, Cowchock, Marquette, Mulgrew, and Kramer (1982) retrospectively reported on 35 long-term survivors. Using only descriptive statistics, the authors found that 17 percent of the children were mentally retarded and that the incidence of mental retardation was greater in those children under the age of 3 years at diagnosis. Statistically significant risks of a young age at treatment have been reported in three studies (Ellenberg et al., 1987; Mulhern & Kun, 1985; Packer et al., 1989). The relationship between age at diagnosis and IQ level reported in other investigations was purely descriptive. Of the studies that did *not* find age at diagnosis to be related to intellectual functioning, one found a significant relationship between age at diagnosis and selective attention, with younger children performing more poorly than older children (Kun & Mulhern, 1983).

Increasing Time since Treatment

Several investigations found a statistically significant decline in intellectual functioning over time from preirradiation to over 4 years posttreatment. However, in one investigation this was true only for those patients receiving cranial (whole brain) irradiation and those irradiated at a younger age (Packer et al., 1989). Patient IQ changes are often a function of neurologic improvement in the immediate postoperative period and subsequent deterioration due to radiation therapy. Kun and Mulhern (1983) reported that at 3 to 70 months postirradiation, below-normal intellectual functioning was evident in 9 of 18 patients. At 10 to 23 months later IQs were stable in 12 patients, improved in 3, and deteriorated in 3. Further,

6 to 23 months later IQs were stable in 8 and improved in 1 patient. No tests of significance were performed to analyze this trend. Similarly, Kun, Mulhern, and Crisco (1983) evaluated patients following surgery but before irradiation and again at 10 to 26 months later, following irradiation. At the second evaluation, 2 patients improved, 5 were stable, and 3 deteriorated with regard to intellectual status.

Mixed results were found in three investigations. Cavazzuti, Winston, Baker, and Welch (1980) found improvements in verbal memory functioning following surgery in patients with right temporal tumors. In contrast, declines in verbal memory functions were found in patients with left temporal tumors evaluated postoperatively. Ellenberg et al. (1987) reported a significant improvement in IQ from 1 to 4 months posttreatment; IQ declined thereafter. This relationship appeared to be mediated by tumor location. Finally, Mulhern and Kun (1985) evaluated patients postsurgery but preirradiation and again 6 months after irradiation. The relationship between time since treatment and intellectual ability varied for older versus younger children: younger children evidenced a greater decline over time in memory functioning than older children. Furthermore, among the older children, females, but not males, showed improvement on Full-Scale, Verbal, and Performance IQ compared to the immediate postoperative period.

Tumor Location

Ellenberg et al. (1987) examined the IQ scores of third ventricular region, posterior fossa region, and cerebral hemisphere region brain tumor patients at four time intervals. Although the IQ scores of patients with hemispheric tumors were lower than those with third ventricular and posterior fossa tumors over all time intervals, this difference was significant only at the 4-month postdiagnosis evaluation, perhaps due to small sample sizes at the other intervals. Mulhern & Kun (1985) found a greater *increase* in IQ scores over time for patients with posterior fossa tumors compared to those with third ventricle region or hemispheric region tumors, but this relationship held only for younger children. Kun et al. (1983) found that a greater proportion of children with hemispheric than posterior fossa tumors showed clinical deterioration of IQ following irradiation. A study by Danoff et al. (1982) suggested that children whose tumor extended to the hypothalamus had a greater likelihood of mental deficiency following surgery and irradiation.

Investigators from Europe have reported on a cohort of 42 consecutively diagnosed children with benign tumors of the cerebral hemispheres (Hirsch, Rose, Pierre-Kahn, Pfister, & Hoppe-Hirsch, 1989). Since these children were treated with surgery alone, they comprise an important comparison group in evaluating the late effects of CRT. Long-term follow-up revealed that approximately 30 percent of these children had IQ levels below 80 with major problems in school. Although the authors did not associate a 20 percent incidence of poorly controlled postoperative seizures with low IQ or school problems, this additional influence cannot be ruled out.

Hydrocephalus

The association between chronic hydrocephalus (ventricular dilatation and increased intracranial pressure) and mental retardation is well documented. However, the effects of episodic and temporary increases in intracranial pressure are not well understood. Of the four studies that examined the relationship between hydrocephalus and intellectual deficits, three found nonsignificant results (Danoff et al., 1982; Kun et al., 1983; Mulhern & Kun, 1985). In contrast, Ellenberg et al. (1987) reported that patients with a history of hydrocephalus scored significantly lower than those patients without a history of hydrocephalus, both at diagnosis and 4 months later. However, an improvement in IQ over the 4-month interval was noted for patients with and without a history of hydrocephalus. This study also compared patients with hydrocephalus who had normalization of intracranial pressure without the need for surgical intervention by shunting to those who required shunting. No significant IQ differences existed between these groups initially. At the 4-month interval, a significant IQ increase was noted for those patients with shunts but not for those patients without shunts.

Specific Neuropsychological Impairments

Several studies have utilized formal measures of neuropsychological functioning in addition to IQ testing. Broadly speaking, the measures can be categorized into those measuring higher conceptual abilities, those assessing specific memory functions, and those assessing visual-motor, visuographic, or fine motor functions.

Problems with cognitive flexibility and problem-solving skills, as measured by the Category Test and Trails Test, have been noted by LeBaron, Zeltzer, Zeltzer, Scott, & Marlin (1988) among 15 children treated for posterior fossa tumors. These deficits were presumably secondary to irradiation of their cerebral hemispheres as opposed to dysfunction related to the tumor itself. Riva, Pantaleoni, Milani, and Belani (1989) also evaluated eight children previously treated for posterior fossa tumors with surgery and radiation therapy and compared them to seven children treated with surgery alone. The Trail-Making Test (Forms A and B) and a computer-administered Continuous Performance Test of vigilance were given to all patients. Both groups of patients performed significantly worse than sibling controls on Trails but not on the Continuous Performance Test. The authors propose that tumor- or surgically related disturbance of the ascending reticular activating system was the common mechanism for observed deficits in attentional abilities because of the close neuroanatomic proximity of these structures to the posterior fossa.

Cavazzuti et al. (1980; Cavazzuti, Fischer, Welch, Belli, & Winston, 1983) have extensively evaluated long-term survivors of temporal lobe tumors. In the first study (Cavazzuti et al., 1980), 20 children with temporal lobe tumors were evaluated with the Weschler Memory Scale and Wisconsin Card Sorting Test. Of the 20 patients, 19 displayed cognitive disturbances commonly associated with both dominant and nondominant cerebral hemisphere insults. Pre- to postoperative improvements in verbal memory were noted in most patients with right temporal lobe tumors; however, all these patients performed worse after surgery on measures of nonverbal memory. Two patients demonstrated preoperative impairment of frontal lobe function as measured by the Wisconsin Card Sorting Test; this impairment persisted postsurgery. Among those patients with left temporal lobe tumors, verbal memory problems following surgery seemed inversely proportional to the severity of these deficits seen prior to surgery but most showed some deterioration. Most patients with left temporal lobe tumors had improvement in nonverbal memory function following surgery.

Using the same tests, Cavazzuti et al. (1983) examined patients who had been treated for craniopharyngioma, a common tumor of the pituitary region, with radical surgical resection using a subfrontal approach or with conservative surgery and local irradiation. Memory function and IQ were equivalent in both groups but patients who received radical surgical resection showed significantly poorer performance on the Wisconsin Card Sorting Test, a measure of problem solving.

Three independent investigations using either the Halstead-Reitan Neuropsychological Battery (Duffner, Cohen, & Thomas, 1983; LeBaron et al., 1988) or the Luria-Nebraska Neuropsychological Battery (Mulhern, Kovnar, Kun, Crisco, & Williams, 1988) with survivors of posterior fossa area tumors have found common problems associated with damage to the cerebellum. A high frequency of visual-motor and visuospatial deficits as well as problems with fine and gross motor steadiness, speed, and coordination were noted. These deficits were probably associated with cerebellar dysfunction secondary to tumor and/or surgical resection. Specific tests of visual-motor functions given independently of these batteries (e.g., Developmental Test of Visual-Motor Integration, Wisconsin Motor Steadiness Battery, Bender Visual Motor Gestalt Test) yield similar findings. Packer et al. (1989) reported poor performance on these tasks among irradiated children with malignant posterior fossa tumors as well as nonirradiated children with benign posterior fossa tumors. Spunberg, Change, Goldman, Auricchio, and Bell (1981) reported that 12 of 13 children with posterior fossa tumors had deficient visual-motor skills.

Specific deficits have seldom been attributed to surgical intervention or chemotherapy. In a prospective study of 16 children treated with surgery and CRT *with or without* chemotherapy, Duffner et al. (1983) found a greater incidence of learning disabilities among children treated with all three modalities. Clopper and colleagues (1977) have reported significantly lower Performance IQ levels than Verbal IQ levels in children receiving surgical resection only for craniopharyngioma.

There is at least one report of the use of neuropsychological testing in the diagnosis of a brain tumor (Mulhern, Wasserman, Kovnar, Williams, & Ochs, 1986). In this case report, a 10-year-old boy had successfully completed his treatment for leukemia 5 years previously. He had been followed with annual neuropsychological evaluations as part of an institutional study of the late cognitive effects of treatment for leukemia. On the basis of an abnormal sensory-perceptual exam, the patient was referred for neuroimaging. Specifically, the child had exhibited normal tactile perception of his right digits with marked imperception on the left, implicating the posterior right parietal lobe. A subsequent CT scan revealed a right posterior parietal brain tumor as a second malignancy.

Summary

Psychological outcomes following treatment for brain tumors in childhood appear to be a multifactorial process, although only one published prospective study has been able to address potential interactions among risk factors (Ellenberg et al., 1987). The optimal study design would prospectively evaluate patient function in important psychological domains (intelligence, academic achievement, personal-social adjustment, adaptive behavior) and analyze changes in patient performance as a function of radiation therapy parameters, age at treatment, time since treatment, tumor location, and the patient's neurological status.

Not surprisingly, many children with brain tumors, especially those with lowered IQ and/or sensory and motor deficits, will also have problems with their school progress. Several studies have noted an incidence of placement in special educational programs of more than 40 percent because of inability to keep pace with age peers in terms of achievement (Duffner et al., 1983; Kun et al., 1983; Spunberg et al., 1981). Among children treated for posterior fossa tumors, academic achievement problems may relate to slow psychomotor speed or to the effects of radiation therapy on other structures remote to the site of the tumor (LeBaron et al., 1988). A concurrent decline in IQ scores and academic achievement relative to normal expectations for age observed by several investigators has been attributed to declining attentional and memory abilities, which impede the acquisition of new knowledge (Mulhern et al. 1988; Silverman et al., 1984). However, learning problems among children treated for brain tumors can also occur despite normal IQ (Duffner et al., 1983).

A high proportion of children treated for brain tumors may have chronic problems with their emotional adjustment, although it is difficult to ascertain whether the symptoms are a direct causal effect of the tumor and treatment on the central nervous system, a direct effect on the central nervous system which makes the children more vulnerable to normal life stresses, or more of an indirect effect of the children having problems in accepting limitations of function following treatment. Estimates of the incidence of clinical maladjustment have been at least 50 percent (Kun et al., 1983; Mulhern & Kun 1985; LeBaron et al., 1988), with most the serious problems among children treated for tumors of the temporal lobe with poorly controlled seizure disorders (Mulhern, Kovnar, et al., 1988).

Mostow, Byrne, Connelly, and Mulvihill (1991) recently published a retrospective comparison of survivors of pediatric brain tumor with their siblings and found a significantly greater likelihood of unemployment, chronic health conditions, and an inability to drive an automobile among the former patients. Those patients with a history of tumors of the cerebral hemispheres and radiation therapy were at greatest risk for adverse outcomes.

Conclusion
Issues Relating to Patient Care

Treating physicians, most often pediatric oncologists and radiation oncologists, at major medical centers are aware of the risks for intellectual and other neuropsychological problems among children with ALL and brain tumors. However, considerable variability among institutions exists as to how these risks affect patient care. The following recommendations are based on the clinical experience of the author and the present review of the literature.

First, available knowledge about the potential for adverse neuropsychological effects of disease and various treatment options must be made explicit to the parent and child, if he or she is old enough to assist in decision making. This is especially important in situations when the child is not receiving treatment on a research study approved by a human subjects review board, which monitors how the risks and benefits are described to patients on forms requiring written informed consent.

Second, a formal plan of surveillance of neuropsychological development should be set forth for each child based on known or suspected risk for problems. This assumes that a qualified psychologist has been identified as a consultant to the institution. Such plans should not depend on the presentation of symptoms because presymptomatic assessments often allow for early interventions that will minimize deficits. For example, a school-aged child with ALL receiving no CRT should have a neuropsychological evaluation scheduled at the completion of therapy and 3 to 5 years later, whereas an infant with a brain tumor should probably be evaluated every 6 months until the age of 3 or 4 years and then yearly until 5 years posttherapy.

Third, formal consultative arrangements should be made between the treating physician and the psychologist in order to clarify methods of information exchange. As obvious as this may seem, problems with the timely communication of patient information can limit the quality of patient care.

Last, a social worker from the cancer center or psychologist should be designated as a liaison with the child's school and other community service agencies. For children with complex medical conditions and concurrent neuropsychological problems, timely communication of accurate information can avoid misunderstandings that have important implications for the child's quality of life.

Future Research

The bulk of neuropsychological studies conducted thus far in the area of pediatric oncology have been retrospective and epidemiologic in nature. That is, the investigators have sought to identify specific subgroups of children at especially high risk for certain types of deficits and to associate these with disease- or treatment-related factors, usually in cross-sectional designs using long-term survivors of cancer. With some limitations, this line of research has been profitable in defining the risks associated with various disease presentations and treatment alternatives. Similar research studies will continue to comprise an important part of neuropsychological research as newer treatment approaches are developed.

Conspicuously absent from the literature are neuropsychological intervention studies with children treated for ALL or brain tumors. Can any of the neuropsychological deficits incurred by treatment for cancer be remediated? I am unaware of any published studies on cognitive rehabilitation with children surviving ALL or brain tumors. Are traditional special educational programs (learning disabled, other health impaired) effective for these children or do they need more specialized programs? These questions raise the prospect that psychologists can directly improve the ultimate quality of life of children surviving cancer even if one cannot control the incidence of cancer or the adverse consequences of its treatment.

Acknowledgment

Preparation of this chapter was supported in part by the American Lebanese Syrian Associated Charities.

References

Bleyer, W. A. (1981). Neurologic sequelae of methotrexate and ionizing radiation: A new classification. *Cancer Treatment Reports, 65,* 89–98.

Bourgeouis, B. F. D., Prensky, A. L., Palkes, H. S., Talent, B. K., & Busch, S. G. (1983). Intelligence in epilepsy: A prospective study in children. *Annals of Neurology, 14,* 438–444.

Brouwers, P., Riccardi, R., Fedio, P., & Poplack, D. G. (1985). Longterm neuropsychologic sequelae of childhood leukemia: Correlation of CT brain scan abnormalities. *Journal of Pediatrics, 106,* 723–728.

Cavazzuti, V., Fischer, E. G., Welch, K., Belli, J. A., & Winston, K. R. (1983). Neurological and psychophysiological sequelae following different treatments of craniopharyngioma in children. *Journal of Neurosurgery, 59,* 409–417.

Cavazzuti, V., Winston, K., Baker, R., & Welch, K. (1980). Psychological changes following surgery for tumors in the temporal lobe. *Journal of Neurosurgery, 53,* 618–626.

Clopper, R. R., Meyer, W. J., Udverhelyi, G. B., Money, J., Aarabi, B., Mulvihill, J. J., & Piasio, M. (1977). Postsurgical IQ and behavioral data on 20 patients with a history of childhood craniopharyngioma. *Psychoneuroendocrinology, 2,* 365–372.

Cohen, M. E., & Duffner, P. K. (1984). Principles of diagnosis. In M. E. Cohen & P. K. Duffner (Eds.), *Brain tumors in children: Principles of diagnosis and treatment* (pp. 9–21). New York: Raven Press.

Copeland, D. R., Fletcher, J. M., Pfefferbaum-Levine, B., Jaffe, N., Ried, H., & Maor, M. (1985). Neuropsychological sequelae of childhood cancer in long-term survivors. *Pediatrics, 75,* 745–753.

Danoff, B. F., Cowchock, S., Marquette, C., Mulgrew, L., & Kramer, S. (1982). Assessment of the long-term effects of primary radiation therapy for brain tumors in children. *Cancer, 49,* 1582–1586.

Duffner, P. K., Cohen, M. E., & Freeman, A. I. (1985). Pediatric brain tumors: An overview. *Ca—A Cancer Journal for Clinicians, 35,* 287–301.

Duffner, P. K., Cohen, M. E., & Parker, M. S. (1988). Prospective intellectual testing in children with brain tumors. *Annals of Neurology, 23,* 575–579.

Duffner, P. K., Cohen, M. E., & Thomas, P. (1983). Late effects of treatment on the intelligence of children with posterior fossa tumors. *Cancer, 51,* 233–237.

Ellenberg, L., McComb, J. G., Siegel, S. E., & Stowe, S. (1987). Factors affecting intellectual outcome in pediatric brain tumor patients. *Neurosurgery, 21,* 638–644.

Fletcher, J., & Copeland, D. (1988). Neurobehavioral effects of central nervous system prophylactic treatment of cancer in children. *Journal of Clinical and Experimental Neuropsychology, 10,* 495–538.

Hirsch, J. F., Rose, C. S., Pierre-Kahn, A., Pfister, A., & Hoppe-Hirsch, E. (1989). Benign astrocytic and oligodendritic tumors of the cerebral hemispheres in children. *Journal of Neurosurgery, 70,* 568–572.

Ivnik, R. J., Colligen, R. C., Obetz, S. W., & Smithson, W. A. (1981). Neuropsychological performance among children in remission from acute lymphocytic leukemia. *Developmental and Behavioral Pediatrics, 2,* 29–34.

Jannoun, L. (1983). Are cognitive and educational development affected by age at which prophylactic therapy is given in acute lymphoblastic leukaemia? *Archives of Diseases of Childhood, 58,* 953–958.

Jannoun, L., & Chessells, J. M. (1987). Long-term psychological effects of childhood leukemia and its treatment. *Pediatric Hematology and Oncology, 4,* 293–308.

Kun, L. E. (1984). Principles of radiation therapy. In M. E. Cohen & P. K. Duffner (Eds.), *Brain tumors in children: Principles of diagnosis and treatment* (pp. 47–70). New York: Raven Press.

Kun, L. E., Camitta, B. M., Mulhern, R., Lauer, S., Kline, R., Casper, J., Kamen, B., Kaplan, B., & Barber, S. (1984). Treatment of meningeal relapse in childhood acute lymphoblastic leukemia: I. Results of craniospinal irradiation. *Journal of Clinical Oncology, 2,* 359–364.

Kun, L. E., & Mulhern, R. K. (1983). Neuropsychologic function in children with brain tumors: II. Serial studies of intellect and time after treatment. *American Journal of Clinical Oncology, 6,* 651–665.

Kun, L. E., Mulhern, R. K., & Crisco, J. J. (1983). Quality of life in children treated for brain tumors: Intellectual, emotional and academic function. *Journal of Neurosurgery, 58,* 1–6.

LeBaron, S., Zeltzer, P. M., Zeltzer, L. K., Scott, S., & Marlin, A. E. (1988). Assessment of quality of survival in children with medulloblastoma and cerebellar astrocytoma. *Cancer, 62,* 1215–1222.

Leviton, A. (1984). Principles of epidemiology. In M. E. Cohen & P. K. Duffner (Eds.), *Brain tumors in children: Principles of diagnosis and treatment* (pp. 22–46). New York: Raven Press.

Longeway, K. L., Mulhern, R., Crisco, J., Kun, L. E., Lauer, S., Casper, J., Camitta, B., & Hoffman, R. G. (1990). Treatment of meningeal relapse in childhood acute lymphoblastic leukemia: II. A prospective study of intellectual loss specific to CNS relapse and therapy. *American Journal of Pediatric Hematology/Oncology, 12,* 45–50.

Meadows, A. T., & Evans, A. E. (1976). Effects of chemotherapy on the central nervous system: A study of parenteral methotrexate in longterm survivors of childhood acute lymphoblastic leukemia. *Cancer, 37,* 1079–1085.

Meadows, A. T., Massari, D. J., Fergusson, J., Gordon, J., Littman, P., & Moss, K. (1981). Declines in IQ scores and cognitive dysfunctions in children with acute lymphocytic leukemia treated with cranial irradiation. *Lancet, 2,* 1015–1018.

Moore, I. M., Kramer, J. H., Wara, W., Halberg, F., & Ablin, A. R. (1991). Cognitive function in children with leukemia: Effect of radiation dose and time since irradiation. *Cancer, 68,* 1913–1917.

Moss, H. A., Nannis, E. D., & Poplack, D. G. (1981). The effects of prophylactic treatment of the central nervous system on the intellectual functioning of children with acute lymphocytic leukemia. *American Journal of Medicine, 71,* 47–52.

Mostow, E. N., Byrne, J., Connelly, R. R., & Mulvihill, J. J. (1991). Quality of life in long-term survivors of CNS tumors of childhood and adolescence. *Journal of Clinical Oncology, 9,* 592–599.

Mulhern, R. K., Crisco, J. J., & Kun, L. E. (1983). Neuropsychological sequelae of childhood brain tumors: A review. *Journal of Clinical Child Psychology, 12,* 66–73.

Mulhern, R. K., Fairclough, D., & Ochs, J. (1991). A prospective comparison of neuropsychologic performance of children surviving leukemia who received 18-Gy, 24-Gy or no cranial irradiation. *Journal of Clinical Oncology, 9,* 1348–1356.

Mulhern, R. K., Horowitz, M. E., Kovnar, E. H., Langston, J., Sanford, R. A., & Kun, L. E. (1989). Neurodevelopmental status of infants and young children treated for brain tumors with pre-irradiation chemotherapy. *Journal of Clinical Oncology, 7,* 1660–1666.

Mulhern, R. K., Kovnar, E. H., Kun, L. E., Crisco, J. J., & Williams, J. M. (1988). Psychologic and neurologic function following treatment for childhood temporal lobe astrocytoma. *Journal of Child Neurology, 3,* 47–52.

Mulhern, R. K., Kovnar, E. H., Langston, J., Carter, M., Fairclough, D., Leigh, L., & Kun, L. E. (1992). Longterm survivors of leukemia treated in infancy: Factors associated with neuropsychological status. *Journal of Clinical Oncology, 10,* 1095–1102.

Mulhern, R. K., & Kun, L. E. (1985). Neuropsychologic function in children with brain tumors: III. Interval changes in the six months following treatment. *Medical and Pediatric Oncology, 13,* 318–324.

Mulhern, R. K., Ochs, J., Fairclough, D., Wasserman, A., Davis, K., & Williams, J. M. (1987). Intellectual and academic achievement status after CNS relapse: A retrospective analysis of 40 children treated for ALL. *Journal of Clinical Oncology, 5,* 933–940.

Mulhern, R. K., Wasserman, A. L., Fairclough, D., & Ochs, J. (1988). Memory function in disease-free survivors of childhood acute lymphocytic leukemia given CNS prophylaxis with or without 1,800 cGy cranial irradiation. *Journal of Clinical Oncology, 6,* 315–320.

Mulhern, R. K., Wasserman, A. L., Kovnar, E. H., Williams, J. M., & Ochs, J. (1986). Serial neuropsychological studies of a child with acute lymphoblastic leukemia and subsequent glioblastoma multiforme. *Neurology, 36,* 1534–1538.

Neglia, J. P., & Robison, L. (1988). Epidemiology of the childhood leukemias. *Pediatric Clinics of North America, 35,* 675–692.

Ochs, J., Rivera, G., Aur, R. J. A., Hustu, H. O., Berg, R., & Simone, J. (1985). Central nervous system morbidity following an initial isolated central nervous system relapse and its subsequent therapy in childhood acute lymphoblastic leukemia. *Journal of Clinical Oncology, 3,* 622–625.

Packer, R. J., Sutton, L. N., Atkins, T. E., Radcliffe, J., Bunnin, G. R., D'Angio, G., Siegel, K. R., & Schut, L. (1989). A prospective study of cognitive function in children receiving whole brain radiotherapy and chemotherapy: Two year results. *Journal of Neurosurgery, 70,* 707–713.

Poplack, D. G., & Reaman, G. (1988). Acute lymphoblastic leukemia in childhood. *Pediatric Clinics of North America, 35,* 903–932.

Price, R. A., & Birdwell, D. A. (1978). The central nervous system in childhood leukemia: III. Mineralizing microangiopathy and dystrophic calcification. *Cancer, 35,* 717–728.

Riva, D., Pantaleoni, C., Milani, N., & Belani, F. F. (1989). Impairment of neuropsychological functions in children with medulloblastomas and astrocytomas in the posterior fossa. *Child's Nervous System, 5,* 107–110.

Robison, L. L., Nesbit, M. E., Sather, H. N., Meadows, A. T., Ortega, J. A., & Hammond, G. D. (1984). Factors associated with IQ scores in long-term survivors of childhood acute lymphoblastic leukemia. *American Journal of Pediatric Hematology/Oncology, 6,* 115–121.

Rowland, J. H., Glidewell, O. J., & Sibley, R. F. (1984). Effects of different forms of central nervous system prophylaxis on neuropsychological function in childhood leukemia. *Journal of Clinical Oncology, 2,* 1327–1335.

Rubenstein, C. L., Varni, J. W., & Katz, E. R. (1990). Cognitive functioning in longterm survivors of childhood leukemia: A prospective analysis. *Developmental and Behavioral Pediatrics, 11,* 301–305.

Said, J. A., Waters, B. G. H., Cousens, P., & Stevens, M. M. (1989). Neuropsychological sequelae of central nervous system prophylaxis in survivors of childhood acute lymphoblastic leukemia. *Journal of Consulting and Clinical Psychology, 57,* 251–256.

Schlieper, A. E., Esseltine, D. W., & Tarshis, M. A. (1989). Cognitive function in longterm survivors of childhood acute lymphoblastic leukemia. *Pediatric Hematology and Oncology, 6,* 1–9.

Silverman, C. L., Palkes, H., Talent, B., Kovnar, E., Klouse, J. W., & Thomas, P. R. M. (1984). Late effects of radiotherapy on patients with cerebellar medulloblastoma. *Cancer, 54,* 825–829.

Spunberg, J. J., Change, C. H., Goldman, M., Auricchio, E., & Bell, J. J. (1981). Quality of long-term survival following irradiation for intracranial tumors in children under the age of two. *International Journal of Radiation Oncology and Biological Physics, 7,* 727–736.

Waber, D. P., Urion, D. K., Tarbell, N. J., Niemeyer, C., Gelber, R., & Sallan, S. E. (1990). Late effects of central nervous system treatment of acute lymphoblastic leukemia in childhood are sex-dependent. *Developmental Medicine and Child Neurology, 32,* 238–248.

Whitt, J. K., Wells, R. J., Laurie, M. M., Wilhelm, C., & McMillan, C. W. (1984). Cranial radiation in childhood acute lymphocytic leukemia: Neuropsychologic sequelae. *American Journal of Diseases of Children, 138,* 730–736.

Williams, J. M., & Davis, K. S. (1986). Neuropsychological effects of central nervous system prophylactic treatment for childhood leukemia. *Cancer Treatment Review, 13,* 113–127.

6

Sibling Adaptation to the Family Crisis of Childhood Cancer

PAUL J. CARPENTER AND CARLA S. LEVANT

A diagnosis of childhood cancer is a catastrophic crisis that poses significant challenges to the stability and adaptive functioning of the entire family system. Following diagnosis, families are not only faced with the difficult tasks of helping a child cope with the physical and emotional stressors of the medical treatments, they must also struggle, both collectively and individually, with the ambiguity associated with the short- and long-term prognosis of this disease and the side effects of treatment. Consequently, it is not unusual for the family system and its individual members to experience intermittent states of acute and/or chronic emotional crisis in their efforts to realign family priorities and meet one another's needs. These crises can trigger an array of emotional, behavioral, and somatic symptoms of distress. The achievement of medical milestones (e.g., remission) and the discovery of devastating setbacks (e.g., relapse) in the patient also present potential crises for families that further challenge their adaptive functioning. Because families are neither isolated from the larger social systems in which they participate nor immune to the stressors and strains of everyday life, other non–illness-related events also pose additional stress on the family system.

Advances in the multimodal treatment of many childhood cancers (e.g., surgery, chemotherapy, radiology, bone marrow transplantation) during the past three decades have significantly altered the prognoses for many of these diseases yet they also have dramatically increased the intensity and duration of treatment (Holland, 1989). In turn, health-care professionals in pediatric oncology have had to change their approach patient care. Given the dismal prognoses a few decades ago for children who had cancer, the emphasis in pediatric oncology was on palliative treatment and comfort of the patient and providing emotional support for parents coping with their children's terminal disease and inevitable death. The psychosocial studies during this period were influenced by models of psychopathology which emphasized the "individual" (Stehbens, 1988). Because recent studies have not supported this approach, there is a need for new conceptual models (Kupst & Schulman, 1988).

The emphasis in pediatric oncology has shifted in the past decade to the medical treatment and supportive care of children with chronic life-threatening diseases that are potentially curable. While acknowledging the acute psychosocial difficulties that patients and their families experience, this shift in focus emphasizes adaptation and resiliency rather than psychopathology (Leonard, 1991; Kupst, Chapter 2, this volume). More aggressive and lengthy medical regimens for treating many childhood cancers have placed new demands on pediatric oncology health-care professionals to provide interventions for a range of complex psychosocial issues among not only patients but their families as well (Kellerman, 1980).

Focus on Siblings

Research findings have consistently indicated that the family crisis of childhood cancer can have a profound impact on siblings' psychosocial functioning (e.g., Carr-Gregg & White, 1987; Sahler et al., 1992). In a review of research on the psychological adjustment of siblings of children with chronic illness, Drotar and Crawford (1985) offered the following recommendations: (1) research should focus on individual differences among siblings; (2) research should focus on the complexities of adjustment rather than dysfunction; (3) research should be conceptualized within a family-centered framework and designed to test alternative models of the relationship between family factors and sibling adjustment; (4) research should compare the siblings of children who have cancer to similar children from a healthy population with regard to the strategies that help siblings cope with a brother or sister's cancer; (5) research needs to define the role of disease and treatment variables in sibling adjustment; and (6) research needs to empirically evaluate specific interventions for facilitating sibling adaptation. Studies and methodological strategies addressing these recommendation are appearing (Daniels, Moos, Billings, & Miller, 1987; Leonard, 1991; Lobato, Faust, & Spirito, 1988)

This chapter seeks to shed light on sibling adaptation and to promote further research in this area by (1) summarizing findings about siblings of childhood cancer patients, (2) discussing approaches for assessing siblings' adjustment, and (3) considering a range of intervention strategies. The relevance of family systems theory for promoting studies in these areas is considered.

Conceptual Issues

Family Systems Model

The work of McCubbin and his colleagues (McCubbin, M. A., & McCubbin, 1991; Patterson & McCubbin, 1983) has focused on the theoretical formulation, refinement, and empirical validation of a family systems model for conceptualizing the etiology and adaptation of families' efforts to adapt to crisis (T-Double

ABCX Model of Family Adjustment and Adaptation). This model provides a way of conceptualizing the crisis of catastrophic childhood illnesses in terms of the entire family system and its subsystems. It conceptualizes the family's efforts to manage the demands associated with the stressors and strains of everyday life and normal transitions as well as unexpected crises. The model considers the family's ability to meet these demands (resources and coping), the family's appraisal of demand characteristics (situational and schematic), and the family's ability to achieve a realignment in its style of functioning (adjustment and adaptation). There are two distinct phases in the model, an adjustment phase and an adaptation phase. Three levels of family functioning—the individual, the family unit, and the community—are considered; each is characterized by both demands and resources. There are dynamic interactions among members within the family as well as trans-actions between the family unit and community resources that reflect a family's struggle to adjust to the crisis.

Critical dimensions of the Family Systems Model as they apply to health and illness are (1) a pileup of demands, that is, of stressors and strains; and (2) family capabilities for coping and appraising the crisis. The "piled up demands" are conditions which produce changes in the family system—a collection of threats or challenges to the family's existing functions. These demands might come from individual family members (work pressures, etc.) or from the family unit (marital conflicts, etc.), and they might take the form of discrete stressors (i.e., events which occur at a discernible point in time) or strains (i.e., tensions associated with a residual unresolved problem from the past or need or desire to change some-thing). These demands produce tension in the family system, and if the tension is not reduced by the family's resources, a state of stress arises. Because demands accumulate and interact with each other, it does not necessarily require a single event to push a family's demand load beyond the family's threshold to manage it. What is implied in this concept of a "pileup" is the dynamic nature of family demands in which stressors and strains are constantly changing over the course of time.

Family capabilities are understood in terms of the potential the family has to meet its demands. These capabilities are defined as characteristics, traits, compe-tencies, or tangible items which can serve to reduce the impact of demands. They may be tangible (e.g., money) or intangible (e.g., self-esteem), and they may come from individual members (innate intelligence, personality characteristic, es-teem, etc.), from the family unit (cohesiveness, flexibility, communication, etc.), or from the community (esteem support, network support, medical care, etc.).

Coping is another kind of capability that can reduce the impact of demands. Although coping most often has been conceptualized at the individual level, it also can be considered at the family and even community levels. Because the family is a dynamic system, coping may be conceptualized as the simultaneous management of competing demands and thus it includes a combination of the following strategies: (1) reducing the number and/or intensity of demands (e.g., doing home treatments for the child with cerebral palsy); (2) acquiring additional resources not already available to the family (e.g., medical assistance and diagnosis, respite care); (3) maintaining or strengthening existing resources so they can be allocated and reallocated to meet demands (e.g., doing things together as a family to maintain cohesiveness); (4) managing tension associated with ongoing strains (exercising, using humor, engaging in enjoyable activities, etc.); and (5) reframing the situation to make it more tolerable or manageable (lowering expectations in the home while caring for an ill member, emphasizing spiritual beliefs to build hope, etc.).

Family Systems Model and Sibling Adaptation to Childhood Cancer

In an adaptation of the family systems model (McCubbin, H. I., & McCubbin, 1991; McCubbin, M. A., & McCubbin, 1991), the family's ability to appraise the interactions between the demands associated with the crisis of childhood cancer and the family's capacity to cope with these demands is considered in conceptualizing the etiology and adaptation of siblings' adjustment (Carpenter & Sahler, 1991). This family systems model is presented in Figure 6.1.

In Figure 6.1, the parent and child are depicted as subsystems of a larger network of extended family, work, and social relationships. Each family has a characteristic style of functioning which can be evaluated on a continuum from highly adaptive to highly maladaptive functioning relative to existing demands, individual perceptions of the family, self and life circumstances, and the repertoire of available coping resources (psychological, interpersonal, community, and material). This dimension of the model conceptualizes the prediagnostic etiological factors that influence a family's initial and ongoing response to the crisis of childhood cancer.

The second major dimension of the model conceptualizes the postdiagnostic etiological factors that predict the range of possible adaptations for a family and its members. Specifically, when a child is diagnosed with cancer, a family crisis ensues that places many new demands on the family system (e.g., hospitalizations and frequent clinic visits, changes in parental roles, increased responsibilities that are physically and emotionally exhausting). In addition, the family develops perceptions of the impact of the family crisis. These perceptions may be idiosyncratic to an individual or they may be shared collectively by all family members. The family's adaptation to this crisis is also a function of the manner in which the family uses new and existing resources to accommodate to the added physical and emotional demands imposed by the stress and to integrate the differing perceptions of each family member of how the crisis has affected her or him.

The third major dimension of the family systems model conceptualizes the potential range of successful and unsuccessful adaptations that families and their members might experience in response to the family crisis of childhood cancer and their associated symptoms and characteristics. This conceptual framework is a useful method for investigating sibling adaptation to childhood cancer and interpreting the findings of studies in this area.

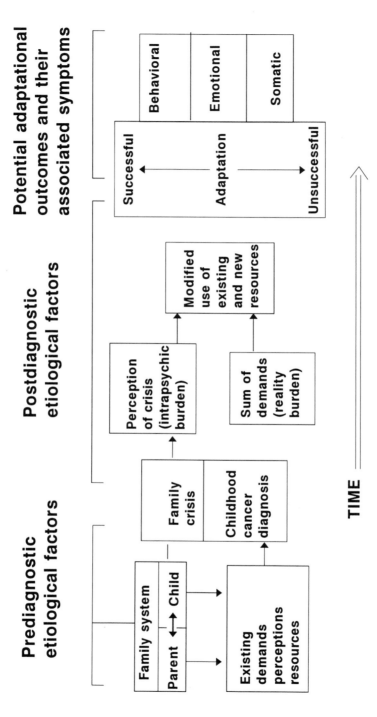

Figure 6.1. Family systems framework for conceptualizing sibling adaptation to the family crisis of childhood cancer. Adapted from the work of McCubbin and colleagues (see McCubbin, M.A. & McCubbin, H.I. 1991).

Research Findings

Although studies about siblings of children with cancer date as far back as the 1950s (Schulman, 1980), a significant body of research has emerged in the last decade (Carpenter & Onufrak, 1985; Sourkes, 1993). Many of these studies are summarized in Table 6.1.

Prevalence of Adjustment Problems

Several studies have reported that approximately 50 percent of the siblings of children who have cancer experience adjustment problems (Binger et al., 1969; Cain, Fast, & Erickson, 1964; Peck, 1979; Sahler & Carpenter, 1987; Walker, 1988). However, these studies do not take into account the rate of adjustment problems among the siblings prior to the diagnosis of cancer. An exception was a study by Sahler and Carpenter (1988) of 82 siblings of children with cancer which found that 22 percent of the siblings were reported by their parents as having had adjustment problems prior to the cancer diagnosis. Thirty-nine percent of the siblings had no prior adjustment problems but were reported by parents to have had adjustment problems following diagnosis, and the remaining 39 percent were reported to have had no adjustment problems either prior to or following the diagnosis of cancer. While studies have found that the prevalence of adjustment problems among siblings diminishes with time, differences between siblings with preexisting problems and those with no preexisting problems have not been established.

Emotional, Behavioral, and Somatic Symptoms

Feelings of guilt, loneliness, rejection, jealousy, anger, sadness, and depression were among emotional symptoms of distress found among siblings (Bendor, 1990; Binger et al., 1969; Carpenter & Sahler, 1991; Hogan, 1988; Spinetta & Deasy-Spinetta, 1981). Symptoms of externalized behavioral distress among siblings included decrements in academic performance, increased acting out at school, isolation from friends and family, acting out at home, and anger directed at parents and the sibling with cancer (Cairns, Clark, Smith, & Lansky, 1979; Carpenter & Sahler, 1991; Horwitz & Kazak, 1990; Sahler & Carpenter, 1987). Somatic symptoms included enuresis, headaches, stomach aches, and changes in sleeping and eating habits (Binger et al., 1969; Carpenter & Sahler, 1991; Koch-Hattem, 1986). Although the studies summarized in Table 6.1 report common clusters of behavioral, emotional, and somatic symptoms among siblings of children with cancer, they do not identify a specific symptom profile.

Etiological Factors

Several of the studies in Table 6.1 provided direct or indirect evidence of the etiological factors associated with successful and unsuccessful adaptation among

Table 6.1. Studies of Siblings of Children with Cancer

	Study Characteristics		Major Findings and Inferences	
Study	Objective	Methods	Symptomatology	Etiological Factors
Cobb (1956)	To characterize the psychological impact of children's death to cancer on the other members of the family	Sibling sample: N = not reported; age at study = not reported Informant: Parent Assessment: Clinical review with parents.	Profound loneliness	Loss of parental availability
Cain et al. (1964)	To characterize siblings' disturbed reactions to the death of their brother or sister to cancer	Sibling sample: N = 58; age at study = 2 to 14 years Informant: sibling Assessment: psychotherapeutic work with siblings in an inpatient setting	Feeling responsible for their brother or sister's death; low self-esteem; feelings of guilt; poor school performance; low self-worth; death phobia; distorted concepts of illness and death	Unavailability of parents during hospitalization and period of mourning
Binger et al. (1969)	To study the impact of a child's death to cancer on his or her siblings' lives	Sibling sample: N = 20; age at study = not reported Informant: parents Assessment: structured interview of parents	Enuresis; poor school performance; depression; headaches; separation anxiety; feelings of rejection; abdominal pain; fear of becoming ill	Not reported
Cairns et al. (1979)	To explore the impact of childhood cancer on healthy siblings	Sibling sample: N = 71; age at study = 6 to 16 years Informant: sibling Assessment: standardized questionnaires	Anxiety; depression; social isolation	Parents do not recognize sibling's concerns (e.g., isolation from parents, other family members, and friends)

128

Study	Purpose	Sample and Assessment	Findings	
Peck (1979)	To investigate the problems experienced by families of long-term survivors of ALL and Wilms tumor	Sibling sample: $N = 20$; age at study = not reported. Informant: parent. Assessment: structured interview; standardized questionnaires on family structure	Jealousy: behavioral problems; school problems; somatic symptoms	Problems began while mother was living in hospital with sick brother or sister
Iles (1979)	To investigate siblings' perceptions of the pediatric cancer experience	Sibling sample: $N = 5$; age at study = 7 to 11 years. Informant: sibling. Assessment: semistructured interview; family drawings	Feelings of resentment, anger, anxiety, and separation from parents	Loss of time with parents; need for social support; limited information about brother or sister's cancer
Sourkes (1980)	To examine siblings' experience of having a brother or sister with cancer	Sibling sample: $N =$ not reported; age at study = not reported. Informant: sibling. Assessment: psychotherapeutic sessions	Fear of also getting sick; guilt for causing illness or not getting it; shame that family is different; change in academic performance; change in social/peer relationships; increased somatic complaints; ambivalent feelings toward brother or sister	Change in sibling-parent relationship
Spinetta and Deasy-Spinetta (1981)	To study siblings of childhood cancer patients within the context of and in relation to the family system	Sibling sample: $N = 102$; age at study = 3 to 18 years. Informant: sibling. Assessment: standardized questionnaires on family systems	4 to 6 years: lower self-esteem and negative toward self; 7 to 12 years: anxiety; depression; 13 to 18 years: perceived family as experiencing conflict and less cohesion	4 to 12 years: psychological distance of parents; 13 to 18 years: loss of family cohesion

Table 6.1. Studies of Siblings of Children with Cancer (*Continued*)

Study	Study Characteristics		Major Findings and Inferences	
	Objective	Methods	Symptomatology	Etiological Factors
Gogan and Slavin (1981)	To investigate the childhood cancer experience of survivors' siblings	Sibling sample: $N=101$; age at study = 1 to 34 years Informant: sibling Assessment: structured interview; standardized questionnaires	Feelings of being left out, jealousy, resentment; preoccupation with own health; parental isolation; sibling rivalry	A closed communication system; maintaining family cohesiveness; siblings' access and perceived closeness to brother or sister with cancer; development of new coping skills
Lansky et al. (1982)	To examine the prevalence of failure to thrive among infant siblings of pediatric cancer patients	Sibling sample: $N=9/$ 65 determined to have failure to thrive; age at study = 3 months to 11 years Informant: parents/ hospital records Assessment: chart reviews/standardized questionnaires	Failure to thrive	Emotional isolation from mother
Kramer (1984)	To determine healthy siblings' perceptions of what it is like to live with a brother or sister with cancer	Sibling sample: $N=11$; age at study = 36 months Informant: siblings Assessment: structured interview of sibling	Increased sibling rivalry; anger; frustration; feelings of rejection, guilt, loneliness, sadness, confusion, anxiety	Emotional deprivation; decreased parental tolerance; increased parental expectations; lack of information; decreased family involvement; insufficient social support
Lauer et al. (1985)	To identify variables related to good and poor sibling adaptation and to study siblings' perceptions and involvement	Sibling sample: $N=19$; home care; 17 hospital care; age at study = 5 to 26 years	Siblings who participated in home care described a significantly different experience than those whose	Siblings in the home-care group reported that they were prepared for the impending death, received

Study	Purpose	Sample/Method	Findings	Implications
	during their brother's or sister's terminal care in the home or hospital environment and subsequent adjustment	Informant: sibling Assessment: structured interview	brothers or sisters died in the hospital	consistent information and support from their parents, and were involved in home-care activities
Koch-Hattem (1986)	To study siblings' perceptions of the pediatric cancer experience	Sibling sample: $N=33$; age at study = unknown Informant: sibling Assessment: structured interview	Feeling of being bothered, sad, and scared; difficulties sleeping	Ability to openly and directly express feelings; seeking support from others
Sahler and Carpenter (1987)	To evaluate developmental (age) differences in siblings' perceptions and understanding of the pediatric cancer experience	Sibling sample: $N=112$; age at study = 6 to 17 years Informant: sibling or parent Assessment: standardized questionnaire	Problems sleeping and eating; behavioral difficulties at home; changes in academic performance; frequency and severity of symptoms were related to age (e.g., anger increased with age)	Siblings' cognitive understanding of brother's or sister's cancer is associated with age
Hogan (1988)	To identify the symptoms and reactions that siblings of children with cancer experience at two time periods following the death of their brothers or sisters (≤ 18 months; ≥ 18 months following death)	Sibling sample: $N=40$; age at study = 13 to 18 years Informant: sibling Assessment: standardized questionnaire	≤ 18 months following diagnosis: assign blame to themselves during first 18 months and then to God; difficulty sleeping and concentrating; perceived loss of family cohesion; 18 months following diagnosis: return to normalcy	As time increases, mothers are identified as the principal person to talk to about grief; fathers become more distant and less available as time passed; in general, time tends to heal for bereaved adolescents and mothers but not for fathers
Brett and Davis (1988)	To describe siblings' changing appraisals of the significance of childhood leukemia ≥ 5 years following diagnosis	Sibling sample: $N=10$; age at study = ≥ 9 Informant: sibling or parent Assessment: structured interview	10 to 14 years: thoughts and worries about the disease and its implications begin to occur	Parental control of information about siblings' brothers or sisters is common and serves as an anxiety-reducing strategy for parents, but because siblings

Table 6.1. Studies of Siblings of Children with Cancer (*Continued*)

Study	Study Characteristics		Major Findings and Inferences	
	Objective	Methods	Symptomatology	Etiological Factors
				lack the external avenues for information and support available to their parents, family communication may contribute to siblings' disease-related ignorance and isolation within the family, so siblings may create their own explanations
Sahler and Carpenter (1988)	To investigate the relationships between the psychosocial functional status of siblings of children with cancer and the functional status of the families of children with cancer	Sibling sample: $N = 82$; age at study = 6 to 7 years Informant: sibling or parent Assessment: standardized questionnaire	Siblings with problems before diagnosis: negativity; feelings of isolation and resentment; illness disrupting usual patterns of family functioning	Interpersonal isolation, lack of support
Walker (1988)	To identify and describe the cognitive and behavioral coping strategies used by siblings of pediatric cancer patients	Sibling sample: $N = 26$; age at study = 7 to 11 years Informant: sibling or parent Assessment: structured interview	Somatic, social, affective, and behavioral symptoms reported	Perception difficulties between parents and siblings.
Hogan and Balk (1990)	To investigate the relationship and congruence between perceptions of self-concept and grief reactions of bereaved adolescent siblings of pediatric	Sibling sample: $N = 14$; age at study = 13 to 18 years Informant: sibling or parent	Changes in self-concept	Parental inaccuracy in evaluating siblings' reactions and level of distress (fathers more accurate than mothers)

	Purpose	Sample/Assessment	Findings
	cancer patients and their parents following a child's death	Assessment: structured interview standardized questionnaire	Emotional isolation from parents during hospitalization
Martinson et al. (1990)	To identify the reactions of family members to the experience of having a child with cancer	Sibling sample: $N = 9$ living brothers/sisters; $N = 7$ with deceased brothers/sisters; age at study = 6 to 12 years; Informant: sibling-parent; Assessment: structured interview	Similarities: Living—inability to reveal feelings; feelings of powerlessness and rejection Dead—depersonalization within the family
Rollins (1990)	To gain an understanding of siblings through an analysis of their drawings	Sibling sample: $N = 20$; age at study = 3 to 11 years; Informant: sibling; Assessment: structured drawing methodology	Confusion about the family; self-image; emotional confusion; Mothers frequently appeared exhausted and unavailable; close-aged siblings important source of support for one another; lack of communication among family members
Bendor (1990)	To report the findings of a group program for siblings of children with cancer	Sibling sample: $N = 0$; age at study = 8 to 9 years; Informant: sibling; Assessment: recorded group sessions	8 to 13 years: isolation and depersonalization with the family; confusion and anxiety; reluctant to express emotions; feelings of isolation from friends; worries about becoming sick; feelings of anger, loneliness, and vulnerability 14 to 19 years: worries about brother or sister dying; worries about effects on parents; feels responsible for family members; feelings of guilt for desiring; Emotional deprivation and loss of parental attention; Reluctance to communicate concerns with parents

Table 6.1. Studies of Siblings of Children with Cancer (*Continued*)

Study	Study Characteristics			Major Findings and Inferences	
	Objective	Methods		Symptomatology	Etiological Factors
				independence from family; fears of death and vulnerability	
Horwitz and Kazak (1990)	To describe the predominant patterns in families of children with cancer, integrating a family systems view with sibling adjustment and a normative development perspective	Sibling sample: $N=25$; age at study = 3 to 6 years Informant: sibling or parent Assessment: structured interviews standardized questionnaires (CBCL)		Siblings showed no major behavioral or social problems in comparison with siblings of healthy children	Families of children with cancer differed from the comparison group with respect to adaptability and cohesion and parental views of similarities or differences in siblings; parents tend to minimize the subjective impact on the other siblings
Carpenter and Sahler (1991)	To examine the relationships between siblings' perceptions of pediatric cancer and parents' perceptions of siblings' postdiagnosis psychosocial adaptation	Sibling sample: $N=112$; age at study = 6 to 17 years Informant: sibling or parent Assessment: standardized questionnaires		Emotional lability; negative attentional behavior; changes in academic performance; somatic complaints; difficulties sleeping; regressive behaviors; less positive and more negative intrapersonal interactions	Sibling adaptation is a function of the degree to which the family (especially parents) are able to maintain the healthy child's perception of him or herself as an integral part of the family unit
Sahler et al. (1992)	To assess the frequency and severity of emotional and behavioral symptoms of distress among siblings of children with cancer from seven institutions throughout the United States participating in a collaborative research project	Sibling sample: $N=254$; age at study = 4 to 18 years Informant: sibling or parent Assessment: structured interviews and standardized questionnaires		In comparison to both the CBCL nonclinical standardization sample and a parent-completed behavioral checklist comprised of CBCL items used in a large national health survey, siblings of children with cancer had significantly higher total behavior problem scores and lower total social competence scores	Not reported

siblings. Three recurring themes emerged: (1) insufficient or infrequent parental communication with siblings about their brother or sister's illness and limited participation of siblings in the treatment and care; (2) siblings' feeling physically and emotionally isolated from their parents (especially their mothers) and depersonalized both within and outside the family system; and (3) insufficient existing resources or the identification of new resources for providing siblings with emotional, social, and peer support.

Communication, Information and Participation

Several studies reported the need for siblings to be able to maintain communication within their families, to receive age-appropriate information about their brother or sister's illness and treatment, and to be active participants in their brother or sister's care (Bendor, 1990; Brett & Davies, 1988; Gogan & Slavin, 1981; Hogan & Balk, 1990; Iles, 1979; Lauer, Mulhern, Bohne, & Camitta, 1985; Martinson, Gilliss, Colaizzo, Freeman, & Bassert, 1990; Sahler & Carpenter, 1987; Walker, 1988). Without the benefit of unambiguous and age-appropriate information about the complexity and uncertainty of their brother or sister's treatment, siblings were found to rely on their own interpretations. These interpretations were based on their parents' reactions and overheard conversations. This often yielded a distorted picture of fear and anxiety about what would happen to the family and the sibling's role within the family system. Siblings also often reported concerns about catching cancer from their siblings and feelings of being left out of their brother or sister's treatment and care (Birenbaum, 1989; Gallo, 1988).

Emotional Isolation and Depersonalization

Another common theme from the studies in Table 6.1 was siblings' feelings of being depersonalized, emotionally isolated, and unimportant both within and outside the family context (Bendor, 1990; Brett & Davies, 1988; Cain et al., 1964; Cairns et al., 1979; Carpenter & Sahler, 1991; Cobb, 1956; Iles, 1979; Kramer, 1984; Lansky, Stephenson, Weller, Cairns, & Cairns, 1982; Lauer et al., 1985; Martinson et al., 1990; Peck, 1979; Rollins, 1990; Sourkes, 1980; Spinetta & Deasy-Spinetta, 1981). Children rarely asked spontaneous questions and left it to their parents to initiate communication about their understanding and feelings. Also, siblings rarely expressed negative feelings toward their other family members, particularly their parents, which seemed to reflect their insecurity about their precarious position in the family.

Emotional, Social, and Peer Support

Siblings' need for emotional, social, and peer support was the third major theme that emerged from the studies in Table 6.1 (Brett & Davies, 1988; Cairns et al.,

1979; Hogan, 1988; Hogan & Balk, 1990; Horwitz & Kazak, 1990; Iles, 1979; Koch-Hattem, 1986; Lauer et al., 1985; Rollins, 1990; Walker, 1988). Siblings cope with a host of confusing questions and emotional reactions resulting from their brother or sister's illness. It was found that they often were reluctant to discuss their own concerns and feelings with their parents so as not to further burden or worry them. Consequently, many siblings lacked a consistent support network. They often felt blamed for their brother or sister's illness and guilty about engaging in normal activities.

Strategies for Assessment and Intervention

Assessment

Early assessment provides an opportunity to formulate a preventive intervention plan. Soon after a child is diagnosed with cancer, an assessment of the family's psychosocial functioning should be made. The assessment should consider how the family typically copes with crises, how the experience of having a child with cancer relates to preexisting family problems, what existing sources of emotional and social support the family has, and the family's previous experiences with illness and medical issues. The assessment should focus less on the specific symptoms of distress that siblings manifest and more on the etiological factors that can explain these symptoms. Because similar symptoms have different etiologies, interventions based solely on symptom reduction are not generally effective. Instead, assessments are most effective when they address individual differences among siblings within the context of a family systems model (Carpenter & Sahler, 1991; Leventhal, Leventhal, & Von Nguyen, 1985; McCubbin, H. I., & McCubbin, 1991).

In many divisions of pediatric oncology at major medical centers, patients and their families routinely are seen by a psychosocial team consisting of a clinical psychologist, social worker, child life specialist, education specialist, and one or more parent advocates. This team assesses the strengths, vulnerabilities, and problems that the patient and his or her family bring to the treatment process (Carpenter, 1989; Carpenter et al., 1992; Kellerman, 1980). Based on this assessment, the team draws up a patient-family systems profile which provides a comprehensive overview of the family's current level of understanding and style of coping as well as the family's available resources and concurrent stressors. Using such a profile, the team is able to anticipate family problems so that the focus can be on crisis prevention rather than crisis intervention.

Patient-family systems profiles developed at the University of Rochester Medical Center, according to the nomenclature of McCubbin and his colleagues (McCubbin & Thompson, 1991), suggested four different types of family profiles:

1. *Regenerative*. Families with successful functioning prior to the diagnosis of childhood cancer who are capable of quickly mobilizing the necessary resources and strategies that facilitate the family crisis of childhood cancer.

2. *Secure*. Families with successful functioning prior to the childhood diagnosis who experience initial difficulties adapting to the crisis of childhood cancer.
3. *Durable*. Families who, at the time of diagnosis, are concurrently struggling with other family crises and who experience extended difficulties adapting to the additional stressors and demands associated with the family crisis of childhood cancer.
4. *Vulnerable*. Families who were in a chronic state of crisis prior to the diagnosis of childhood cancer and who will require extensive support in coping with the additional stressors and demands of having a child with cancer.

Approximately 30 percent of families were classified as regenerative, 35 percent as secure, 25 percent as durable, and 15 percent as vulnerable. Different types of family systems required different intervention strategies by health-care professionals.

Intervention

Research findings suggest several intervention strategies for facilitating sibling adaptation: (1) strategies for the effective dissemination of age-appropriate information to siblings about their brother or sister's illness and treatment; (2) strategies for minimizing siblings' emotional isolation from family members and depersonalization; (3) strategies for involving siblings in the care of their brother or sister; and (4) strategies for mobilizing existing resources and identifying new resources to help siblings adjust to the family crisis.

According to Walker (1990), sibling interventions can be categorized as educational, interpersonal, and distractional. Educational types of interventions address siblings' need for information about their brother or sister's illness, treatment, effects, and prognosis. Interpersonal types of interventions address siblings' need for emotional support, outlets to express their feelings, and their need for recognition as an important and useful family member. Distraction types of interventions address siblings' need for a timeout, or escape, from their families' preoccupation with issues of childhood cancer.

Schorr-Ribera (1991) and Bendor (1990) considered several strategies that parents can follow to help healthy siblings cope with the family crisis of childhood cancer. These included (1) providing information about cancer and its treatment in terms that the child can understand; (2) sharing feelings with children, thereby making it easier for the child to express his or her feelings; (3) including siblings, as much as possible, in family decisions; (4) acknowledging siblings' efforts to take on additional responsibilities in the family; (5) allowing siblings to be involved in the medical aspects of a brother or sister's treatment; (6) encouraging siblings to ask questions of parents and medical staff; (7) maintaining a positive outlook; (8) connecting with the siblings in little ways when parents are away and when their energy is limited; (9) alerting teachers to the family situation and encouraging feedback; (10) maintaining, as much as practical, a balance of attention among all the children in the family; and (11) calling upon significant relatives, adult friends, and parents of friends to spend time with the healthy siblings to help them feel cared about.

Specific Interventions for Siblings

Lauer and her colleagues (1985) studied the effects home-care programs for children dying of cancer in terms of their influence on the siblings of the dying child. They found that siblings who participated in a home-care program, compared to siblings whose brother or sister died in a hospital, were better prepared for the impending death, received consistent information and support from their parents, and viewed their own involvement as an important aspect of the experience.

Sahler and Carpenter (1989) and Carpenter, Sahler, and Davis (1990) evaluated a camping program for the siblings of children with cancer. Objectives that were realized through the camp experience included (1) creating an environment for siblings that gave them time out from the family crisis and an opportunity for peer support, (2) enhancing siblings' knowledge and correction of their misconceptions about childhood cancer, and (3) providing opportunities for peer support for siblings to share their experiences, feelings, and frustrations.

A one-day hospital-based program (Adams-Greenly, Shiminski-Maher, McGowan, & Meyers, 1986) for siblings of pediatric cancer patients also has been found to be helpful in facilitating siblings' adjustment. This program emphasized education and support. The educational component provided siblings with a lesson about treatments for childhood cancer and their side effects as well as a tour of the hospital. The support component of the intervention had siblings view a videotape of other siblings discussing their feelings, experiences, and strategies for coping. This was followed by a group discussion.

Family Systems–Oriented Interventions

A family systems–oriented assessment provides important information in identifying or developing the most appropriate kinds of interventions for siblings and identifying the most appropriate providers (e.g., hospital-based or community-based). Initiating interventions that effectively meet siblings' needs requires a clear understanding of the etiology of a sibling's distress, the family's dynamics, the existing resources being utilized by the family, a determination of whether the resources available to the treatment team are appropriate for addressing the issues, and knowledge of support groups and professional services that are available in the community. In addition, each health-care provider in pediatric oncology needs to realistically evaluate whether his or her skills and training are appropriate for providing any or all components of a recommended intervention. Although it is generally assumed that all siblings can benefit from preventive, family-centered interventions in minimizing distress, the specific issues that need to be addressed and the required resources for minimizing distress vary across families so that a standardized intervention for all siblings undermines the efficiency of psychosocial resources. For example, families that conform to the *regenerative* or *durable* profile, as described earlier, would benefit from a single-session intervention program with both immediate and extended family members meeting with the members of the pediatric oncology team. During such a session, etiological factors that contribute to sibling distress (e.g., siblings' sense of emotional isolation from their parents) could be discussed with the family and strategies that would maximize family cohesion, communication, emotional connectedness and overall adaptability could be planned.

In contrast, families that conform more to the *vulnerable* profile, as described earlier, often experience multiple psychosocial problems that create a persistent state of crisis requiring more intensive and comprehensive services than can be provided by the hospital-based treatment team. For these kinds of families, referrals to community agencies usually are necessary.

Conclusion

A diagnosis of childhood cancer constitutes a catastrophic family crisis that critically challenges the existing adaptive capabilities of the entire dynamic system and its individual members. Because of the sudden and unavoidable fragmentation of the family system and the added stressors and demands placed on parents, healthy siblings often experience emotional isolation from their parents, depersonalization, and loss of identity as well as heightened ambivalence regarding their feelings about their brother or sister's medical condition and its effect on the family. Unless interventions are initiated which focus on the siblings' adjustment to the family crisis of childhood cancer, siblings develop a range of emotional and somatic symptoms. Such symptoms are best treated in terms of their underlying causes as understood from a family systems approach.

Further research is needed to better understand what factors in family systems predict successful and unsuccessful modes of sibling adjustment. Other issues that warrant further study have to do with how a family's adjustment to childhood cancer differs from other kinds of family crises, such as divorce, the death of a parent, or family abuse. Research also is needed to better understand the relationship between siblings' means of adjusting to the crisis of childhood cancer in the family and their prediagnostic psychosocial functioning.

References

Adams-Greenly, M. T., Shiminski-Maher, N., McGowan, N., & Meyers, P. A. (1986). A group program for helping siblings of children with cancer. *Journal of Psychosocial Oncology, 4,* 455–467.

Bendor, S. J. (1990). Anxiety and isolation in siblings of pediatric cancer patients: The need for prevention. *Social Work in Health Care, 14,* 17–35.

Binger, C. M., Ablin, A. R., Feuerstein, C., Kushner, J. H., Zoger, S. & Mikkelsen, C. (1969). Childhood leukemia: Impact on patient and family. *New England Journal of Medicine, 280,* 414–418.

Birenbaum, L. K. (1989). The relationship between parent-sibling communication and coping of siblings with death experience. *Journal of Pediatric Oncology Nursing, 6,* 86–91.

Brett, K. M., & Davies, E. M. B. (1988). What does it mean? Sibling and parental appraisals of childhood leukemia. *Cancer Nursing, 11,* 329–338.

Cain, A., Fast, I., & Erickson, M. (1964). Children's disturbed reactions to the death of a sibling. *American Journal of Orthopsychiatry, 34,* 741–752.

Cairns, N. U., Clark, G. M., Smith, S. D., & Lansky, S. B. (1979). Adaptation of siblings to childhood malignancy. *Journal of Pediatrics, 95,* 484–487.

Carpenter, P. J. (1989). Establishing the role of the pediatric psychologist in a university-based oncology service. *Journal of Training and Practice in Professional Psychology, 3,* 21–28.

Carpenter, P. J., & Onufrak, B. (1985). Pediatric psychosocial oncology: A compendium of the current professional literature. *Journal of Psychosocial Oncology, 2,* 119–136.

Carpenter, P. J. & Sahler, O. J. Z. (1991). Sibling perception and adaptation to childhood cancer: Conceptual and methodological considerations. In J. H. Johnson & S. B. Johnson (Eds.), *Advances in child health psychology* (pp. 193–205). Gainesville: University of Florida Press.

Carpenter, P. J., Sahler, O. J., & Davis, M. S. (1990). Use of a camp setting to provide medical information to siblings of pediatric cancer patients. *Journal of Cancer Education, 5,* 21–26.

Carpenter, P. J., Vattimo, C. J., Messbauer, L. J., Stolnitz, C., Bell-Isle, J., Stutzman, H., & Cohen, H. J. (1992). Development of a parent advocate program as part of a pediatric hematology/oncology service. *Journal of Psychosocial Oncology, 10,* 27–38.

Carr-Gregg, M., & White, L. (1987). Siblings of pediatric cancer patients: A population at risk. *Medical and Pediatric Oncology, 15,* 62–68.

Cobb, B. (1956). Psychological impact of long illness and death of a child on the family circle. *Journal of Pediatrics, 49,* 746–751.

Daniels, D., Moos, R. H., Billings, A. G., & Miller, J. J. (1987). Psychosocial risk and resistance factors among children with chronic illness, healthy siblings, and healthy controls. *Journal of Abnormal Psychology, 15,* 295–308.

Drotar, D., & Crawford, P. (1985). Psychological adaptation of siblings of chronically ill children: Research and practice implications. *Journal of Developmental and Behavioral Pediatrics, 6,* 355–367.

Gallo, A. M. (1988). The sibling relationship in chronic illness and disability: Parental communication with well siblings. *Holistic Nursing Practice, 2,* 28–37.

Gogan, J. L., & Slavin, L. A. (1981). Intervening with brothers and sisters. In G. P. Koocher & J. E. O'Malley (Eds.), *The Damocles Syndrome* (pp. 101–111). New York: McGraw-Hill.

Hogan, N. S. (1988). The effects of times on the adolescent sibling bereavement process. *Pediatric Nursing, 14,* 333–335.

Hogan, N. S., & Balk, D. E. (1990). Adolescent reactions to sibling death: Perceptions of mothers, fathers, and teenagers. *Nursing Research, 39,* 103–106.

Holland, J. C. (1989). Historical overview. In J. C. Holland & J. H. Rowland (Eds.), *Handbook of psychooncology* (pp. 3–12). New York: Oxford University Press.

Horwitz, W. A., & Kazak, A. E. (1990). Family adaptation to childhood cancer: Sibling and family systems variables. *Journal of Clinical Child Psychology, 19,* 221–228.

Iles, P. J. (1979). Children with cancer: Healthy siblings' perceptions during the illness experience. *Cancer Nursing, 2,* 371–377.

Kellerman, J. (1980). Comprehensive psychosocial care of the child with cancer: Description of a program. In J. Kellerman (Ed.), *Psychological aspects of childhood cancer* (pp. 195–214). Springfield, IL: Charles C Thomas.

Koch-Hattem, A. (1986). Siblings' experience of pediatric cancer: Interviews with children. *Health and Social Work, 11*, 107–117.

Kramer, R. F. (1984). Living with childhood cancer: Impact on the healthy siblings. *Oncology Nursing Forum, 11*, 44–51.

Kupst, M., & Schulman, J. (1988). Long-term coping with pediatric leukemia: A six-year follow-up study. *Journal of Pediatric Psychology, 13*, 7–22.

Lansky, S. B., Stephenson, L., Weller, E., Cairns, G. F., & Cairns, N. V. (1982). Failure to thrive during infancy in siblings of pediatric cancer patients. *American Journal of Pediatric Hematology/Oncology, 4*, 361–366.

Lauer, M. E., Mulhern, R. K., Bohne, J. B., & Camitta, B. M. (1985, February). Children's perceptions of their sibling's death at home or in the hospital: The precursors of differential adjustment. *Cancer Nursing*, 21–27.

Leonard, B. J. (1991). Siblings of chronically ill children: A question of vulnerability versus resilience. *Pediatric Annals, 20*, 501–506.

Leventhal, H., Leventhal, E. A., & Von Nguyen, T. (1985). Reactions of families to illness: Theoretical models and perspectives. In D. C. Turk & R. D. Kerns (Eds.), *Health, illness, and families* (pp. 108–145). New York: Wiley.

Lobato, D., Faust, D., & Spirito, A. (1988). Examining the effects of chronic disease and disability on children's sibling relationships. *Journal of Pediatric Psychology, 13*, 389–407.

Martinson, I. M., Gilliss, C., Colaizzo, D. C., Freeman, M., & Bassert, E. (1990). Impact of children's cancer on healthy school-age siblings. *Cancer Nursing, 13*, 183–190.

McCubbin, H. I., & McCubbin, M. A. (1991). Family system assessment in health care. In H. I. McCubbin & A. I. Thompson (Eds.), *Family assessment interventions for research and practice* (pp. 63–80). Madison: University of Wisconsin Press.

McCubbin, H. I., & Thompson, A. I. (1991). Family topologies and family assessment. In H. I. McCubbin & A. I. Thompson (Eds.), *Family assessment interventions for research and practice* (pp. 35–62). Madison: University of Wisconsin Press.

McCubbin, M. A., & McCubbin, H. I. (1991). Family stress theory and assessment: The T-Double ABCX Model of family adjustment and adaptation. In H. I. McCubbin & A. I. Thompson (Eds.), *Family assessment interventions for research and practice* (pp. 3–34) Madison: University of Wisconsin Press.

Patterson, J. M., & McCubbin, H. I. (1983). Chronic illness: Family stress and coping. In C. R. Figley & H. I. McCubbin (Eds.), *Stress and the family: Coping with catastrophe* (pp. 21–36). New York: Brunner/Mazel.

Peck, B. (1979). Effects of childhood cancer on long-term survivors and their families. *British Medical Journal, 1*, 1327–1329.

Rollins, J. A. (1990). Childhood cancer: Siblings draw and tell. *Pediatric Nursing, 16*, 21–27.

Sahler, O. J., & Carpenter, P. J. (1987). Developmental differences among siblings' perceptions of the pediatric cancer experience. *Journal of Developmental and Behavioral Pediatrics, 8*, 121.

Sahler, O. J., & Carpenter, P. J. (1988). Relationship between family functioning and sibling adaptation to the pediatric cancer experience. *Journal of Developmental and Behavioral Pediatrics, 9*, 106–107.

Sahler, O. J., & Carpenter, P. J. (1989). Evaluation of a camp program for siblings of children with cancer. *American Journal of Diseases of Children, 143*, 690–696.

Sahler, O. J., Roghmann, O., Carpenter, P. J., Mulhern, R., Dolgin, M. J., Sargent, J. R., Barbarin, O. A., Copeland, D. R., & Zeltzer, L. K. (1992). Adaptation to childhood cancer: Sibling psychologic distress. *Pediatric Research, 31,* 137.

Schorr-Ribera, H. (1992). Caring for siblings during diagnosis and treatment. *Candlelighters, 16,* 1–2.

Schulman, J. C. (1980). Psychosocial aspects of childhood cancer: A bibliography. In J. C. Schulman & M. J. Kupst (Eds.), *The child with cancer* (pp. 86–105). Springfield, IL: Charles C Thomas.

Sourkes, B. M. (1980). Siblings of the pediatric cancer patients. In J. Kellerman (Ed.), *Psychological aspects of childhood cancer* (pp. 47–69). Springfield, IL: Charles C Thomas.

Sourkes, B. M. (1993). Psychological aspects of leukemia and other hematologic disorders. In D. G. Nathan & F. A. Oski (Eds.), *Hematology of infancy and childhood* (pp. 1754–68). Philadelphia: Saunders.

Spinetta, J. J., & Deasy-Spinetta, P. (1981). The siblings of the child with cancer. In J. J. Spinetta & P. Deasy-Spinetta (Eds.), *Living with childhood cancer* (pp. 133–142). St. Louis: Mosby.

Stehbens, J. A. (1988). Childhood cancer. In D. K. Routh (Ed.), *Handbook of pediatric psychology* (pp. 135–161). New York: Guilford Press.

Walker, C. L. (1988). Stress and coping in siblings of childhood cancer patients. *Nursing Research, 37,* 208–212.

Walker, C. L. (1990). Siblings of children with cancer. *Oncology Nursing Forum, 17,* 355–360.

7

Bone Marrow Transplantation

SEAN PHIPPS

The use of bone marrow transplantation (BMT) to treat pediatric malignancies has grown enormously over the past decade and is likely to see continued growth in the coming years. It has become standard therapy for some of the most high-risk leukemias, and it is generally the preferred option after leukemic relapse (Parkman, 1986; Sullivan, 1989). There has been rapid growth in the number of transplant centers, stimulated by developments in the field of BMT that have led to an increase in the number of potential transplant recipients and donors. In the past, many patients could not be transplanted unless they had a fully compatible sibling donor based on HLA (human lymphocyte antigen) typing, which occurs only in approximately one-third of cases (Thomas et al., 1975). Today, with the advent of bone marrow registries in North America and Europe, HLA-matched unrelated volunteer donors may be found for many patients (Beatty, 1991). In addition, technical improvements in T-cell depletion of donor marrow and other prophylactic treatments for prevention of graft versus host disease (GVHD), one of the most common and problematic complications of transplant, allow for use of related donors who are not fully HLA compatible (Beatty et al., 1985). Finally, autologous transplantation (in which the patient's own bone marrow is harvested and reinfused after treatment) is being used for an increasing number of nonhematologic malignancies (Parkman, 1986; Sullivan, 1989). Concurrent with the increased use of the procedure, technical advances in supportive care have led to improvements in outcome, and thus to a growing number of long-term survivors of BMT.

Perhaps owing to the very rapid development of BMT, we have been left with a gap in our understanding of the psychological sequelae of the procedure, as well-designed psychological studies have lagged behind the medical advances. Much of the psychological literature to date has been descriptive and anecdotal, involving small numbers of subjects and case study approaches (Atkins & Patenaude, 1987; Bradlyn & Boggs, 1989; Kaleita, Shields, Tessler, & Feig, 1989; Linn, Beardslee, & Patenaude, 1986). Studies of survivorship have typically been limited to the immediate posttransplant period. There have been only a few empirical reports of long-term survivors, and those involved primarily adult and late adolescent patients (Heugeveld, Houtman, & Zwann, 1988; Pot-Mees, 1989; Wolcott, Wellisch, Fawzy, & Landsverk, 1986a). Empirical research on many aspects of pediatric BMT has been difficult because of the relatively small numbers of patients transplanted at each center, the high mortality of the procedure, and the difficulty in follow-up when patients who have traveled a great distance for transplant return to their local communities. Clearly, large-scale collaborative studies are needed, but none have yet been reported.

Given the paucity of published empirical data, this chapter will provide an overview of the clinical issues related to transplant, outlining the salient research questions raised and exploring ways in which these might lend themselves to empirical study in the future.

Medical Overview and Bone Marrow Transplantation Sequence

Despite the technical advances, BMT remains a very high-risk procedure, involving a prolonged aversive treatment regimen with high levels of morbidity and mortality. The procedure invariably involves multiple stresses and taxes the coping capacity of the patient and family. The transplant process can be conceptualized in three phases. The *pretransplant* or *anticipatory* phase involves the weeks and months prior to admission for transplant, in which the decision to undergo transplant is made and the search for a suitable donor occurs. The *acute* phase involves the inpatient hospitalization for transplant, generally lasting from 1 to 3 months. For those who survive, there is the *posttransplant* follow-up phase, where treatment of chronic GVHD and other posttransplant complications may be required for several months. This is followed by a period of several years of intermittent monitoring for medical and neuropsychological late effects.

Pretransplant Phase

Even limiting our focus to only those patients with malignancies, the population of patients who are candidates for BMT can be a very heterogeneous group. Some patients will have had extensive previous treatment, where transplant represents a dramatic and heroic final effort, whereas others may be recently diagnosed, facing transplant as a standard component of treatment for their disorder. The sequence and demands of pretransplant evaluations will vary accordingly and will determine the nature of the stressors for patient and family. Consideration of transplant initiates a sequence of events, beginning with blood typing of all immediate family members for HLA compatibility.

Identification of a suitable donor within the family can be a mixed blessing. Although the medical risks of the bone marrow harvest procedure are exceedingly small, the parents must nevertheless consent to putting a healthy child through a surgical procedure involving general anesthesia; they may experience considerable conflict about this. The compatible sibling may also experience considerable anxiety and ambivalence about the procedure yet feel there is no choice, even in the absence of any overt coercion by the family (Patenaude, 1990). In those instances where there is more than one suitably matched sibling, there may be no compelling medical reason for choosing one over the other. This leaves the family and transplant team to negotiate the issue of how to make the decision. A unilateral decision by the transplant physicians absolves the parents from having to make such a difficult choice, yet it denies the autonomy of the family. Occasionally there are compelling psychosocial issues that suggest that one sibling is a more appropriate choice, and psychological evaluation prior to choosing the donor may be helpful. The patient may feel beholden to the chosen sibling or guilty for having placed him or her in such a predicament. Siblings not chosen may feel disappointed and ignored. Thus even the "best-case scenario" of a fully matched sibling creates the potential for family tensions and conflicts. Experience suggests that the majority of families manage these issues without great difficulty, but there is an absence of empirical data to document the frequency and magnitude of problems with this process. Again, prospective research on this issue is made difficult by the fact that in many cases the process of choosing and preparing a donor may begin in one location (the local cancer center) and end in another (the transplant center).

If a suitable donor is not found within the family, a search of the bone marrow registries may begin. Although the efficacy of these searches is improving, the delay may still be from 1 to 6 months (Howard, Hows, Gore, & Bradley, 1991). The anxiety of this waiting period is magnified when it involves a vulnerable patient with a tenuous remission status at high risk to relapse at any time or to develop some other medical complication that could preclude transplant. The relief and gratitude that families sometimes experience when a donor is located may create the mistaken impression that the battle has been won, when the worst of the burden is still ahead (Patenaude, 1990). There have been no studies reporting the attitudes of pediatric patients toward their unrelated donor, although some have suggested that patient fantasies that they will take on characteristics of the donor are common (Lesko, 1990). At St. Jude Children's Research Hospital an adolescent patient was about to undergo a transplant with a donor from London. The transplant physician was also from London, and his accent left little doubt about this. During a pretransplant interview the patient joked: "I don't care where the donor is from, as long as it doesn't make me start to talk funny, like Dr. B." Such humor may mask underlying anxieties regarding what the transplant process may do to one's identity. Issues of sexual identity may be of particular concern to some patients when donor and recipient are of different gender.

The Acute Phase

Although the search for and choice of a donor may have been stressful for the family, it is merely a prologue to the intense and demanding ordeal that begins as they enter the acute phase, with admission for transplant. The milieu which the patient enters may vary considerably from center to center. At one extreme are the laminar airflow units, involving complete reverse isolation and the concomitant physical restrictions, with sterilization of all the patient's belongings and supplies that enter the room, limitations on visitors, and the use of sterile gowns and masks by all those entering the room (Lindgren, 1983; Marshall, 1985). Other centers use regular rooms and are less stringent in their precautions. All, however, impose a high degree of isolation of the patient, whose world will be almost entirely delimited by the four walls of the hospital room, from admission through discharge.

The acute phase involves three components: the pretransplant conditioning, the actual transplant procedure, and the engraftment period. Upon admission, the patient undergoes 1 week to 10 days of pretransplant conditioning, involving high-dose chemotherapy, with or without total body irradiation (TBI) (Parkman, 1986; Sullivan, 1989). The conditioning regimen has a dual purpose: it provides maximal destruction of any remaining malignant cells and it ablates the recipient's bone marrow and immune system to allow for engraftment of donor marrow and prevent rejection. During this phase acute cardiorespiratory responses or other acute organ toxicities occur rarely and chemotherapy-induced seizures occur occasionally (Sullivan, 1989). Otherwise, this is a period that may be characterized by a variable degree of discomfort, but generally no major medical complications for the patient. The most common complaints are those well recognized with other forms of chemotherapy, including nausea and vomiting, fatigue, malaise, and fevers and chills. With the advent of more effective antiemetic therapies, many pediatric patients get through this phase with surprisingly little difficulty (Carden, Mitchell, Waters, Tiedeman, & Ekert, 1990; Hewitt, Cornish, Pamphilon, & Oakhill, 1991).

Following completion of the conditioning regimen, the actual transplantation of tissue occurs. Although this may be imbued with great medical and symbolic significance and anxiously anticipated by patient and family, the procedure is relatively simple and safe, involving a direct transfusion of donor marrow through the central venous catheter. (All patients will have an indwelling venous catheter surgically placed prior to the transplant, to facilitate administration of intravenous medications, fluids, and nutrition.) The relief expressed by many patients and parents upon completion of the marrow transfusion belies the fact that the period of greatest risk for complications is still ahead.

Now begins the waiting period between transplant and the first signs of engraftment, which generally lasts between 2 and 4 weeks. This is a time when the side effects of conditioning often become most pronounced and distressing. Mucositis can be particularly severe, often requiring the use of narcotic analgesics. Nausea and vomiting may continue to be problematic, both as a result of conditioning and as a side effect of multiple other medications, such as those used prophylactically against GVHD (e.g. cyclosporine, methylprednisolone). Even when nausea and vomiting are not problematic, some degree of anorexia is frequently seen. Most patients are unable to maintain adequate oral intake and require some form of intravenous nutritional support (total parenteral nutrition, or TPN) during this period.

The patient is most severely immunocompromised, and thus at high risk for a multitude of bacterial, fungal, and viral infections, during this immediate post-transplant period (Engelhard, Marks, & Good, 1986; Meyers, 1986). Much of the medical care during this period is focused on prevention, surveillance, and early aggressive treatment at the first sign of infection. In addition to the environmental prevention provided by the laminar airflow room and/or other techniques utilized to maintain the patient in sterile isolation, the patient must also be protected from endogenous organisms, particularly those of the oral mucosa and gastrointestinal tract (Lindgren, 1983; Marshall, 1985). This requires frequent administration of oral antibiotics and mouth rinses, an aspect of the treatment regimen many patients find to be particularly aversive. Because of the urgency for early, aggressive treatment of suspected infections in this population, most patients will receive some combination of IV antibiotic and antifungal therapy during the course of their transplant hospitalization, which can add to their malaise and discomfort, even in the absence of an underlying infection (Engelhard, Marks, & Good, 1986; Meyers, 1986). Those patients who develop infections can become critically ill with remarkable rapidity. Fatal infectious complications will occur in 10 to 20 percent of this population (Meyers, 1986).

As patients begin to show signs of engraftment, they enter the period of risk for the other major complication of transplant, GVHD. The skin, gut, and liver are the most common symptomatic sites of GVHD (Cheson & Curt, 1986; Parkman, 1986). Patients may develop a measleslike skin rash; frequent diarrhea, which can be accompanied by considerable abdominal discomfort; or jaundice. Because so much effort is focused on prevention of this disorder, the onset of GVHD symptoms can be psychologically debilitating to patients and families, in addition to the physical distresses entailed. More aggressive treatments are initiated, arousing further anxieties in patients and families as they wait to see whether the progression of symptoms can be reversed. Not only may the GVHD be life-threatening of itself, but its treatment necessitates the use of further immunosuppressive agents, leaving the patient at increased risk for latent viral infections, particularly cytomegalovirus (CMV), which is also associated with very high mortality (Engelhard, Marks, & Good, 1986).

Posttransplant Phase

Discharge from the inpatient unit for those patients who engraft successfully and do not develop major complications will typically occur 3 to 6 weeks posttransplant. This often elicits mixed emotions among patients, whose initial joy upon "escaping" their confinement is tempered by anxiety over their lost protection and their reexposure to the outside world. The joy is tempered further with the realization that although their environment has changed, their physical and social isolation has not ended. Patients may regain adequate neutrophil counts within 4 to 6 weeks, but they will remain in a severely immunocompromised state for several months (Parkman, 1986). Thus they remain at high risk for opportunistic infections, and many precautions must be maintained. Close contact is typically limited to immediate family members, and patients may be required to wear masks and gloves any time they must be in public. Close outpatient follow-up is maintained, and readmission to the hospital for fever or other complications is not uncommon but can be extremely disappointing and anxiety producing for the patient and family.

Development of chronic GVHD will generally occur within the first 6 months posttransplant, but this is an age-dependent phenomenon, with pediatric patients being affected much less frequently (Parkman, 1986). The pediatric patients at highest risk for GVHD are those who survived severe acute GVHD earlier in their treatment. The physical stigmata of this disorder, in combination with the effects of the high-dose steroid treatment it necessitates, can leave the patient with a rather grotesque appearance, lasting for several weeks or months. This can have an obviously damaging effect on the patient's self-esteem, particularly among adolescents.

In summary, the BMT process is associated with a series of intense and often unique stressors for the patient and family. The technical advances which have improved medical outcome have not eliminated the psychosocial dilemmas; rather, they have created many new ones. The rapidity of medical advances has made study of the psychological sequelae of many of these stressors difficult. The following sections review the psychological research that has been done and suggest areas in which additional studies are needed.

Psychological Responses of the Patient

In one of the earliest papers to address the psychological issues of pediatric BMT, Gardner, August, and Githens (1977) described a number of problems typical of BMT patients, including affective disturbance, with increased anxiety and depression; overdependence associated with feelings of helplessness; anger toward staff and parents; reduced tolerance for medical procedures; and periodic refusal to cooperate. As was typical of the initial publications regarding BMT, these conclusions were based on the clinical experience of the authors with a small number ($N = 7$) of patients. Other early papers provided some corroboration of these findings, and all stressed the need for intensive psychosocial intervention as part of the BMT program (Patenaude, Szymanski, & Rappeport, 1979; Pfefferbaum, Lindamood, & Wiley, 1977).

These papers were helpful in providing a narrative description of the BMT process and the difficult psychological demands it produced, but none provided any substantial empirical support for their conclusions. This was a time when those working in the area were pioneers traversing uncharted territories, and their anecdotal impressions provided a necessary first step in developing our understanding of the process. Unfortunately, the state of the art has not progressed much since then. To date, there has been little empirical evidence to confirm or dispute the conclusions made by Gardner et al. (1977) in their original paper. The literature continues to consist predominantly of case reports that illustrate a chronology of psychosocial events for individual patients over the course of the transplant process (Atkins & Patenaude, 1987; Bradlyn & Boggs, 1989) or focus on specific issues, such as specialized intervention techniques (Linn et al., 1986) or the immediate transitional problems of survivors (Freund & Siegel, 1985; Patenaude & Rappeport, 1982). When case reports from different sources appear to confirm each other, we begin to develop a knowledge base. However, this is a slow process and is fraught with subjectivity. Thus, although in the past 15 years we have seen a gradual accumulation of clinical knowledge regarding BMT, most of this must be considered tentative and still awaiting empirical confirmation.

The following sections address a number of psychological issues and problems commonly faced by BMT clinicians. In some instances there is a significant body of literature available to review, while in others we are left to describe the problem from clinical experience. The issues covered include the prolonged isolation of the patient; compliance problems commonly encountered; pharmacologic issues; acute care issues; and survivorship, including late effects of BMT treatment.

Response to Prolonged Protected Isolation

One of the major stressors that patients experience during the course of BMT is the prolonged and often extensive restrictions of protected isolation. There have been a few pediatric studies addressing this issue, and additional inferences can be obtained from adult studies and literature on related areas of sensory deprivation and extreme social isolation (Lesko, Kern, & Hawkins, 1984). Studies of adults experiencing prolonged sensory deprivation indicate that problems with concentration, affective liability, and predominantly negative mood states are common; and more severe cognitive impairment and paranoidlike delusions are occasionally seen (Lesko et al., 1984). However, in a study of adult cancer patients treated in laminar airflow rooms, Holland et al. (1977) found that such symptoms were rare, and that emotional stability was generally maintained. Psychological symptoms appeared to be directly related to the physical status of the patient.

The pediatric literature includes a number of case reports of infants raised in sterile isolation necessitated by immune deficiency. These generally suggest that adequate cognitive and social development can occur in these circumstances, and any delays that are seen are transitory, disappearing after return to a normal environment (Lesko et al., 1984). In a pediatric oncology setting, where patients were isolated and separated from parents by a glass partition in a manner similar to laminar airflow rooms for BMT, Powazek, Goff, and Schuyling (1978) found that patients showed increased levels of anxiety and depression. This was influenced by age, with younger patients showing more severe affective disturbances. Kellerman et al. (1976; Kellerman, Rigler, & Siegel, 1979) studied pediatric patients with advanced solid tumors who were treated in a laminar airflow unit. They found that intellectual functioning measured with standard psychometric instruments remained stable during this period. They also used a Likert-type daily rating scale consisting of 63 behavioral items, which was completed by nursing staff. They found no instances of severe psychological disturbance; they commented on the generally positive adaptation of patients to this environment and concluded that children adapt more easily to protected environments than do adults (Kellerman et al., 1979). However, a closer look at their findings suggests a less benign outcome, with a number of adverse responses. For example, at least half of their subjects reported some hallucinatory experiences. There were also regressive disturbances in mood state, activity, and social-communicative behavior over time. This symptomatology was seen despite the presence of a strong program of psychosocial supportive care. It should be noted, however, that the average length of stay in this study was 90 days, which is somewhat longer than is typical for a BMT patient today, and most of the behavioral disturbances were observed after 6 weeks or more in isolation.

None of the studies reported thus far involved BMT patients. At present there are no empirical data that address whether there are unique aspects of BMT which might impact specifically on the patients' experience of protected isolation. Clinical experience appears to support the conclusion of Holland et al. (1977) that psychological state in this setting is largely dependent on the physical status and comfort of the patient. From that perspective, one might be able to predict times of greater psychological disturbance according to the sequence of transplant, for example, conditioning, infusion, or onset of GVHD. However, confirmation of such an association awaits empirical demonstration. It is curious that such a basic and relatively straightforward research question has yet to be addressed.

Compliance with Aversive Regimen

Gardner et al. (1977) first commented on the refusal to cooperate commonly seen among BMT patients, and others have confirmed this (Bradlyn & Boggs, 1989; Patenaude, 1990; Phipps & Decuir-Whalley, 1990). BMT may be unique in the degree of cooperation that is required from the patient and/or the patient's family over an extended period of time. The patient will experience a multitude of discomforts, and many of these cannot simply be passively tolerated but require the patient's active participation. Fortunately, most patients are highly motivated at the outset of the BMT procedure. However, their initial enthusiasm is likely to wane as the demands of the procedure increase in parallel with the increases in their physical discomfort. In some instances, patients may become generally uncooperative and oppositional, but more often problems develop with specific aspects of the treatment regimen. One of the most common areas of difficulty involves the taking of oral medications and the regimen of antibiotic mouth care.

It is not surprising that a patient suffering from severe oral mucositis along with frequent nausea and vomiting might develop an aversion to the large number of oral medications administered and the unpalatable antibiotic mouth rinses required several times daily. In an earlier paper, Phipps and DeCuir-Whalley (1990) demonstrated that some difficulty with oral medications is almost universal in this population, and significant compliance problems requiring intervention occur in over 50 percent of cases. A high incidence of noncompliance was found in all but the youngest group of patients. A variety of behavioral interventions were utilized to improve compliance, including education, cueing, modeling, operant conditioning, and various forms of desensitization. Aversion to the treatment regimen was often so intense that compliance problems were resistant to intervention. Furthermore, aspects of the BMT milieu also provided obstacles to intervention. The following case illustrates the magnitude of the problem and the multicomponent interventions that are necessary to improve compliance.

The patient was a 3-year-old girl with acute myelogenous leukemia who had a strong negative response to the medication regimen upon admission to the BMT unit. She was noted to cry and cover her face with a blanket whenever mouth care was presented. There was frequent screaming, fighting, and spitting out of medications at the nurse. When she was able to take the medication, this was often followed by gagging and vomiting, so that the process would have to be repeated. Her mother attempted to help in setting limits, but this often progressed to a frustrated pleading, which was thought to be counterproductive.

A treatment plan with four components was developed. First, the medication times were handled entirely by nursing staff, and the mother was asked to briefly leave the unit during these times. She was to return only after successful compliance had been obtained. Second, an operant reinforcement program was initiated, involving a sticker chart and small prizes. The administration of stickers was handled by nursing staff, while the giving of prizes was handled by the mother, and both were encouraged to supplement this with praise and support. The third component involved a type of desensitization, pairing medication presentation with enjoyable activities for the patient. The nurse entered the patients' room and read the patient a favorite story while administering the medication. The final component involved therapeutic play, in which the patient could work through some of her feelings regarding the medications. She was provided with the materials so that she could enact giving medication to her Raggedy Ann doll prior to receiving her own medication. This appeared to have a significant impact in reducing the anxiety she experienced when she was informed that medication time was approaching. The psychologist also expanded on this therapeutic play approach during their scheduled sessions. The patient's compliance improved significantly in response to the intervention plan, and, just as important, her distress regarding the issue was also reduced. (Case reported by Phipps & Decuir-Whalley, 1990.)

This case was somewhat atypical in the degree of success that was achieved. In general, it appears that the great majority of BMT patients continue to experience some compliance difficulties despite intervention. Clearly, further research is needed on techniques to improve compliance in this population. In particular, it would be helpful to explore determinants of patient response (e.g., age, gender, previous treatment history, coping styles) that might lead to a differential response to various interventions.

Pharmacologic Issues

BMT patients are exposed to a large number of medications during the course of their treatment, and many of these may affect their mental status. This can make it very difficult to distinguish among the etiological factors responsible for any affective or behavioral changes observed in a patient.

The chemotherapeutic agents used in conditioning may have acute effects on the central nervous system (CNS), causing delirium or encephalopathy, but such effects are rare and generally transient (Young & Posner, 1980). More significant are the physical side effects of these agents, such as nausea, vomiting, and oral mucositis, which necessitate the use of additional medications to achieve symptomatic relief. Thus patients frequently receive one or more antiemetic agents including phenothiazines and benzodiazepines, as well as narcotic analgesics for pain. The multiple potential CNS side effects of these agents when used individually are well documented, and the situation becomes even more confusing when several agents are used simultaneously. An action that all have in common is a prominent sedative effect. In addition there are the frequent injections of diphenhydramine hydrochloride, which patients receive as a premedication for transfusions or other medications, providing further sedation. Not infrequently, psychological consultation is requested on a patient who is lethargic, withdrawn, and sleeping excessively, and questions of depression are raised. Evaluation in this context must consider at least three etiological factors—a normal physical response to the illness and effects of conditioning, a drug-induced response to the multiple sedating agents, and a "true" affective disturbance. In many cases, it is difficult to differentiate between these factors, but the effects of this "polypharmacy" on the patient must always be considered in the evaluation.

The problem of multiple medications often becomes more pronounced as the acute phase of BMT continues, particularly for those patients who develop GVHD or other complications. High-dose corticosteroids are used very frequently for GVHD treatment, and the CNS effects of these agents are well documented, presenting a continuum from mild affective liability to frank psychoses (Lewis & Smith, 1983; Ling, Perry, & Tsuang, 1981). Cyclosporin, another agent used commonly for GVHD prophylaxis, has been associated with a number of adverse CNS side effects, including delirium and an encephalopathic presentation (Canafax & Ascher, 1983; deGroen, Aksamit, Rakela, Forbes, & Krom, 1987). In addition to the direct effects of these agents on the CNS, they are often acutely toxic to other organs such as kidney and liver, which in turn may produce metabolic disturbances affecting the CNS (Wolcott, Fawzy, & Wellisch, 1987). The development of such organ failure may necessitate the introduction of additional medications with potential neurotoxicity, in a cycle quite familiar in the management of complicated BMT patients.

A recent example illustrates the phenomenon of polypharmacy in BMT patients with multiple medical complications and the difficulties this poses for evaluation of behavioral disturbance.

The patient was a 20-year-old with relapsed acute myelocytic leukemia (AML) who received an allogeneic transplant from his HLA-matched sibling. His posttransplant course was relatively uncomplicated with signs of early engraftment, and he was preparing for discharge when he developed acute GVHD of the gut. He had frequent severe diarrhea, which was accompanied by intense abdominal pain. He was placed on high-dose corticosteroids, which had little effect, and the pain remained difficult to control despite continuous-infusion narcotics administered through the use of a patient-controlled analgesia pump. The patient began to display unusual behaviors that were of concern to the nursing staff, including many compulsive checking, cleaning, and self-care behaviors (e.g., meticulously retaping his Hickman catheter for hours at a time). He was intermittently confused and disoriented, and at times he appeared to be hallucinating. When he was found one night on his hands and knees washing the floor of his room with towelettes, this was labeled as psychotic behavior and psychologic evaluation was requested on an emergent basis. When seen by the psychologist, the patient was tense and agitated but clearly oriented and coherent. It appeared that his mental status was tenuous and highly variable but with definite periods of lucidity. He justified his behavior of the previous evening in a very compelling manner, describing how, since development of his gut GVHD, he had become intermittently incontinent while on narcotics, and he was quite humiliated by this. That night he had awakened at the onset of an episode of diarrhea, tried to reach the commode, and in the process left a mess on the floor. He immediately began to clean it up, both to save himself from the embarrassment of being "found out", and because he felt that this was his responsibility and he wanted to take care of it. Many of his behaviors reflected his pressing need to be actively involved in taking care of himself. He expressed some anger at the nursing staff for "making such a big deal out of it," and he reiterated his wish to be left alone.

A review of his chart revealed that he had received 17 different medications in the prior 48 hours, including oral and IV antibiotics, antifungals, anti-GVHD steroids, premedications for transfusions, benzodiazepines, and narcotic and non-narcotic analgesics. The patient had a grossly distended abdomen and blood chemistries suggestive of early liver failure. His wife confirmed that he did seem to hallucinate at times, and she felt that this followed as a direct response to boosts of narcotics. There were also many significant social issues, but none more pressing than the basic reality that this was his eighth week of hospitalization and isolation in the same room, a stay which included Christmas, New Year, his birthday, and the couple's first wedding anniversary.

One can readily appreciate the complexities of clinical evaluation and intervention in such circumstances, and this may be approached as a problem in differential diagnosis or as an illustration of the overdetermined nature of symptoms, where there are multiple interrelated etiological factors contributing to the presentation. For example, a typical differential diagnosis might consider the possibilities of steroid-induced psychosis versus a hepatic encephalopathy (see Balthazar, 1991). Although in some instances such differentiation can be fairly straightforward, in the BMT milieu this is often exceedingly difficult. Even when a specific diagnosis or etiology can be determined, primary intervention may be precluded, because tapering of the steroid dose or a quick reversal of the metabolic disturbance may not be medically feasible. Moreover, when focusing on a specific diagnosis, it is important that one not neglect the multiple collateral stressors inherent in this context and thereby miss the global or ecological perspective.

Thus in the preceding case illustration several etiological factors were considered. Undoubtedly there were a number of metabolic disturbances, both endogenous and medication-induced, that may have been influencing the patient's behavior and increasing the risk for a more serious decompensation. In addition, the stresses of prolonged isolation, multiple disappointments with loss of holidays, uncertain prognosis, chronic pain, and loss of bodily functions coupled with loss of privacy and dignity, precipitated an agitated depression that left him close to the threshold of psychosis. Normally the patient coped in an obsessive-compulsive style, which may not have been the most adaptive but helped him maintain some degree of psychological integration. His intermittent decompensations appeared to be triggered by the narcotic analgesics, which reduced his tenuous ability to hold himself together. Lowering the steroid dose was not an option. Neuroleptic or antidepressant medications were considered, but these would only expand the polypharmacy, and their impact in combination with such a large number of other medications was uncertain. The plan in this case included changing the narcotic analgesia and lowering the dose, reducing the stress of isolation by encouraging the patient to leave his room for brief periods, and reinterpreting some of the patient's behaviors to staff while reinforcing his need for as much privacy as possible. The patient's mental status showed some improvement, but he continued to have occasional episodes of confusion and disorientation. As his GVHD proved resistant to therapy and became progressively worse, his confusion was replaced by periods of somnolence, which grew longer until he eventually entered the terminal phase of his illness.

Other Acute-Care Issues

Related to the issue of multiple medications is the use of hyperalimentation, or total parenteral nutrition (TPN), for patients with reduced or absent oral intake. In practice, this will be necessary for nearly 100 percent of patients receiving allogeneic transplants as well as the majority of autologous transplants. This may be less significant for those patients with a long history of chemotherapeutic treatment who have been previously exposed to intermittent use of TPN. But for others this loss of control over nutritional intake can be very threatening (Malcolm, Robson, Vanderveen, & Mahlen, 1980). Some patients who try unsuccessfully to maintain adequate oral intake view the initiation of TPN as a personal failure or a sign that their treatment is not going well. This may be avoided if TPN is utilized routinely for all BMT patients.

Initiation of TPN or subsequent changes in the nutrient concentrations can be complicated by the development of metabolic disturbances, which in rare instances may produce a transient encephalopathy (Lesko, 1990). More common are the affective disturbances associated with the loss of this basic bodily function and a concern over the return of appetite and the ability to eat adequately once the physical impediments to oral intake have resolved. Consider the patient who may have developed a negative taste for many previously favorite foods, and whose only oral intake for weeks consists of taking pills and unpalatable liquid medications. It is not surprising that this patient might experience some anxiety and resistance to demands that he or she increase oral intake. Although it seems reasonable to assume that the longer patients are maintained on TPN, the more difficulty they would have with the transition back to normal nutrition, there are no empirical data to confirm this association. Similarly, it seems reasonable to assume that patients who continue some oral intake while on TPN will be better prepared to maintain their caloric requirements when TPN is discontinued, but once again, few data are available to support this. This is another area in need of investigation, including studies of interventions designed to promote oral intake.

A general problem for all patients, but particularly those who develop complications which extend their hospitalization, might be labeled "endurance" or the ability to tolerate the BMT milieu for an extended period. Sackett (1979) used the term "decay" to describe the decline in compliance that occurs when treatment regimens are extended over time. This phenomenon need not be limited specifically to compliance but can relate to declines in general affective status and behavior when the BMT stay is prolonged. Thus even patients who were coping quite well initially are likely to develop disturbances in the face of setbacks that extend their hospital stay. For patients who are not experiencing a great deal of physical distress, boredom and agitation may predominate, while depression and withdrawal appear more likely among those in greater pain. This nonspecific problem is the primary issue that necessitates the prophylactic intervention of a multidisciplinary psychosocial staff.

Another unique aspect of the BMT process is the prolonged period in which the patient may be in an imminently life-threatening situation while the outcome remains uncertain. The nature of BMT is such that consent to transplant generally implies a commitment to aggressive treatment of complications, even when the prognosis is poor. Thus despite the high mortality of the procedure, few BMT patients will actually enter a phase of terminal care before they die. Every complication that develops during the BMT process serves to heighten the precarious prognosis for the patient, while at the same time the increasingly aggressive interventions signal that there is hope for a medical victory. This uncertainty and ambiguity is pervasive for the critically ill BMT patient, the family, and the medical staff, who must struggle to find the positions that allow them to cope with different potential outcomes simultaneously. Does the aggressive medical support deprive the patient and family of an opportunity to prepare for death and saving goodbye? This issue, which we know very little about, is difficult to study from an observational perspective. Such agendas often remain unspoken, navigated silently by the individual participants. Occasionally children may verbalize death-related concerns and express their wish to continue or to stop treatment, but more often such wishes are left unexpressed. The tensions and conflicts that can develop about whether to continue or discontinue treatment are discussed further in the section on staff issues.

Survivorship

The survivor of BMT today is akin to the survivor of childhood cancer two decades earlier in terms of the odds that have been overcome and the unknown risks that lie ahead. From that perspective, much of what has already been written about cancer survivors will be directly applicable to the survivors of BMT (Koocher & O'Malley, 1981; Kazak, Chapter 8, this volume). To date, only a few empirical studies of BMT survivors have been reported (Pot-Mees, 1989 , Wolcott et al., 1986a). This discussion focuses on two aspects of BMT survivorship, the transition and social reintegration of the posttransplant period and the medical and/or neuropsychological late effects of transplant conditioning.

Postdischarge Transition

Discharge from the BMT hospitalization marks the passing of a major hurdle and is imbued with great significance by the patient and family. This is often celebrated by family and staff, and there may be exchanges of gifts or photographs or other acts symbolizing transition (Atkins & Patenaude, 1987; Freund & Siegel, 1986; Lesko, 1990). Although the patient is by no means out of danger, such celebrations may reinforce that perception, with the theme of the party being "I survived." The intense feelings of relief may be heightened if the patient was aware of the deaths of any other transplant patients who were hospitalized

during the same time. On the other hand, considerable ambivalence and a type of "survivor guilt" develops for some patients, although such feelings are often covered by massive denial at the time of discharge (Patenaude & Rappeport, 1982).

The elation of the patient and family at discharge is likely to be followed by some degree of disappointment due to subsequent setbacks and readmission, the degree of isolation that continues to be required, or the painful realities of a gradual readjustment to normal functioning. Many patients, including those who display good adjustment during the transplant hospitalization, often show an increase in affective disturbance in the early weeks and months posttransplant. In the only empirical study addressing this issue, the data of Pot-Mees (1989) appear to support this impression. She reported an increase in affective and behavioral disturbance, particularly depression, measured 6 months posttransplant, in comparison to pretransplant.

This finding could be related to the continued use of high-dose steroids during the posttransplant period. However, what is more frequently observed is a type of "crash" that occurs, in the relative calm after the ordeal of the acute phase of BMT has past. During the transplant hospitalization, patients must mobilize high levels of psychic defense against intense and continuous stressors of a life-threatening nature. After discharge, when the most intense threat has diminished, their defenses may begin to relax, thereby making them more susceptible to affective disturbance. This occurs a a time when they are just beginning to end their isolation and must adjust to reintegration into normal school and social interactions, often while still carrying many of the physical stigmata of transplant, such as skin GVHD, patchy bald heads, and markedly cushingnoid appearance, with swollen, hirsute faces. The stresses of reintegration, while perhaps more mundane than those of the transplant, often prove problematic for patients. Further research is necessary to improve our understanding of the nature and determinants of posttransplant adjustment, particularly regarding the temporal relationship to medication schedules, physical symptomatology, and social events (e.g., school reentry).

In a note of optimism, Pot-Mees (1989) did report a slight improvement in affective status between 6 and 12 months postransplant.

Late Effects

Survivors of BMT are at risk to develop complications in a number of organ systems. The major late effects that have been the focus of study thus far involve endocrine dysfunction, affecting both growth and gonadal development, ophthalmologic abnormalities, and CNS abnomalities (Sanders, 1990; Sanders et al., 1989). As all of these have obvious implications for psychological functioning, they are discussed briefly here.

Across organ systems, the deleterious long-term outcomes appear largely dependent on whether the conditioning regimen included total body irradiation (TBI). Furthermore, many studies differentiate between the more deleterious effects of single-dose versus fractionated TBI (Thompson, Sanders, Flournoy, Buckner, & Thomas, 1986). In practice, most centers have abandoned the use of single-dose TBI, but for some organ systems, long-term outcome data on fractionated TBI are unavailable.

Regarding the endocrine system, thyroid dysfunction has been found in approximately 50 percent of children who received single-dose TBI, 15 to 20 percent of children who received fractionated TBI, and less than 1 percent of children conditioned with chemotherapy alone (Sanders et al., 1989). Growth velocity has been normal in children transplanted without TBI but decreased in nearly all children receiving TBI, regardless of fractionation (Sanders et al., 1989). This growth delay is exacerbated in patients with chronic GVHD. Furthermore, patients with GVHD who did not receive TBI showed catachup after discontinuation of GVHD therapy, but patients who received TBI did not. Growth following transplant also appears related to the therapy received prior to transplant, particularly cranial radiation. Growth hormone deficiency in children receiving TBI was found in 90 percent of those who had prior cranial radiation, compared to only 42 percent of those who had not (Sanders et al., 1989).

Onset of puberty and development of secondary sexual characteristics appear to be normal in BMT survivors who did not receive TBI. Among those who received TBI, approximately 50 percent show delay or absence of sexual development and require some hormonal supplementation (Sanders, 1990). Regarding fertility, the outcome is similar, with permanent gonadal failure occurring in nearly all patients who receive TBI. For those conditioned with high-dose cyclophosphamide and no radiation, nearly all females show eventual recovery of normal gonadal function. Males may show some reduction in fertility, but it appears that the majority will recover normal spermatogenesis. To date, no studies have been reported relating attitudes and affective status of post-BMT patients to issues of fertility or other neuroendocrine outcomes.

The eye is another common target organ for late toxicities of BMT, particularly the development of cataracts (Sanders et al., 1989). Early studies suggested that over 80 percent of patients conditioned with TBI would require cataract repair. It now appears that this was related to single-dose TBI, and the incidence of cataracts among those exposed to fractionated TBI is approximately 20 percent, roughly the same as the incidence among those transplanted without TBI (Sanders, 1990). Treatment for these patients is the same as for cataracts of other etiologies. With proper monitoring and ophthalmological intervention, few patients will develop significant visual impairment.

Late effects of transplant conditioning on the CNS have begun to be documented (Thompson et al., 1986; Wiznitzer, Pacher, August, & Burky, 1984). To date, reports have been limited to physical findings on diagnostic imaging or to the incidence of gross neuropathology; no large-scale empirical studies of neuropsychological outcomes have been published. Thompson et al. (1986) reported an incidence of multifocal leukoencephalopathy of 7 percent in patients (both adults and children) transplanted with TBI. Leukoencephalopathy occurred only among those patients who had previous CNS therapy (either radiation or intrathecal chemotherapy), and there were no cases among those without prior CNS therapy or without TBI. Most discussions of this issue reflect the reports of neuropsychological deficits in pediatric survivors of conventional leukemia treatment with cranial radiation, implying that an analogous set of outcomes may be expected for BMT survivors of TBI (Copeland, Fletcher, & Pfefferbaum-Levine, 1985; Said, Waters, Cousens, & Martens , 1989; Mulhern, Chapter 5, this volume). However, no such findings have been documented relating specifically to TBI (Barret, 1982; Sanders et al., 1989). Although GVHD may exacerbate the late effects found in other organ systems, there is no evidence of chronic GVHD involving the CNS or having any direct impact on CNS function (Patchell, White, Clark, Beschorner, & Santos, 1985).

Some anecdotal evidence has been presented suggesting that survivors of pediatric BMT who received TBI may have a higher incidence of school problems than those transplanted without TBI, but this awaits confirmation with standardized psychoeducational assessments (Sanders, 1990). One study presenting long-term follow-up of a small cohort of patients transplanted in infancy revealed normal neurodevelopmental functioning 2 1/2 to 6 years following BMT (Kaleita et al., 1989). Three of four patients received TBI, but none had any previous CNS therapy.

In a larger study of 44 survivors of pediatric BMT followed for 12 months posttransplant, Pot-Mees (1989) found no significant changes in cognitive abilities. In fact, the observed trend suggested a slight improvement in scores at 12 months in comparison to pretransplant, a phenomenon which the author attributed to pretransplant anxiety.

In contrast, Pot-Mees also reported academic achievement significantly below age expectations at 12 months posttransplant. However, these findings might have been confounded by the inclusion of a subset of patients transplanted for genetic storage diseases that are associated with cognitive impairment, where a successful transplant would be expected to improve cognitive function. Such patients must be analyzed separately from those transplanted for leukemia or other malignancies, in order to obtain an unbiased picture of neuropsychological outcome. In addition, it is unlikely that 12 months would allow enough time for any neuropsychological changes associated with TBI to become manifest. Nevertheless, the striking contrast between cognitive performance and academic achievement may reflect heightened difficulties in school reintegration for this population.

From the limited data available regarding survivors both of BMT and of conventional treatments for childhood leukemia, one might hypothesize that TBI in the fractionated doses typical of current conditioning regimens will have a relatively benign impact on neurocognitive function, but such treatment may potentiate or exacerbate cognitive deficits in patients with previous CNS therapy. This calls for prospective longitudinal neuropsychological assessments of a cohort of BMT survivors large enough to allow for analysis in a two (+ and − prior CNS treatment) by two (+ and − TBI) quasi-experimental design.

Donor Issues

There is very little in the literature relating specifically to the psychological problems of BMT donors, and even less empirical information from this population. There is some anecdotal evidence to suggest that sibling donors are more likely than nondonor siblings to develop new behavioral problems in the peritransplant period (Pot-Mees & Zeitlin, 1987). The only published empirical study involved 18 adult BMT sibling donors evaluated 2 to 7 years after transplant (Wolcott, Wellisch, Fawzy, & Landsverk, 1986b). Utilizing a series of self-report questionnaires assessing affect, self-esteem, and life satisfaction, the authors found no differences from a normative population. These donors also reported little change in their relationship with their recipient siblings since transplant. A major limitation of this study was that only donors whose recipient was still alive were included. Given the continued high mortality of the BMT procedure, it is important to include donors of deceased recipients in future studies. Intuitively, it is among this group where we would expect to find donors at greater risk for psychological difficulties.

There is a fairly extensive literature addressing the psychosocial sequelae of kidney donation, but this also is limited by a largely adult focus. In a landmark study, Simmons reported on the outcome of 230 living related kidney donors 2 years posttransplant, in comparison to a group of matched controls (Simmons, Klein, & Simmons, 1977). The donor group reported higher self-esteem than did controls, and 95 percent of donors reported some psychological benefit and expressed positive feelings about donation. Only 5 percent demonstrated any evidence of negative sequelae. A follow-up study found that most of the positive impact was maintained 5 to 9 years following transplant (Simmons, 1983). Subsequent reports have confirmed these findings but also have pointed out the higher risk for negative sequelae when the transplant fails, particularly if the recipient dies (Burley & Stiller, 1985; Hirvas, Enckell, Kuhlback, & Pasternak, 1980; Sharma & Enoch, 1987). A recent paper highlighted this in striking fashion, reporting on the suicides of two related kidney donors following the recipients' deaths (Weizer, Weizman, Shapira, Yussim, & Munitz, 1989). Both donors had undergone psychiatric screening prior to donation, and no psychopathology was identified. The authors described the multiple traumas experienced by the donor when the transplant fails, and lamented that psychiatric support for the donor was generally not provided, since there was no routine medical contact with the donors following transplant surgery. They concluded that psychiatric evaluation and follow-up are indicated for all related donors whose recipient dies.

These findings raise questions regarding the psychological adjustment of pediatric BMT sibling donors, who often are quite young, and this highlights the need for analogous studies in pediatric populations. The physical risks to the BMT donor and the losses involved—replaceable tissue (bone marrow) instead of nonreplaceable organ (e.g., kidney)—suggest that the threat of BMT donation might not be as great as that faced by the organ donor. However, an aspect unique to BMT compared to organ transplants, which might potentiate higher levels of stress, is the development of GVHD in the recipient. In renal transplants, failures may occur when the recipient rejects the donor's organ. With GVHD, it is the donor's tissue which attacks the recipient and may be directly responsible for the recipient's death. Thus it would seem that the risk for guilt reactions may be greater in this group, at least among those child donors who can comprehend the meaning of GVHD. Anecdotal evidence has been presented to support this (Gardner et al., 1977; Patenaude et al., 1979). For now, this remains a hypothesis, but one which can be tested in future studies if donor outcome is analyzed according to the outcome for the recipient.

Much of the remaining literature relating to donors has focused on issues of informed consent and other ethical and legal concerns. This is addressed in a later section, with only brief mention made here of the role of the psychologist in donor evaluations. In the past, the parents of a potential sibling donor who was a minor may have been required to make a court appearance to gain legal approval prior to proceeding with transplant. The court would then order psychological evaluation as part of the procedure. Other centers utilized a court-appointed child advocate (Serota, August, O'Shea, Woodward, & Koch, 1981). Today these practices have been dispensed with in most centers, but psychological evaluation of donors prior to transplant continues to be a routine part of the pretransplant workup. At St. Jude Children's Research Hospital routine psychological evaluations are undertaken to (1) assess whether the donor has an age-appropriate understanding of the bone marrow harvest and transplant procedures; (2) explore the child's attitude toward donation and uncover any undue anxieties about the procedure; and (3) ensure that the child is not being unduly coerced. This can be very difficult to accomplish in one or two interviews with an often anxious and highly defended child; moreover, the absence of a body of literature or any normative data on these issues makes this a highly subjective process. In practice, such interviews are often helpful for identifying and correcting any misconceptions the child may have about the procedure, and to begin the process of preparing the child, using a model of anticipatory guidance. Preparation for the harvest procedure may then be supplemented by child life specialists or surgical nurses (Kinrade, 1987; Ruggiero, 1988). Follow-up is often limited to the peritransplant period by default, since donors are generally not available beyond that period.

Family Issues

The multiple stresses of the BMT process present a unique challenge to the maintenance of family cohesion and integration, while the prolonged nature of the procedure may deplete the family's physical, emotional, and financial resources over time. Yet, despite the obvious burden of BMT for all family members, there have been no studies specifically on family functioning during BMT. Ironically, one of the major stressors for the family has also been one of the major obstacles to family studies—the frequent geographic separation of family members during transplant.

When transplant occurs in a setting far removed from the family's home community, parents are frequently separated, with one remaining at the hospital with the patient while the other remains at home with siblings. This arrangement may promote an unusual closeness between the patient and "resident parent" while isolating them from the remainder of the nuclear family (Freund & Siegel, 1986; Pot-Mees, 1989). An alternative arrangement often seen has both parents staying at the hospital during the acute phase, while the remaining siblings are cared for by extended family or friends. Whatever the final arrangements, compromises must be made which may promote tension, guilt, or alienation among subsets of family members. Even when family communication is optimal, differences in perspective are inevitable between the resident family members and those at home. Some families have recently used exchanges of videotapes to help reduce the effect of separation. However, as described by one mother, a videotape may help nonresident family members appreciate the physical confines of a laminar airflow unit, but "it doesn't begin to convey the realities of being here on a day to day basis."

Another frequently observed phenomenon is that family members who stay with the patient tend to rely on hospital staff and other patient families for support, while the extended family and previously established social networks become less significant (Freund & Siegel, 1986; Patenaude et al., 1979). A feeling may develop among families that only those who are actively involved can begin to understand their experience. What effect does this have on the support available to families when they return to their home communities and begin to reintegrate into their social networks? Unfortunately, little is known about this process.

Although carrying out family-focused research on the immediate and long-term sequelae of BMT can be logistically daunting, it is extremely important to our understanding of the process. Collaborative studies that involve transplant centers and those that frequently refer to them would provide one approach to the problem that has not been reported. Also, the use of telephone and mail follow-up, despite some disadvantages, has not been fully exploited. Circumventing the logistical obstacles to family-based studies of BMT is not impossible but will demand unusual creativity and persistence of investigators.

Impact of Bone Marrow Transplantation on Medical Staff

Some of the early descriptive papers regarding BMT commented on the stresses of the staff working in this milieu, with its prolonged intensive care and high mortality rates (Brown & Kelly, 1976; Patenaude et al., 1979; Pfefferbaum et al., 1977). Observations were made regarding the intense relationships that often develop between BMT staff (particularly nurses) and patients and families, which can magnify the staff's sense of frustration, guilt, or self-blame and the impact of grief and loss should the patient die. Although this has not been the subject of any programmatic research, these themes continue to be discussed in recent papers, with the general conclusion that BMT team members are a group at high risk for "burnout" (Brack, LaClave, & Blix, 1988; Rappaport, 1988; Wolcott et al., 1987). This highlights the need for routine supportive services for team members. It has been suggested that such services should be built into the regular team processes, perhaps as part of weekly psychosocial rounds which address both patient and staff issues (Patenaude et al., 1979).

The emotional closeness that develops between patients and staff can be problematic. On one hand, because of the intensity and length of care involved, a certain degree of closeness is inevitable and desirable. The supportive relationships that develop can be very helpful to patients and families and can be useful to staff in gaining compliance and cooperation from patients under difficult circumstances. On the other hand, a situation of closeness which blurs boundaries, where a staff member is perceived (or perceives himself or herself) as a member of the family, may interfere with the objectivity necessary to provide optimal medical care; ultimately this is likely to become problematic for both parties, particularly if the patient dies. Every staff member (including the mental health professionals) is susceptible to crossing these boundaries with a given patient. Therefore, it becomes necessary for staff to regularly monitor their attitudes, feelings, and relationships with patients. Supportive group meetings, with input from mental health professionals, can help staff maintain their perspective, so that they can achieve an optimal level of closeness that will foster a flexible balance between intimacy and objectivity.

In the only published study addressing BMT staff issues, Brack et al. (1988) assessed patterns of communication between patients and staff. They reported on the incongruence between the staff's outwardly optimistic behavior with patients and their actual pessimism about the patient's prognosis. Although the staff endorsed providing accurate information, they tended to behave in an increasingly optimistic manner as the patient's conditioned worsened, a form of paradoxical, or double-binding, communication. Such communication inhibits the patient from frank expression of concerns. Although this report was concerned with the double-binding communications of staff vis-à-vis the patient, one can also appreciate the analogous double bind for the staff in caring for these patients and the tremendous strain this places on the caregivers. This is especially true when patients begin to deteriorate and, although staff expectations for their survival diminish, life-saving supportive measures are intensified.

As mentioned earlier, the patient with a progressively downhill course may create growing tensions among staff as conflicts arise regarding whether it is fruitful to continue aggressive therapy. Disagreements may be openly verbalized, which perhaps allows for a more healthy resolution. Unfortunately, such disagreements often go "underground," being discussed secretly in small factions that create dissension or can lead to a more major splitting among the team. It is not uncommon for differences to be observed between attitudes of attending physicians and primary nursing staff. This can create an untenable double-bind situation for nurses, who must carry out aggressive therapy, which they feel is inappropriate, on a patient they feel is likely to die anyway.

The appropriate line of transition between aggressive supportive care and terminal care has always been blurred in BMT, and recent technological advances have added to this ambiguity. Consequently, a great tolerance for ambiguity is demanded of all those involved with transplant—patients, families, and staff. This involves another paradox, in that although many BMT patients will die, one rarely has the opportunity to work with the "dying patient." Although our understanding of the needs of terminally ill patients has grown considerably in recent decades, as has our ability to provide both medical and psychosocial care, much of this is not directly applicable to the BMT patient who is deteriorating. Therefore, we may need to develop a new model for working with these patients, who are "dying in limbo"—one that allows for acknowledgment and communication regarding good and bad outcomes simultaneously, that allows a reasonable opportunity to ascertain the patient's attitude regarding continuation of therapy, and that allows us to help the patient prepare for the worst, without interfering with the patient's hope and struggle for survival.

Ethical and Legal Issues

The practice of bone marrow transplantation is fraught with ethical issues and potential legal dilemmas. Although a comprehensive consideration of these is beyond the scope of this chapter, a brief review follows of the most salient issues. The central issue which forms the basis for all subsequent discussion involves the principle of informed consent, particularly as it relates to minors.

Informed consent involves two related processes: the legally mandated procedure of signing research protocol consent forms, and the less formal but more extensive informing that needs to occur in the days and weeks preceding signed consent, which allows for autonomous decision making by the patient and family. The elements of informed consent proper are dictated by federal regulations and must include descriptions of the nature and purpose of the study, including which procedures are experimental, the reasonably foreseeable risks along with the potential benefits to the subject and to others, and the available alternative treatments (Fletcher, van Eys, & Dorn, 1988; King & Cross, 1989). This is to be accompanied by a written document, evaluated for its ease of comprehension by an institutional review board (IRB). However, some literature relating specifically to pediatric BMT suggests that for practical purposes, the true informed consent occurs prior to the actual consent signing session.

Chauvenet and Smith (1988) surveyed 21 pediatric oncology centers not performing BMT, regarding their experiences referring patients elsewhere for transplant. Although ostensibly each BMT center performed an extensive psychosocial evaluation prior to transplant, followed by lengthy discussion and obtaining of informed consent, in practice, 100 percent of patients who arrived at the BMT center were transplanted. In no instance among 146 patients did the psychosocial evaluation or subsequent discussion at the transplant center alter the decision to proceed with transplant. The authors argued that since the decision-making process occurs in the home community, the onus for providing informed consent falls on the referring physician. This process occurs without any standardized forms or documentation, highlighting the often superfluous nature of the consent signing session in terms of it's role in promoting informed decision making. This makes it imperative that referring physicians remain fully informed regarding the risks and benefits of transplant. The risk inherent in this situation is that there is a diffusion of responsibility between the referring center and the BMT center, which could promote less than fully informed decisions about the process. Unfortunately, no survey was made of the patients and families to assess their satisfaction with the process.

Such a survey was done by Lesko et al. (1989) assessing the attitudes of adult patients, parents of pediatric patients, and physicians toward the consent process at a major transplant center. They found that patients and parents generally viewed the process and the consent document quite favorably and appeared to retain the major points of information, although they had difficulty recalling specifics, such as side effects of treatment. The physicians, however, had a much less favorable view of the process, particularly regarding the consent document, which they felt was overly technical and complex. Patients and parents did not share this view. Despite the authors' generally positive conclusions about the process, some of their findings were disturbing. Regarding the decision-making process, 74 percent of patients and parents acknowledged difficulty in making a decision and over 90 percent stated that they relied heavily on the physicians' advice in making their decision, yet almost all respondents (95 percent) perceived the physician as strongly wanting them to accept treatment. By design, all participants in this study had already consented to transplant and there was no mention of whether any patients decided against transplant after the consent session. Another finding of concern was that over 40 percent of patients and 60 percent of parents reported having questions they had not asked despite having been given opportunities to do so. Similarly, from the physician's perspective, 90 percent of patients and 73 percent of parents were viewed as withholding doubts or concerns about the treatment. This raises questions about how "informed" such consents actually are, and how freely the decision to transplant is made.

Consent as a legal concept implies the act of a competent adult making an autonomous decision regarding her or his own affairs, whereas in pediatrics one must rely on the approval of parents or legal guardians, which might be more appropriately labeled permission rather than consent (Bell, 1986; Fletcher et al., 1988; Williams, 1984, 1990). This has led to the development of the concept of "assent," implying the informed agreement of the child participant, in contrast to a legally valid consent. Federal regulations now require that an IRB ensure that adequate provisions are made for soliciting the assent of child subjects, where the IRB determines that such children are capable of providing assent. Although it is unclear at what age a child might be capable of making a meaningful assent, a cutoff of 7 years has often been used (Fletcher et al., 1990). The IRB also has the right to waive the assent requirement where there is evidence of direct benefit to the child. Presently, the IRB of the National Cancer Institute (NCI) waives the assent requirement on each pediatric cancer project with therapeutic intent. Given that all BMT protocols have therapeutic intent, documenting the agreement of the pediatric BMT recipient is generally not a major concern. This will be left to the clinical judgment of the physician, who presumably would be disinclined to proceed with transplant over the vigorous objections of a child, if those objections were at all reasonable.

The situation is quite different, however, when one considers the potential child donor, because there is clearly no direct medical benefit to the donor in this situation. With kidney donations involving minors, it has been customary to ask for a court order before proceeding (Brant, 1984; Holder, 1990). This is generally obtained without difficulty if no objections are verbalized by the child. In practice, cases involving minor BMT donors rarely are taken to court any longer (Holder, 1990). This presupposes an evaluation that has failed to uncover any objections from the donor. In the event that evaluation revealed clear evidence of coercion of the child, a court order would need to be sought. As far as can be ascertained, no such court cases have been reported.

The circumventing of court appearances has saved the families of BMT patients an added burden, but it has created potential ethical dilemmas for the psychologists and social workers who must do the in-house evaluations. At St. Jude's, several potentially problematic scenarios have transpired, including a child who assented initially but later expressed objections after transplant conditioning had started, and a very young child (age 6) who vacillated about his intentions from moment to moment. To date the courts are not involved, but these situations can create some personal discomfort and insecurity regarding the ethical and legal duty of medical staffs to protect patients.

The very young child highlights another ethical conundrum. If the notion of assent implies that the child actually has a choice about whether to undergo donation, then the infant and toddler who are incapable of providing any meaningful assent are denied the same protection as the older child. This becomes particularly salient in those instances where parents conceive a child for the express purpose of providing bone marrow for an older sibling. This is a phenomenon which is occurring and has begun to receive exposure in the popular press (Morrow, 1991). An extension of this is the use of fetal tissue for transplantation (Clarke, Fletcher, & Petersen, 1989; Durbin, 1988). A recent case highlights the potential difficulties. A family sought prenatal diagnosis, with their intention being to produce a healthy child to serve as a bone marrow donor for their son affected with Wiskott-Aldrich syndrome (Clarke et al., 1989). They planned to abort any HLA-incompatible fetuses that would have been unsuitable donors. However, after considerable deliberation, the prenatal diagnostic center refused the family's request. Continued technical developments are likely to produce more such dilemmas in the future and raise new questions about how we protect our "most uninformed and uninformable potential donors" (Durbin, 1988).

Regarding adult donors, the law has been very clear and consistent, holding that the word "donation" means "gift," and one cannot obtain court orders to compel gifts (Bell, 1986; Brant, 1984; Holder, 1990). In several cases where petitioners attempted to force their relatives to be tested for compatibility, such requests have always been denied. Conversely, the national bone marrow registries for unrelated donors will not allow persons under 18 to be enrolled, even with parental permission (Durbin, 1988). Thus children other than relatives are denied the opportunity to voluntarily donate marrow.

Conclusion

Bone marrow transplantation continues to be associated with multiple and intense psychological stresses that challenge patients, families, and staff, thus providing a fertile field for psychological research. Our knowledge base in this arena has accumulated slowly, and empirical studies have been lacking. Some of the obstacles to systematic empirical research that were unavoidable in past years, such as small sample size, can be overcome today, particularly with the development of collaborative studies. This chapter has enumerated multiple relevant research questions. It is hoped that well-designed research studies will begin to provide some answers in the coming decade.

References

Atkins, D., & Patenaude, A. F. (1987). Psychosocial preparation and follow-up for pediatric bone marrow transplantation patients. *American Journal of Orthopsychiatry, 57,* 246–252.

Balthazar, J. E. (1991). Steroid psychosis and hepatic encephalopathy in liver transplant patients. *Critical Care Nursing Quarterly, 14,* 51–55.

Barret, A. (1982). Total body radiation before bone marrow transplantation in children: A review. *Clinical Radiology, 33,* 131–135.

Beatty, P. G. (1991). The world experience with unrelated donor transplants. *Bone Marrow Transplantation, 7* (Suppl. 1), 54–58.

Beatty, P. G., Clift, R. A., Mickelson, E. M., Nisperos, B. B., Flourney, N., Martin, P. J., Sanders, J. E., Stewart, P., Buckner, C. O., Storb, R., Thomas, E. D., & Hansen, J. A. (1985). Marrow transplantation from related donors other than HLA identical siblings. *New England Journal of Medicine, 313,* 765–771.

Bell, C J. (1986, Fall). Children as organ donors: Legal rights and ethical issues. *Health and Social Work,* 291–300.

Brack, G., LaClave, L., & Blix, S. (1988). The psychological aspects of bone marrow transplant: A staff's perspective. *Cancer Nursing, 11,* 221–229.

Bradlyn, A. S., & Boggs, S. R. (1989). Bone marrow transplantation in children: A case study. In M. C. Roberts & C. E. Walker (Eds.), *Casebook of child and pediatric psychology.* New York: Guilford Press.

Brant, J. (1984). Legal issues involving bone marrow transplants to minors. *American Journal of Pediatric Hematology/Oncology, 6,* 89–91.

Brown, H. N., & Kelly, M. J. (1976). Stages of bone marrow transplantation: A psychiatric perspective. *Psychosomatic Medicine, 38,* 439–446.

Burley, J. A., & Stiller, C. R. (1985). Emotionally related donors and renal transplantation. *Transplantation Proceedings, 17,* 123–127.

Canafax, D. M., & Ascher, N. L. (1983). Cyclosporin immunosuppression. *Clinical Pharmacy, 2,* 515–524.

Carden, P. A., Mitchell, S. L., Waters, K. D., Tiedemann, K., & Ekert, H. (1990). Prevention of cyclophophamide/cytarabine-induced emesis with ondansetron in children with leukemia. *Journal of Clinical Oncology, 8,* 1531–1535.

Chauvenet, A. R., & Smith, N. M. (1988). Referral of pediatric oncology patients for marrow transplantation and the process of informed consent. *Medical and Pediatric Oncology, 16,* 40–44.

Cheson, B. D., & Curt, G. A. (1986). Bone marrow transplantation: Current perspectives and future directions. *Journal of the National Cancer Institute, 76,* 1265–1267.

Clarke, R. D., Fletcher, J., & Petersen, G. (1989). Conceiving a fetus for bone marrow donation: An ethical problem in prenatal diagnosis. *Prenatal Diagnosis, 9,* 329–334.

Copeland, D., Fletcher, J., & Pfefferbaum-Levine, B. (1985). Neuropsychological sequelae of childhood cancer in long term survivors. *Pediatrics, 75,* 745–753.

deGroen, J. R., Aksamit, A. J., Rakela, J., Forbes, G. S., & Krom, R. A. F. (1987). Central nervous system toxicity after liver transplantation: The role of cyclosporin and cholesterol. *New England Journal of Medicine, 317,* 861–866.

Durbin, M. (1988). Bone marrow transplantation: Economic, ethical and social issues. *Pediatrics, 82,* 774–783.

Engelhard, D., Marks, M. I., & Good, R. A. (1986). Infections in bone marrow transplant recipients. *Journal of Pediatrics, 108,* 335–346.

Fletcher, J. C., van Eys, J., & Dorn, L. D. (1988). Ethical considerations in pediatric oncology. In P. A. Pizzo & D. G. Poplack (Eds.), *Principles and practice of pediatric oncology.* Philadelphia: Lippincott.

Freund, B. L., & Siegel, K. (1985). Problems in transition following bone marrow transplantation: Psychosocial aspects. *American Journal of Orthopsychiatry, 56,* 244–252.

Gardner, G. G., August, C. S., & Githens, J. (1977). Psychological issues in bone marrow transplantation. *Pediatrics, 60,* 625–631.

Heugveld, M. V., Houtman, R. B., & Zwann, F. E. (1988). Psychological aspects of bone marrow transplantation: A retrospective study of 17 long term survivors. *Bone Marrow Transplantation, 3,* 69–75.

Hewitt, M., Cornish, J., Pamphilon, D., & Oakhill, A. (1991). Effective emetic control during conditioning of children for bone marrow transplantation using ondansetron, a 5-HT3 antagonist. *Bone Marrow Transplantion, 7,* 31–434.

Hirvas, J., Enckell, M., Kuhlback, B., & Pasternak, B. (1980). Psychological and social problems encountered in active treatment of chronic uraemia: III. Prediction of the living donor's psychological reaction. *Acta Medica Scandinavica, 208,* 285–287.

Holder, A. R. (1990). Legal issues in bone marrow transplantation. *Yale Journal of Biology and Medicine, 63,* 521–525.

Holland, J., Plumb, M., Yates, J., Harris, S., Tuttolomondo, A., Holmes, J., & Holland, J. F. (1977). Psychological response of patients with acute leukemia to germ-free environments. *Cancer, 40,* 871–879.

Howard, M. R., Hows, J. M., Gore, S. M., & Bradley, B. A. (1991). Unrelated donor marrow transplantation: An interim analysis of the International Marrow Unrelated Search and Transplant (IMUST) study. *Bone Marrow Transplantation, 7* (Suppl. 1), 126–127.

Kaleita, T. A., Shields, W. D., Tesler, A., & Feig, S. (1989). Normal neurodevelopment in four young children treated for acute leukemia or aplastic anemia. *Pediatrics, 83,* 753–757.

Kellerman, J., Rigler, D., & Siegel, S. E. (1979). Psychological response of children to isolation in a protected environment. *Journal of Behavioral Medicine, 2,* 263–274.

Kellerman, J., Rigler, D., Siegel, S. E., McCue, K., Poposil, J., & Uno, R. (1976). Psychological evaluation and management of pediatric oncology patients in protected environments. *Medical and Pediatric Oncology, 2,* 353–360.

King, N. M., & Cross, A. W. (1989). Children as decision makers: Guidelines for pediatricians. *Journal of Pediatrics, 115,* 10–16.

Kinrade, L. C. (1987). Preparation of sibling donor for bone marrow transplant harvest procedure. *Cancer Nursing, 10,* 77–81.

Koocher, G. P., & O'Malley, J. E. (1981). *The Damocles syndrome: Psychological consequences of surviving childhood cancer.* New York: McGraw-Hill.

Lesko, L. M. (1990). Bone marrow transplantation. In J. C. Holland & J. H. Rowland (Eds.), *Handbook of psychoonocology.* New York: Oxford University Press.

Lesko, L. M., Dermatis, H., Penman, D., & Holland, J. C. (1989). Patient's, parents' and oncologists' perceptions of informed consent for bone marrow transplantation. *Medical and Pediatric Oncology, 17,* 181–187.

Lesko, L. M., Kern, J., & Hawkins, D. R. (1984). Psychological aspects of patients in germ-free isolation: A review of child, adult and patient management literature. *Medical and Pediatric Oncology, 12,* 43–49.

Lewis, D., & Smith, R. (1983). Steroid induced psychiatric syndromes. *Journal of Affective Disorders, 5,* 319–332.

Lindgren, P. S. (1983). The laminar airflow room: Nursing practices and procedures. *Nursing Clinics of North America, 18,* 553–561.

Ling, M. H., Perry, P. J., & Tsuang, M. T. (1981). Side effects of corticosteroid therapy: Psychiatric aspects. *Archives of General Psychiatry, 38,* 471–477.

Linn, S., Beardslee, W., & Patenaude, A. F. (1986). Puppet therapy with pediatric bone marrow transplant patients. *Journal of Pediatric Psychology, 11,* 37–46.

Malcolm, R., Robson, J., Vanderveen, T. W., & Mahlen, P. (1980). Psychosocial aspects of parenteral nutrition. *Psychosomatics, 21,* 115–123.

Marshall, D. (1985). Care of the pediatric oncology patient in a laminar air flow setting. *Nursing Clinics of North America, 20,* 67–81.

Meyers, J. D. (1986). Infection in bone marrow transplant recipients. *American Journal of Medicine, 81,* 27–36.

Morrow, L. (1991, June 17). When one body can save another. *Time,* 54–58.

Parkman, R. (1986). Current status of bone marrow transplantation in pediatric oncology. *Cancer, 58,* 569–572.

Patchell, R. A., White, C. L., Clark, A. W., Beschorner, W. E., & Santos, G. W. (1985). Neurologic complications of bone marrow transplant. *Neurology, 35,* 300–306.

Patenaude, A. F. (1990). Psychologic impact of bone marrow transplantation: Current perspective. *Yale Journal of Biology and Medicine, 63,* 515–519.

Patenaude, A. F., & Rappeport, J. M. (1982). Surviving bone marrow transplantation: The patient in the other bed. *Annals of Internal Medicine, 97,* 915–918.

Patenaude, A. F., Szymanski, L., & Rappeport, J. (1979). Psychological costs of bone marrow transplantation in children. *American Journal of Orthopsychiatry, 49,* 409–422.

Pfefferbaum, B., Lindamood, M. M., & Wiley, F. (1977). Pediatric bone marrow transplantation: Psychosocial aspects. *American Journal of Psychiatry, 134,* 1299–1301.

Phipps, S., & DeCuir-Whalley, S. (1990). Adherence issues in pediatric bone marrow transplantation. *Journal of Pediatric Psychology, 15,* 459–475.

Pot-Mees, C. C. (1989). *The psychological effects of bone marrow transplantation in children*. Delft, Netherlands: Eburon.

Pot-Mees, C. C., & Zeitlin, H. (1987). Psychosocial consequences of bone marrow transplantation in children: A preliminary communication. *Journal of Psychosocial Oncology, 5*, 73–81.

Powazek, M., Goff, J. R., & Schuyling, J. (1978). Emotional reactions of children to isolation in a cancer hospital. *Journal of Pediatrics, 92*, 675–678.

Rappaport, B. S. (1988). Evaluation of consultation-liaison services in bone marrow transplantation. *General Hospital Psychiatry, 10*, 346–351.

Ruggiero, M. R. (1988). The donor in bone marrow transplantation. *Seminars in Oncology Nursing, 4*, 9–14.

Sackett, D. L. (1979). Methods for compliance research. In R. B. Haynes, D. W. Taylor, & D. L. Sackett (Eds.), *Compliance in health care* (pp. 323–333). Baltimore: Johns Hopkins University Press.

Said, J. A., Waters, B., Cousens, P., & Martens, M. M. (1989). Neuropsychological sequelae of central nervous system survivors of childhood acute lymphoblastic leukemia. *Journal of Consulting and Clinical Psychology, 57*, 251–256.

Sanders, J., Sullivan, K., Witherspoon, R., Doney, K., Anasetti, C., Beatty, P., & Petersen, F. B. (1989). Long term effects and quality of life in children and adults after marrow transplantation. *Bone Marrow Transplantation* (Suppl. 4), 27–29.

Sanders, J. E. (1990). Late effects following marrow transplantation. In F. L. Johnson & C. Pochedly (Eds.), *Bone marrow transplantation in children*. New York: Raven Press.

Serota, F. T., August, C. S., O'Shea, A. T., Woodward, W. T., & Koch, P. A. (1981). Role of a child advocate in the selection of donors for pediatric bone marrow transplantation. *Journal of Pediatrics, 98*, 847–850.

Sharma, V. K., & Enoch, M. D. (1987). Psychological sequelae of kidney donation. A 5–10 year follow-up. *Acta Psychiatrica Scandinavica, 75*, 264–267.

Simmons, R. G. (1983). Social-psychological problems in living donor transplantation. In N. Levy (Ed.), *Psychonephrology II*. New York: Plenum.

Simmons, R. G., Klein, S. D., & Simmons, R. L. (1977). *The social and psychological impact of organ donation*. New York: Wiley.

Sullivan, K. (1989). Current status of bone marrow transplantation. *Transplantation Proceedings, 21*, 41–50.

Thomas, E. D., Storb, R., Clift, R. A., Fefer A., Johnson, F. L., Nieman, P. E., Lerner, K. G., Glucksberg, H., & Buckner, C. D. (1975). Bone marrow transplantation. *New England Journal of Medicine, 292*, 895–902.

Thompson, C. B., Sanders, J. E., Flournoy, N., Buckner, C. D., & Thomas, E. D. (1986). The risks of central nervous system relapse and leukoencephalopathy in patients receiving marrow transplants for acute leukemia. *Blood, 67*, 195–199.

Weizer, N., Weizman, A., Shapira, Z., Yussim, A., & Munitz, H. (1989). Suicide by related kidney donors following the recipients' death. *Psychotherapy and Psychosomatics, 51*, 216–219.

Williams T. E. (1984). Ethical and medicolegal issues in bone marrow transplantation. *American Journal of Pediatric Hematology/Oncology, 6*, 83–88.

Williams, T. E. (1990). Ethical and psychosocial issues in bone marrow transplantation in children. In F. L. Johnson & C. Pochedly (Eds.), *Bone marrow transplantation in children*. New York: Raven Press.

Wiznitzer, M., Packer, R., August, C., & Burky, E. D. (1984). Neurological complications of bone marrow transplantation. *Annals of Neurology, 16*, 569–576.

Wolcott, D. L., Fawzy, F. I., & Wellisch, D. K. (1987). Psychiatric aspects of bone marrow transplantation: A review and current issues. *Psychiatric Medicine, 4,* 299–317.

Wolcott, D. L., Wellisch, D. K., Fawzy, F. I., & Landsverk, J. (1986a). Adaptation of adult bone marrow transplant recipient long term survivors. *Transplantation, 41,* 478–484.

Wolcott, D. L., Wellisch, D. K., Fawzy, F. I., & Landsverk, J. (1986b). Psychological adjustment of adult bone marrow transplant donors whose recipient survives. *Transplantation, 41,* 484–488.

Young, D. F., & Posner, J. B. (1980). Nervous system toxicities of the chemotherapeutic agents. In P. J. Vinken & G. W. Bruyn (Eds.), *Handbook of clinical neurology.* New York: Elsevier.

8

Implications of Survival: Pediatric Oncology Patients and Their Families

ANNE E. KAZAK

With increasing rates of survival from childhood cancers, many important psychological questions related to the implications of survival are emerging. This chapter reviews empirical research on psychological adjustment in survivors of childhood cancer, with three specific emphases: (1) a focus on research designs and methodologies with discussion of new models and methodologies that pediatric psychologists can bring to this field; (2) a concern for developmental issues with respect to the age and developmental stage of the child and family and in terms of link between child and family experiences during treatment and long-term effects; and (3) a contextual approach which emphasizes families and other systems that interact with children cured of cancer.

Existing research is organized by type of question asked. A large body of psychological research concerns questions that emerge related to sequelae of the *treatments* used to cure cancer (e.g., "What are the implications of irradiation and/or chemotherapy on intelligence and academic performance?"). Other treatment-related sequelae such as growth, metabolic, or fertility problems may have psychological sequelae that have not been investigated empirically. Another literature examines long-term *individual adjustment*—emotional, social, and vocational—of survivors (e.g., "Is childhood cancer related to later psychological disturbances?"). Less well understood are the implications of childhood cancer survival on the *family* (e.g., "Does the family of origin return to 'normal' after mobilizing to cope with the demands of serious childhood illness? What are the long-term effects on parents as individuals? How do survivors function later as parents and spouses?"). Broader still are concerns that emanate from our *society* (e.g., "How will cancer survivors be treated with respect to employment, insurance, and positions of leadership?").

Van Eys (1987) proposed three components of cure: a biological cure (disease eradication); a psychological cure ("the acceptance of having had cancer as a past event without interference with normal development and schooling''; p. 114); and a social cure (''incorporation of the person cured of cancer into society, without consideration of this past history of cancer and its therapy''; p. 114). These distinctions provide a framework for understanding the complexity of survival, particularly in terms of what it means to survivors and their parents. Most research clearly focuses on the biological cure and views psychological adjustment secondary to biological cure. This approach, however, neglects the possibility of related but autonomous psychological and social processes necessary for full adjustment to survival. For example, if psychological and social cures were investigated explicitly, relatively lower rates of ''cure'' may be found than for biological cure. Throughout this chapter, the need to distinguish among biological, social, and psychological cures with respect to long-term psychological adjustment is emphasized.

Most psychological research on childhood cancer survival is in early stages of development. This chapter reviews research on psychological issues related to survival of childhood cancer and is organized in terms of studies that look predominantly at disease and treatment sequelae, adjustment of individual survivors, family adaptation, and broader concerns. The focus is on empirical reports. Studies in which children completing treatment were combined with those receiving treatment are not included, unless the groups were analyzed separately.

The Disease and Survival

Much of medicine is geared toward eradicating disease. Fortunately, for increasing numbers of children with cancer, medical knowledge and treatments have resulted in elimination of biological disease. When no evidence of disease has been detected for a period of time that is specific to the diagnosis, from a medical standpoint, the child is considered ''cured.'' Beginning in the mid-1970s a significant number of children, primarily with leukemia and some solid tumors, began to achieve long-term remissions and were identified as the first group of childhood cancer survivors. At present, approximately 60 percent of currently diagnosed children with cancer will survive. The number of childhood cancer survivors is estimated to be about 1 in every 1000 young adults (Meadows & Hobbie, 1986).

Improvements in treatment and survival have also altered the developmental framework for understanding family adjustment. With an average age of onset of 5 years and treatment duration of 1 to 3 years, childhood cancer frequently affects the family system during early child-rearing years and results in a population of long-term survivors who are still children. Family concerns during treatment (e.g., how young siblings in the family were cared for during early stages of treatment; how the patient's behavior may be affected by hospitalizations or medication during treatment; how parents' educational and career objectives may be altered) may have long-term implications. In addition, some survivors of childhood cancer will relapse and have had two or more distinct treatment regimes. Developmentally the family will be at a different stage, but it still may be a relatively young family facing the impact of illness at two or more distinct points.

As noted previously, the notion of "cure" is multifaceted. In pediatric or health psychology research, close attention to disease and treatment variables is integral to meaningful research. However, in order to fully understand psychological variables, it is important to augment the predominant medical model. In the case of childhood cancer, the medical point of cure is unquestionably a landmark for the individual and family. Its full psychological meaning is not known, however. Similarly, the thinning out of visits to the oncologist is based on a decreased *medical* need to evaluate patients frequently. There are few data to suggest that these changes have meaning psychologically in terms of the patient's overall well-being and return to normal health.

With treatment spanning several years and survival, possibly with substantial medical "late effects," an increasingly common outcome, childhood cancer has become more akin to a chronic rather than acute illness. While cancer cells may have been eradicated, treatment continues, sequelae remain, and the possibility looms of yet undetectable disease. Given the chronic nature of the diseases, treatments, and their sequelae, and commonalities with other serious pediatric conditions (e.g., concern for cognitive impairment; sequelae that require ongoing medical care), closer associations with models of other chronic pediatric illness and childhood cancer survivors should be beneficial (see Kazak, 1989; Wallander, Varni, Babani, Banis, & Wilcox, 1989).

From a medical standpoint, even for patients in remission and those with less frequent medical visits, the risk of recurrence is very real. The risk of relapse is considered low after 7 or 8 years of continuous remission, although very late recurrences have been documented (Salloum et al., 1989). In addition, survivors of childhood cancer are generally believed to be at 10 to 20 times greater risk of a second malignancy than a first malignancy in age-matched individuals in the general population (Meadows, 1991). Koocher and O'Malley (1981) turned to Greek mythology to aptly label the dilemma that children and families feel when medically cured but worried about future recurrence and/or new tumors the *Damocles syndrome.* While being honored at a banquet, Damocles looked up and noted a sword suspended above his head by a horsehair; to be happy to be a survivor but justifiably frightened of the future captures one important aspect of childhood cancer survival.

Most existing research on childhood cancer survival is based on survivors of leukemia. As survival curves change for other cancers, additional research will be necessary to understand the medical sequelae of particular diseases and treatments. Psychological research on a broader group of survivors will help to understand the more general principles of childhood cancer survival while also clarifying the role that specific types and intensities of treatment may play in long-term psychological outcome.

In general, there has been a lack of clarity regarding the role that illness factors play in psychological outcome. Although it is likely that there are commonalities in the impact of chronic childhood illness on families, different illnesses and treatments do have specific and unique impacts as well. Rolland (1984, 1987) has outlined four characteristics of illnesses (onset, course, outcome, and degree of incapacitation) that may affect psychological outcome differentially. This model could be tested even with different types of childhood cancer, both during treatment and as a model of long-term follow-up.

Treatment-Related Sequelae

Effects on Intelligence

Treatment advances, including intrathecal chemotherapy and cranial irradiation for leukemia, have played a major role in increasing rates of survival. They have also been documented to play a role in the cognitive impairments seen in some survivors of childhood cancer. In the determination of the "cost-benefit" ratio, with cost being the extent of learning and cognitive impairment pursuant to cancer therapy, the long-term impact of deficits and complications related to treatment is not fully understood. Miller (1988) raised the troublesome thought that malpractice litigation could possibly be tied to long-term treatment-related sequelae. In the area of neuropsychological sequelae, such treatment and long-term impairment are closely associated.

Declines in intellectual ability in children treated for leukemia with cranial irradiation at the dose of 24 Gy have been shown; the impact on short-term memory, attention, and cognitive processing is particularly noticeable (c.f., Eiser & Lansdowne, 1987; Meadows et al., 1981; Pfefferbaum-Levine et al., 1984). In an effort to balance survival with psychological morbidity (i.e., IQ decline), irradiation doses have been reduced when equal efficacy has been documented. The impact of a lower dose (18 Gy) appears to be less on intellectual ability, although specific deficits related to learning have been found (Himmelberg, Kazak, & Meadows, 1992; Mulhern, Fairclough, & Ochs, 1991; Mulhern, Wasserman, Fairclough, & Ochs, 1988). In addition to cranial irradiation, the effects of other treatments for childhood leukemia on cognitive functioning, specifically methotrexate, are being identified as causes of later learning problems (c.f., Ochs et al., 1991). Methodological complications in this body of research are discussed in detail by Madan-Swain and Brown (1991) and by Mulhern (Chapter 5, this volume).

Survival has increased for other childhood cancers and the impact of treatment on long-term intellectual abilities for other groups now warrants further investigation. For example, children with brain tumors are surviving with greater frequency. The higher level of irradiation that they receive, coupled with surgery, can have striking neuropsychological impacts, often combined with physical disabilities. Mulhern and colleagues reviewed literature on neuropsychological functioning in children with brain tumors pointing to the high levels of risk for learning problems, associated in particular with younger children and those who receive whole-brain irradiation (Mulhern, Hancock, Fairclough, & Kun, 1992). Because the full effects of radiation often are not seen within the first 1 to 2 years, ongoing screening and evaluation for survivors of childhood cancers who are at risk for learning problems are necessary.

Mulhern (Chapter 5) provides a thorough discussion of the neuropsychological impact of childhood cancer. Other recent reviews of this field are available (e.g., Eiser, 1991; Madan-Swain & Brown, 1991).

Academic and School Performance

A separate issue related to neuropsychological sequelae concerns the impact of treatment-related factors on academic achievement and general functioning in school. Not surprisingly, neuropsychological difficulties are closely associated with difficulties in academic achievement. Children with leukemia treated with 24 Gy were achieving at an average of two grade levels below their age, with particular difficulties in math and reading (Peckham, Meadows, Bartel, & Marrero, 1988). Special education placements and retention in a grade were common in this sample of long-term survivors.

Most literature on school issues and childhood cancer focuses on school reentry after treatment commences or on concerns about an increased rate of absences by children in treatment. Far less has been written about survivors outside of the neuropsychological literature. Often the cognitive impact of cancer treatment is first observed in the school setting. Using the Child Behavior Checklist with children off treatment for leukemia, their siblings, and a control group, the only significant differences, found consistently across the Youth Self Report, Teacher Report, and Parent Report forms, were on the School Performance scale (Sawyer, Toogood, Rice, Haskell, & Baghurst, 1989).

With some children, the question of learning problems may be raised by the school or the parents. Often school personnel are unaware of the potential academic impact of treatment that a child received many years earlier. The types of subtle learning difficulties that some childhood cancer survivors evidence are often similar to behavioral difficulties. Thus difficulties with attention and memory and a generally discouraged attitude toward school performance may be attributed to laziness, depression, family problems, or other nonspecific emotional distress.

Examination of the academic histories of childhood cancer survivors is an area ripe for psychological research. Such research would necessitate investigations of several different aspects of the survival experience. One aspect is the impact on the individual survivor of school difficulties related to treatment. As an example, Madan-Swain and Brown (1991) suggested that a learned helplessness model explains the sense of frustration and discouragement survivors may feel related to their decreased cognitive capabilities and resulting academic frustration. School-based interventions to address these concerns should be developed.

A second aspect is parental perceptions of learning difficulties in survivors and the ways in which parents process these difficulties for themselves, their children, and the school. In a study of parental perceptions of (1) acute lymphoblastic leukemia (ALL) survivors who received 1800 cGy radiation and intrathecal methotrexate, or intrathecal methotrexate alone, (2) learning-disabled children, and (3) a community control group, the ALL survivors were perceived by their parents as having poor academic skills, which were often attributed to school absences (Williams, Ochs, Williams, & Mulhern, 1991).

Additional attention could be directed toward investigating how schools can be better prepared for the diverse and long-term needs of childhood cancer survivors. Related to this is the impact of federal education legislation for childhood cancer survivors and other advocacy work on their behalf. Specifically, under the Education for All Handicapped Children Act (P.L. 94-142) and its downward extension for preschoolers (P.L. 99-457), children who have or have had cancer are eligible for special education services if they experience learning difficulties.

Fertility, Growth, and Other Late Effects

Treatment for childhood cancer can result in other long-term medical consequences including growth deficiencies, problems with sexual maturation, hypothyroidism, scoliosis, dental and facial abnormalities, cardiac disease, pulmonary problems, liver damage, urinary tract problems, and eye difficulties (Meadows & Silber, 1985). Other problems, such as obesity (Zee & Chen, 1986), have also been described.

Amputation is an accepted outcome of treatment for some bone tumors, and psychological adaptation to amputation in childhood generally is considered good. Tyc (1992) provided a thorough review of the literature on childhood limb amputation and considered factors that affect psychological outcome. Specifically, within the context of treatment for childhood cancer, it is important that the patient and family receive emotional preparation and support for the amputation. The meaning attached to the amputation (e.g., tangible removal of the tumor) and family support and coping strategies have been identified as important factors in research on this topic. Tyc also reported studies which suggested an overall lack of difference in functional outcome for patients receiving limb salvage rather than amputation. The need for more rigorous research on psychological outcome in this area is clear, with many studies relying on constructed questionnaires or clinical interviews. In addition, most of the literature on amputation has not studied long-term survivors and has not identified pertinent aspects of the adjustment process over time.

In light of the obvious physical manifestations of some treatment sequelae (e.g., short stature, amputation, enucleation [eye removal]), the effects on body image and psychological adjustment is an important question. Surprisingly, little research has reported on the relationship between more and less severe physical impairment and psychological outcome (including body image) in this population. In general, the literature on childhood chronic illness has documented an inconsistent relationship between severity of disabilities and psychological outcome (Cadman, Boyle, Szatmari, & Offord, 1987; Wallander, Feldman, & Varni, 1989). Most literature on body image in children with cancer focuses on children and adolescents currently in treatment and on short-term body changes such as hair loss and weight gain or loss.

More severe late effects have been associated with poorer psychological adjustment in a sample of long-term survivors (Greenberg, Kazak, & Meadows, 1989). Fritz and Williams (1988) provided detailed data on survivors' self-concept and body image. Although survivors reported normal self-concept scores on a standardized self-report measure, in interviews more than half expressed concerns about their bodies, including worries about relapses, and physical appearance, and they showed inclinations to somatization and hypochondriasis.

In addition, cancer therapy can have significant effects on sexual maturity and fertility (Byrne et al., 1987; Meadows & Silber, 1985). Fertility is often expressed by parents as a critical concern, although the extent to which survivors worry about it is not known. Conceptualized as a family issue, infertility could result in a lack of biological grandchildren and thus threaten continuance of the family's genetic legacy. As a problem faced by adults in the general population, infertility is usually not suspected until difficulties with conception have been identified. For the long-term survivor of childhood cancer, however, the possibility of infertility may loom for many years. Fertility may remain an area in which ambiguity continues for individuals who have had cancer. Clinically, many parents report that they have not discussed fertility concerns with their children, because it is an area in which they feel uncomfortable. In some instances the lack of open discussion of this issue parallels the reluctance to discuss the cancer experience in general. In other cases it reflects the uncertainty and discomfort with this particular topic. However, the likelihood of infertility is very often not defined, and some who have been suspected to be infertile have later successfully conceived children.

Developmental Issues

Several developmental issues that warrant consideration in survivors of childhood cancer have methodological implications for research in this area. The first is the developmental stage of the survivor. As noted, the broad age ranges included in previous studies are troublesome complications in the survivor literature. Survivors who are young children, adolescents, young adults, and in other stages of adulthood have different developmental tasks. An important goal in understanding the adjustment of survivors is the extent to which their development continues normally. Therefore, developmental parameters in studies are necessary.

An underlying concern, and an alternative conceptualization, is the impact of the age of the survivors when they were ill. This is probably of significance equal to or greater than current age. Despite efforts of the treatment team to promote the "normal" growth and development of pediatric oncology patients and their families, cancer is disruptive of normal experiences. The extent to which treatment arrests development temporarily (i.e., language delays or regression in infants and preschoolers, school absences in latency-age children, or limitations on socialization and dating in adolescents) is generally not documented in any systematic way. The long-term differential impact of minor or substantial arrests in development are topics worthy of investigation. Similarly, the extent to which treatment occurred at an age when memories can be recalled "accurately" versus developmental periods when there is no conscious memory is a variable which has not been explored with regard to its long-term impact.

The developmental stage of the family is also of interest. For childhood cancer survivors who are still children or adolescents, the ways in which parents facilitate normal development hinges on the family's stage of development as well. For the family with older children and adolescents, the possibility of loss (separation, divorce, death of a grandparent or family friend) increases, along with the developmentally expected stage of launching children to college, marriage, and/or employment.

One of the most obvious omissions in the research on childhood cancer survivors is that of a developmental perspective on the entire diagnosis–treatment–survival process. Central to this is consideration of the experience of the disease, for the child and family, and the quality of the relationship formed with the treatment team.

The psychological concerns identified as pertinent during treatment (e.g., family disruption, pain, anxiety, compliance) become part of the family's history and are integrated into family development in subtle ways. Every family with a child with cancer must face the fear that their child might die and resolve their own feelings about childhood death generally. Even when resolved, the trauma of facing the prospect of losing a child is likely to continue to influence family patterns. The long-term implications of these issues, and how they were experienced and resolved, influence the long-term survivor in ways that are generally unexplored.

A key issue in the long-term relationship among the patient, family, and treatment team concerns the way in which the cancer diagnosis is communicated. Open communication with the child and family about the diagnosis is a relatively recent standard of care. Even relatively young children understand a great deal about their illness (Bearison & Pacifici, 1989; Claflin & Barbarin, 1991) and studies of long-term survivors indicate that knowledge about their illness was perceived as strongly beneficial (Slavin, O'Malley, Koocher, & Foster, 1982). The emotional bond among the patient, family, and treatment team is an intense one and the nature of this relationship over time warrants attention, particularly with respect to compliance, trust, and boundaries among patient, family, and staff. For long-term survivors, the nature of the earlier working relationship with health-care providers may relate to the survivors' inclination to continue to utilize medical care appropriately and to engage in health-promoting activities.

A related developmental concern pertains to the period of transition from treatment. This period, during which contact with the treatment team decreases, can be a time of anxiety. More attention to the ways in which patients and families reorganize at this time is necessary. At this time, the challenge is to begin to perceive of oneself as an "ex"-cancer patient.

Ebaugh (1988) has described this process of role transition, noting that in our society today becoming "an ex" is much more likely than in previous generations. One may change careers, leave marriages, or survive illnesses that were once fatal. Some of these role changes are relatively common and have established names associated with them (e.g., alumnae, ex-husband or wife, recovering alcoholic). Others, including the survivor of childhood cancer, lack an apt name to characterize the process of ending treatment and becoming a "survivor." We lack an appropriate way to characterize children who have ended treatment but have not reached the 5-year disease-free point to be called cured. We generally do not know what they and their parents call themselves. Survivor in these cases may carry some sense of impermanence or feel somehow undeserved, paralleling Ebaugh's (1988) descriptions of doubt during role transitions. With psychological cure yet to be obtained, the label of survivor may also inhibit children, adolescents, and parents from voicing their uncertainties and troublesome memories.

Impact on the Individual Survivor

Research on disease- and treatment-related sequelae views the implications for survival as essentially linear phenomena. That is, the sequelae that have been studied result *directly* from the disease or its treatment. Although this is appropriate and useful for investigating the relationship, for example, between cranial irradiation dosage and intelligence, it is a reductionistic model that makes other potential effects on outcome more difficult to identify and measure.

The first psychological study of long-term survivors continues to be one of the best known, *The Damocles Syndrome* (Koocher & O'Malley, 1981). It is a comprehensive study of 117 survivors, with extensive data also published in other psychological literature (Gogan, Koocher, Fine, Foster, & O'Malley, 1979; Koocher, O'Malley, Gogan, & Foster, 1980; O'Malley, Foster, Koocher, & Slavin, 1980; O'Malley, Koocher, Foster, & Slavin, 1979; Slavin et al., 1982). This descriptive, retrospective study broke new ground by exploring in detail many aspects of the psychosocial functioning of survivors of childhood cancer (Table 8.1).

By the late 1980s several studies of long-term survivors were published (Cella et al., 1987; Chang, Nesbit, Youngren, & Robison, 1987; Fritz, Williams, & Amylon, 1988; Fritz & Williams, 1988; Greenberg et al., 1989; Kazak & Meadows, 1989; Moore, Glasser, & Ablin, 1987; Mulhern, Wasserman, Friedman, & Fairclough, 1989; Spirito et al., 1990; Tebbi & Mallon, 1987; Teta et al., 1986; Wasserman, Thompson, Wilimas, & Fairclough, 1987). In general, these studies either were based on interviews or involved standardized measures of adjustment or psychopathology. Most studies were of survivors of ALL or Hodgkin's lymphoma and tended to utilize samples across a broad age range. From these studies, strong support for generally normal levels of psychosocial adjustment among long-term survivors of childhood cancer emerges. Despite an overall picture of normal adjustment, there was also consistent evidence for psychological difficulties, especially subclinical anxiety or depression, for a significant percentage of survivors.

One interpretation of findings published to date is that a turning point has been reached. The data are clear in stating that most childhood cancer survivors do not have clinically significant psychological difficulties and most function well. However, a troubling subset of survivors do have significant difficulties, which we do not presently understand very well. Because of the lack of data to explain the nature and causes of psychological morbidity in this group of survivors, the extent to which the phenomena underlying the difficulties may apply to a broader representation of the survivor population is unknown.

Table 8.1. Research on Individual Adjustment of Children Off Treatment

Study	Sample	Design or Method	Major Findings
Koocher and O'Malley (1981)[a]	$N = 117$; age = 5 to 37 years; off treatment, $M = 12$	Control group = 22 patients with other resolved chronic disease; patient structured interview; patient self-report; family, parent, sibling interviews; standardized assessments	Landmark, comprehensive study; first study to show that survivors lead relatively normal lives; also documented evidence of psychological problems in nearly 50%
Teta et al. (1986)	$N = 542$ survivors; young adults at study time	Questionnaire	Surveyed socioeconomic vocational impact and documented evidence for these concerns
Cella et al. (1987)	$N = 42$; age = 18 to 32; off treatment 2 + years; Hodgkin's disease	Self-report staff ratings	1/3 maladjusted
Chang et al. (1987)	$N = 42$; age = 11 to 25 years	Self-report (MMPI, WRAT, PIC)	Learning problems identified; adjustment normal, evidence of anxiety, withdrawal, immaturity
Moore et al. (1987)	$N = 35$, ALL, solid tumors; age = 8 to 17 years; off treatment N/S[a]	Parent, teacher questionnaires; control group = 35 classmates	School and behavior problems in ALL reported
Tebbi and Mallon (1987)	$N = 20$, off treatment 5 to 19 years; amputees included; age = 17 to 37 years	Questionnaire	Overall good adjustment; family support
Wasserman et al. (1987)	$N = 40$; age = 10 to 38 years; Hodgkin's disease	Psychiatric interview	Worst thing about treatment was side effects; good educational achievement; see cancer as benefit
Fritz et al. (1988)	$N = 52$; age = 7 to 21 years; off treatment, $M = 3.7$ years	Comparison group = healthy children; patient structured interview and patient/parent self-report	Good global adjustment; communication, peer support important; disease variables not related to outcome
Fritz and Williams (1988)	$N = 41$ adolescents	Self-report; independent rating or adjustment	Good global adjustment; presence of mild adjustment problems and concerns about relationships; also saw benefits

180

Greenberg et al. (1989)	$N = 138$; to age = 8 to 16 years; off treatment >5 years	Self-report	Overall adjustment normal; more severe late effects related to psychological difficulties
Kazak and Meadows (1989)	$N = 35$; age = 10 to 15 years; off treatment >5 years	Self-report; peer-nominated controls	Scores on CBCL, Harter scales normal; survivors perceived less social support
Mulhern et al. (1989)	$N = 183$; to age = 7 to 16 years; off treatment = 2 to 15 years	CBCL completed by parents	School problems and somatic complaints fourfold increase over age/gender rates
Spirito et al. (1990)	$N = 56$; age = 5 to 12 years; off treatment, $M = 3.5$ years	Comparison group = 52 healthy; patient, parent, teacher self-report and interview	Few differences between patients and controls

[a]NS = not specified.
[a]Also published in Gogan et al. (1979), O'Malley et al. (1979), Koocher et al. (1980), Slavin et al. (1982).

Positive adaptation after a serious illness like childhood cancer supports the notion of resiliency, with most individuals using successful coping strategies. It also raises the question of the role of family systems and other systems (e.g., schools, medical facilities) in supporting children as they end treatment and resume a more nearly normal childhood. Elevated levels of psychological distress, where present, are not unexpected and appear to be consistent with the higher rates of psychopathology and emotional vulnerability in children with other chronic diseases (Cadman et al., 1987; Nelms, 1989).

Ultimately, examining the implications of survival on individuals, families, or the impact of broader societal and cultural issues necessitates a more complex, contextual model. As this review emphasizes, some findings appear relatively superficial and marginally helpful in designing interventions. Many earlier studies were very difficult to conduct. Sample sizes were limited, and choice of variables to study was unclear due to the novelty of survival in this population. Nonetheless, some methodological criticisms may be helpful in the design of research on long-term survivors.

One issue pertains to comparison groups. Although comparison groups have an important role in traditional research designs, their limitations must also be acknowledged. Comparing survivors with children who have never been ill requires using dependent variables which are applicable to both groups. These general outcome measures are affected by a myriad of other factors, which may underestimate or even wash out the effects of the cancer experience. Similarly, a growing body of literature showing "no differences" between children with chronic diseases and other children has brought into question the utility of this comparative design. No differences between survivors and others who have never been ill is not reason to assume that the impact of illness is not detectable or important.

A second issue is a developmental one. Some of the early literature reports on long-term survivors across a wide age range in an effort to obtain adequate sample sizes, mixing adults in their thirties or forties with adolescents. Research which looks at specific developmental issues for discrete age groups will be most meaningful. With increasing numbers of survivors and networks of pediatric oncology centers established for research, psychologists should focus on long-term survivors within strict developmental ranges. Given the overall normal levels of adjustment for long-term survivors, the null hypothesis is that the psychological phenonemon will be distributed as broadly in the general population for that age group as for cancer survivors.

This leads to a third issue, choice of outcome measures, and the implications of choosing measures of psychopathology or those of adjustment. Although most of the standardized instruments utilized in the studies reported in Table 8.1 rely on measures of psychopathology, evidence for positive psychological sequelae of the illness and treatment experience also were found. Existing evidence suggests that psychopathology will be found in a relatively small percentage of long-term survivors. Thus a focus on coping and adaptation may help unravel the unique attributes of cancer survivors, and it will facilitate identification of less adaptive but perhaps not psychopathological coping strategies in this population.

Finally, a lack of theoretically derived research limits the growth of psychological research on long-term survivors. Descriptive survey research has its place in documenting phenomena. However, understanding the complex and indirect effects of coping, family variables, or intervening historical events on psychological adjustment will require the articulation and testing of relevant psychological theories. Research in this area demands hypothesis generation and will benefit from the incorporation of alternative research methodologies.

Families and Survival

Two aspects of the family system warrant further investigation among survivors of childhood cancer. One, the more frequently investigated, concerns the survivor's family of origin, the child's family that experienced the entire spectrum of cancer diagnosis, treatment, and cure. The second concerns the family that the childhood cancer survivor goes on to create and into which he or she enters as an adult. Generally addressed in terms of the survivor's marital and parental status, this is actually a much broader system in which long-term implications of survival become evident.

The Survivor's Family of Origin

The first investigation of the impact of survival on parents was a small study by Peck (1979) in which the parents of children with leukemia and Wilms tumor who

Table 8.2. Research on Family Adjustment of Children Off Treatment

Study	Sample	Design or Method	Major Findings
Peck (1979)	24 parents (ALL, Wilms tumor); off treatment, $M = 5.5$ years	Parent interview	Parental anxiety evident; marital impact mixed; lack of family communications about illness
Wallace et al. (1987)	85 parents; off treatment 1 to 15+ years	Questionnaire	Relief at survival; parental anxiety
Kupst and Schulman (1988)	43 families 6–8 years from diagnosis; M age = 12.8 years	Prospective self-report and interview (includes bereaved)	Generally good coping; documents important coping resources
Spinetta et al. (1988)	$N = 51$ parents; off treatment 5 years	Prospective self-report and interview (includes bereaved)	Consistency in family coping; adaptation and communication important
Kazak and Meadows (1989)	$N = 35$ parents; patient age = 10–15 years; off treatment >5 years; ALL	Self-report; peer-nominated controls	Learning problems associated with parental distress
Speechley and Noh (1992)	63 mothers, 49 fathers; patient age = 3 to 18 years	Self-report matched controls	Parents of survivors with lower levels of social support were more distressed than controls with similar levels of support

had completed treatment for an average of 5¹/₂ years were interviewed. The results of this study continue to be echoed in more recent work with families of long-term survivors. These include parental anxieties and the importance of family and other social support, as illustrated in Table 8.2. Parents repeatedly voiced relief at survival, anxiety about relapse, and painful memories of the treatment, combined with concerns about meeting the long-term medical, psychological, and educational needs of survivors (Kupst & Schulman, 1988; Spinetta, Murphy, Vik, Day, & Mott, 1988; Wallace, Reiter, & Pendergrass, 1987).

Some insights into parental vulnerability among survivors are provided by recent research reports. In a study comparing parental anxiety, depression, and social support between mothers and fathers of patients who had completed cancer treatment with controls, comparable levels of parental adjustment were found (Speechley & Noh, 1992). However, an interaction between level of social support and group was reported, with parents of childhood cancer survivors who had low levels of social support appearing more psychologically distressed than parents in the control group. Parental distress was also found to be greater in families where long-term survivors required special education services than for those who were functioning in regular classrooms (Kazak & Meadows, 1989).

The need for prospective family research in this area is clear. Two prospective studies report data on families of long-term survivors (Kupst & Schulman, 1988; Spinetta et al., 1988). These studies also include data on families whose children died, thus providing comparisons between bereaved families and families of survivors. The results stress the importance of strong family communication and social support and indicate a consistency in coping skills over time.

Conducting longitudinal family research is very difficult, and not without its own problems. Attrition because of families lost to follow-up, deaths, or refusals complicates the results. Changes in the structure of families because of divorce, remarriages, and additional children make it difficult to compare family systems over time. Development of new instruments, or new theories to explain family functioning, can complicate data collection and interpretation, and there is always the risk that funding will be lost when studies continue for several years.

Kazak and Nachman (1991) review some of the issues to be considered in family research in pediatric oncology. Among them are three that are particularly important for families of long-term survivors: (1) conceptualization of what "normal" functioning is for a family with a child with cancer; (2) identification of measures of individual and family coping which proactively help us learn about coping strategies, rather than assuming that the absence of psychopathology indicates good mental health; and (3) consideration of racial and ethnic differences.

Family and Peer Relationships Formed by Survivors

Concerns about disturbed peer and family relationships during treatment often lead to questions regarding the ability of long-term survivors to pursue and maintain intimate relationships as they enter adulthood. Most research in this area has been epidemiological and based on survey methodologies. The results of a large epidemiological study indicate that both men and women childhood cancer survivors are somewhat less likely to "marry or live as married" than sibling controls, that those with central nervous system tumors marry later, and that no overall differences with respect to divorce rates exist between survivors and siblings (Byrne et al., 1989). Koocher and O'Malley (1981) report a lower frequency of marriage among female survivors of cancer with physical disabilities and a higher rate of marriage among male survivors than among female survivors.

As a index of success in adult life, marital status alone is a crude measure. Relatively little is known about the quality of marriages among long-term survivors and of the factors that may affect marital quality. Mutual interest in children and biological ability to have children are likely to have an impact on marital quality. Given the broad spectrum of individual psychological outcome among long-term survivors, the marriages of these individuals are likely to be equally diverse in terms of the roles and dynamics within relationships. This is an area in which essentially no research has yet been conducted.

The impact of cancer diagnosis and treatment on long-term psychological functioning inevitably will also have an impact on marital and family relationships. Partner choice and type of functioning within the relationship (e.g., the ways in which the family is structured and how roles and tasks within the family are distributed), attitudes toward children and health care, handling of anxiety, and communication patterns were learned in the survivor's family of origin during the significant trauma of childhood cancer.

Related to issues of marital quality and relationships are general social networks of close relationships, friendships, and collegial relationships during adulthood. In light of concerns about social isolation of families as they go through treatment and of the potential negative impact of absent peer relationships for the cancer patients themselves, nonmarital relationships are an area in need of further investigation.

Broader Systems and Survival

A contextual approach to childhood cancer survival entails consideration of other systems that relate to survivors and their families. These systems, including the health-care system, the educational system, and broader societal mores and policies, relate to Van Eys's (1987) notion of a ''social cure'' for childhood cancer. The areas in which educational and health-care systems can respond to the needs of long-term survivors were outlined earlier. Somewhat more difficult to remediate are the economic, employment, and insurance problems of survivors, which have been documented (Bloom, Knorr, & Evans, 1985; Cairns, Clark, Black, & Lansky, 1979; Mellette & Franco, 1987; Monaco, 1987). The usual recommendation made in this area is the call for further advocacy work by long-term survivors and their supporters. Further research pertaining to the psychological adjustment of survivors may be helpful in providing information that can educate the public and influence attitudes toward cancer survivors.

Theoretical Approaches

There are three general theoretical approaches (social ecology, coping and adaptation, and posttraumatic stress) which may aid in the conceptualization of future psychological research in pediatric oncology.

Social Ecology

The first approach we review is a social ecological and systems orientation toward childhood chronic illness (Kazak, 1989; Kazak & Nachman, 1991; Michael & Copeland, 1987). Social ecology is the study of the relationships between the developing person and the settings and contexts in which the person is actively involved (Bronfenbrenner, 1979). In this model, the child is figuratively at the center of a series of concentric rings, with the nested circles representing increasingly larger environments with which the child interacts. This model allows for consideration of family, social support, and other systems and considers the reciprocal impact between children, families, and other systems over time (Bronfenbrenner, 1986). Utilization of a social ecological perspective with respect to childhood cancer survival allows for consideration of contextual factors influencing adjustment and shifts the focus away from only disease and treatment variables. With increasing time away from treatment, clearly the role and interaction of child, family, and others, become increasingly more complex and difficult to untangle without a theoretical perspective to guide empirical research.

Stress and Coping

Another useful orientation is a general coping and adaptation perspective toward adjustment. While there are many specific approaches to coping and adjustment, the critical shared element is an emphasis on factors that contribute to successful adaptation and handling of stress. Garmezy (1987) outlined three variables in predicting invulnerability to stress: disposition, supportive family milieu, and an enhancing social support system. For the survivor of childhood cancer, understand of long-term psychological outcome could be furthered by combining research on personality and cognitive ability with consideration of social support, as well as family variables.

Related to coping mechanisms are the psychological "benefits" of childhood cancer survival expressed by survivors and their parents. Altruism, sensitivity to others, and the sense of "being a better person" because of the illness have all been expressed with some regularity in the literature on childhood cancer survival (Fritz et al., 1988). Somewhat more ambiguous in terms of their implications for long-term mental health are attributions of being "special," being "glad" that they had cancer, and use of denial as a coping mechanism among survivors. These are psychological coping mechanisms, elicited clinically, which warrant further empirical investigation.

Posttraumatic Stress

A third perspective that holds promise for understanding the long-term psychological adjustment of childhood cancer survivors is a posttraumatic stress model. In early literature, adjustment to cancer was viewed as following a sequence of loss and grief reactions, similar to the stages of grief outlined by Kubler-Ross (1969). Once one reaches the stage of acceptance, having presumably successfully resolved states of shock, anger, and sadness, the implicit expectation is that lingering painful memories will not haunt the individual. An alternative model is one of posttraumatic stress, in which the individual may reexperience certain distressing aspects of the illness and treatment repeatedly. Such posttraumatic stress is manifested on a continuum of severity and may or may not be of a level to warrant a psychiatric diagnosis.

The diagnosis of posttraumatic stress disorder (PTSD) is contingent on symptoms which include hypervigilance for threat, avoidance of traumatic reminders, recurrent intrusive memories, reckless behavior, regressive dependency, affective blunting, irritability, sense of isolation, and attentional difficulties related to exposure to an event which is beyond usual experiences and which is generally accepted as something that would bother most people (American Psychiatric Association, 1987). These experiences seem consistent with those described by Koocher and O'Malley (1981). Although PTSD is often thought of with regard to disaster or single-event trauma, Terr (1989) proposed two types of PTSD, which are particularly pertinent to children. Type I is a single-incident trauma (e.g., witnessing a shooting); Type II is related to a series of traumas or a prolonged traumatic stressor (e.g., child sexual abuse). It is hypothesized that psychological reactions to these two types of trauma may differ and should be accounted for in the measurement and understanding of PTSD in children (McNally, 1991). Whereas Type I PTSD is associated with reexperiencing, Type II is related to numbing, dissociation, and denial. Viewing childhood cancer as a Type II trauma suggests that the more serious psychological difficulties experienced by some long-term survivors may be understood as PTSD symptomatology.

There are many aspects of childhood cancer and its treatment which can be considered "traumas." The diagnosis itself is shocking and inevitably one of the most difficult stressors a family can face. The process of diagnostic evaluation and early symptoms may have been traumatic. Early phases of treatment can be considered traumatic with sudden onset of short-term side effects of chemotherapy such as nausea and vomiting, hair loss, fatigue, and inability to attend school regularly. Painful repeated procedures such as lumbar punctures, bone marrow aspirates, and bone marrow biopsies, and anticipatory anxiety around them, can also be considered traumatic. Hospitalizations and frightening events observed by the child can also remain traumatic memories (e.g., a child dying on the ward or dramatic medical codes). Other treatments such as irradiation or bone marrow transplantation may also contain uniquely traumatic elements.

Nir (1985) was the first to suggest that children undergoing treatment for cancer might experience posttraumatic stress. Pot-Mees (1989) reported evidence from clinical interviews for PTSD in children undergoing bone marrow transplantation. Using measures developed and utilized in samples of children who had witnessed traumatic events (e.g., sniper shootings), Stuber and colleagues found persistent levels of posttraumatic stress in children up to 1 year after bone marrow transplant (Stuber, Nader, Yasuda, Pynoos, & Cohen, 1991).

In a sample of adults with a relapse of cancer within the past month, posttraumatic stress related to learning of their recurrence was high, with respect to both intrusive thoughts about it and avoidant behaviors (Cella, Mahon, & Donovan, 1990). The data suggested a curvilinear relationship between adjustment and extent to which relapse was accepted as a possibility. The adults who either expected or were completely surprised at relapse were more distressed psychologically than those who had been more prepared for the possibility of relapse. There are several implications of this for the survivor of childhood cancer. For many years beyond treatment, the possibility of relapse or a second malignancy lingers. Acceptance of this possibility and the ability to verbalize this worry may be healthy and might be encouraged. A low level of anxiety regarding recurrence may promote healthy behaviors and avoidance of high-risk behaviors, such as smoking and poor dietary habits. In addition, many childhood cancer survivors have survived more than one bout with the disease. Therefore, posttraumatic responses among relapsed and multiply relapsed patients may differ from those who had one occurrence.

Consistent with a lack of family research on long-term survivors is a lack of attention to posttraumatic stress responses in parents. Parents are likely to have vivid memories of their child's treatment. The extent to which their recall may focus on intrusive or upsetting memories is unknown. Their memories will differ from those of children by virtue of being adults and their parental roles. Their memories may also be different in terms of the types of experiences which are recalled as traumatic. Evidence for parental posttraumatic stress is emerging from ongoing research at the Children's Hospital of Philadelphia and the University of California at Los Angeles. Between 40 and 50 percent of parents of children completing treatment for a minimum of 2 years previously reported posttraumatic stress within the severe range on standardized measures (Kazak et al., 1992).

Conclusion

Early psychological research on survivors of childhood cancer has documented their overall positive adjustment after treatment ends. Research has also clearly documented the presence of more serious adjustment problems in subsets of the survivor population. Existing methodologies—primarily global measures of outcome or interviews—have significant limitations in terms of providing new data to understand the personal meaning of cancer survival for children, adolescents, and their families. It will be important in future research to utilize creative methodologies to explore specific aspects of the cancer survival experience identified from the theoretical models discussed earlier.

Developmentally, the ways in which children and their families end treatment and reorganize their lives warrant further investigation. Family, school, and broader social issues need to be addressed, within a model that looks at individual coping models and contextual variables, and which aims to integrate biological and psychological cures.

The issue of intervention has been overlooked in the literature on childhood cancer survivors except with regard to acute distress and school reentry. Clearer understanding of the variables that contribute to adjustment and use of theoretical approaches with clear implications for treatment strategies will help provide avenues for clinical intervention with survivors and their families.

References

American Psychiatric Association. (1987). *Diagnostic and statistical manual of mental disorders* (3rd ed. rev.). Washington, DC: Author.

Bearison, D., & Pacifici, C. (1989). Children's event knowledge of cancer. *Journal of Applied Developmental Psychology, 10,* 469–486.

Bloom, B., Knorr, R., & Evans, E. (1985). The epidemiology of disease expenses: The costs of caring for children with cancer. *Journal of the American Medical Association, 253,* 2393–2397.

Bronfrenbrenner, U. (1979). *The ecology of human development.* Cambridge, MA: Harvard University Press.

Bronfenbrenner, U. (1986). Ecology of the family as a context for human development: Research perspectives. *Developmental Psychology, 22,* 723–742.

Byrne, J., Fears, T., Steinhorn, S., Mulvihill, J., Connelly, R., Austin, D., Holmes, G., Holmes, F., Latourette, J., Teta, M., Strong, L., & Myers, M. (1989). Marriage and divorce after childhood and adolescent cancer. *Journal of the American Medical Association, 262,* 2693–2699.

Byrne, J., Mulvihill, J., Myers, M., Connelly, R., Naughton, M., Krauss, M., Steinhorn, S., Hassinger, D., Austin, D., Bragg, K., Holmes, G., Homes, F., Latourette, H., Weyer, P., Meigs, J., Teta, M., Cook, J., & Strong, L. (1987). Effects of treatment on fertility in long-term survivors of childhood or adolescent cancer. *New England Journal of Medicine, 317,* 1315–1321.

Cadman, D., Boyle, M., Szatmari, P., & Offord, D. (1987). Chronic illness, disabilities and mental and social well-being: Findings of the Ontario Child Health Study. *Pediatrics, 79,* 805–813.

Cairns, N., Clark, G., Black, J., & Lansky, S. (1979). Childhood cancer: Nonmedical costs of the illness. *Cancer, 43,* 403–408.

Cella, D., Mahon, S., & Donovan, M. (1990). Cancer recurrence as a traumatic event. *Behavioral Medicine, 15,* 15–22.

Cella, D., Tan, C., Sullivan, M., Weinstock, L., Alter, R., & Jow, D. (1987). Identifying survivors of pediatric Hodgkin's disease who need psychological interventions. *Journal of Psychosocial Oncology, 5,* 83–96.

Chang, P., Nesbit, M., Youngren, N., & Robison, L. (1987). Personality characteristics and psychosocial adjustment of long-term survivors of childhood cancer. *Journal of Psychosocial Oncology, 5,* 43–58.

Claflin, C., & Barbarin, O. (1991). Does "telling" less protect more? Relationships among age, information disclosure, and what children with cancer see and feel. *Journal of Pediatric Psychology, 16,* 169–191.

Ebaugh, H. (1988). *Becoming an ex: The process of role exit.* Chicago: University of Chicago Press.

Eiser, C. (1991). Cognitive deficits in children treated for leukemia. *Archives of Diseases of Childhood, 66,* 164–168.

Eiser, C., & Lansdowne, R. (1987). Retrospective study of intellectual development in children treated for leukemia. *Archives of Disease in Childhood, 52,* 525–529.

Fritz, G., & Williams, J. (1988). Issues of adolescent development for survivors of childhood cancer. *Journal of the American Academy of Child and Adolescent Psychiatry, 27,* 712–715.

Fritz, G., Williams, J., & Amylon, M. (1988). After treatment ends: Psychosocial sequelae in pediatric cancer survivors. *American Journal of Orthopsychiatry, 58,* 552–561.

Garmezy, N. (1987). Stress, competence, and development: Continuities in the study of schizophrenic adults, children vulnerable to psychopathology, and the search for stress resilient children. *American Journal of Orthopsychiatry, 46,* 159–174.

Gogan, J., Koocher, G., Fine, W., Foster, D., & O'Malley, J. (1979). Pediatric cancer survival and marriage. *American Journal of Orthopsychiatry, 19,* 423–430.

Greenberg, H., Kazak, A., & Meadows, A. (1989). Psychological functioning in 8–16 year old cancer survivors and their families. *Journal of Pediatrics, 114,* 488–493.

Himmelberg, P., Kazak, A., & Meadows,A. (1992). Neuropsychologic sequelae of methotrexate therapy with and without 18 Gy cranial irradiation in children with leukemia. Manuscript under editorial review.

Kazak, A. (1989). Families of chronically ill children: A systems and social ecological model of adaptation and challenge. *Journal of Consulting and Clinical Psychology, 57*, 25–30.

Kazak, A., & Meadows, A. (1989). Families of young adolescents who have survived cancer: Social-emotional adjustment, adaptability, and social support. *Journal of Pediatric Psychology, 14*, 175–191.

Kazak, A., & Nachman, G. (1991). Family research on childhood chronic illness: Pediatric oncology as an example. *Journal of Family Psychology, 4*, 462–483.

Kazak, A., Stuber, M., Torchinsky, M., Houskamp, B., Christakis, D., & Kasiraj, J. (1992, August). *Post traumatic stress in childhood cancer survivors and their parents.* Paper presented at the annual meeting of the American Psychological Association, Washington, DC.

Koocher, G., & O'Malley, J. (1981). *The Damocles syndrome.* New York: McGraw-Hill.

Koocher, G., O'Malley, J., Gogan, J., & Foster, D. (1980). Psychological adjustment among pediatric cancer survivors. *Journal of Child Psychology and Psychiatry, 21*, 163–173.

Kubler-Ross, E. (1969). *On death and dying.* New York: Macmillan.

Kupst, M., & Schulman, J. (1988). Long-term coping with pediatric leukemia: A six-year follow-up study. *Journal of Pediatric Psychology, 13*, 7–22.

Madan-Swain, A., & Brown, R. (1991). Cognitive and psychosocial sequelae for children with acute lymphocytic leukemia and their families. *Clinical Psychology Review, 11*, 267–294.

McNally, R. (1991). Assessment of post-traumatic stress disorder in children. *Psychological Assessment: A Journal of Consulting and Clinical Psychology, 3*, 531–537.

Meadows, A. (1991). Follow-up and care of childhood cancer survivors. *Hospital Practice, 26*, 91–100.

Meadows, A., Gordon, J., Massari, D., Littman, P., Ferguson, J., & Moss, K. (1981). Declines in IQ scores and cognitive dysfunctions in children with acute lymphocytic leukemia treated with cranial irradiation. *Lancet, 2*, 1015–1016.

Meadows, A., & Hobbie, W. (1986). The medical consequences of cure. *Cancer, 58*, 524–528.

Meadows, A., & Silber, J. (1985). Delayed consequences of therapy for childhood cancer. *Cancer Journal for Clinicians, 35*, 271–286.

Mellette, S., & Franco, P. (1987). Psychosocial barriers to employment of the cancer survivor. *Journal of Psychosocial Oncology, 5*, 97–115.

Michael, B., & Copeland, D. (1987). Psychosocial issues in childhood cancer: An ecological framework for research. *American Journal of Pediatric Hematology/Oncology, 9*, 73–83.

Miller, D. (1988). Editorial: Late effects of childhood cancer. *American Journal of Diseases of Childhood, 142*, 1147.

Monaco, G. (1987). Socioeconomic considerations in childhood cancer survival. *American Journal of Pediatric Hematology/Oncology, 9*, 92–98.

Moore, I., Glasser, M., & Ablin, A. (1987). The late psychosocial consequences of childhood cancer. *Journal of Pediatric Nursing, 3*, 150–158.

Mulhern, R., Fairclough, D., & Ochs, J. (1991). A prospective comparison of neuropsychologic performance of children surviving leukemia who receive 18 Gy, 24 Gy or no cranial irradiation. *Journal of Clinical Oncology, 9*, 1348–1356.

Mulhern, R., Hancock, J., Fairclough, D., & Kun, L. (1992). Neuropsychological status of children treated for brain tumors: A critical review and integrative analysis. *Medical and Pediatric Oncology, 20,* 181–191.

Mulhern, R., Wasserman, A., Fairclough, D., & Ochs, J. (1988).Memory function in disease free survivors of acute lymphocytic leukemia given CNS prophylaxis with or without 1800 cGy cranial irradiation. *Journal of Clinical Oncology, 6,* 315–320.

Mulhern, R., Wasserman, A., Friedman, A., & Fairclough, D. (1989). Social competence and behavioral adjustment of children who are long-term survivors of cancer. *Pediatrics, 83,* 18–25.

Nelms, B. (1989). Emotional behaviors in chronically ill children. *Journal of Pediatric Psychology, 17,* 657–668.

Nir, Y. (1985). Post-traumatic stress disorder in children with cancer. In S. Eth & R. S. Pynoss (Eds.), *Post-traumatic stress disorder in children* (pp. 123–132). Washington, DC: American Psychiatric Press.

Ochs, J., Mulhern, R., Fairclough, D., Parvey, L., Whitaker, J., Ch'ien, L., Mauer, A., & Simone, J. (1991). Comparison of neuropsychologic functioning and clinical indicators of neurotoxicity in long-term survivors of childhood leukemia given cranial radiation or parenteral methotrexate: A prospective study. *Journal of Clinical Oncology, 9,* 145–151.

O'Malley, J., Foster, D., Koocher, G., & Slavin, L. (1980). Visible physical impairment and psychological adjustment among pediatric cancer survivors. *American Journal of Psychiatry, 137,* 94–96.

O'Malley, J., Koocher, G., Foster, D., & Slavin, L. (1979). Psychiatric sequelae of surviving childhood cancer. *American Journal of Orthopsychiatry, 49,* 608–616.

Peck, B. (1979). Effects of childhood cancer on long-term survivors and their families. *British Medical Journal, 1,* 1327–1329.

Peckham, V., Meadows, A., Bartel, N., & Marrero, O. (1988). Educational late effects in long-term survivors of acute lymphocytic leukemia. *Pediatrics, 81,* 127–133.

Pfefferbaum-Levine, B., Copeland, D., Fletcher, J., Reid, H., Jaffe, N., & McKinnon, W. (1984). Neuropsychological assessment of long-term survivors of childhood leukemia. *American Journal of Pediatric Hematology/Oncology, 6,* 123–128.

Pot-Mees, C. C. (1989). *The psychosocial effects of bone marrow transplantation in children.* Delft, Netherlands: Eburon.

Rolland, J. (1984). Towards a psychosocial typology of chronic and life threatening illness. *Family Systems Medicine, 2,* 245–262.

Rolland, J. (1987). Chronic illness and the life cycle: A conceptual framework. *Family Process, 26,* 203–221.

Salloum, E., Pico, J., Herait, P., Bayle, C., Ghosn, M., Moran, A., Friedman, S., & Hayat, M. (1989). Very late recurrence of childhood acute lymphoblastic leukemia treated with chemoimmunotherapy: A report of three cases occurring 19, 11, and 9 years after discontinuation of chemotherapy. *Medical Pediatric Oncology, 17,* 155–158.

Sawyer, M., Toogood, I., Rice, M., Haskell, C., & Baghurst, P. (1989). School performance and psychological adjustment of children treated for leukemia. *American Journal of Pediatric Hematology/Oncology, 11,* 146–152.

Slavin, L., O'Malley, J., Koocher, G., & Foster, D. (1982). Communication of the cancer diagnosis to pediatric patients: Impact on long-term adjustment. *American Journal of Psychiatry, 139,* 179–183.

Speechley, K., & Noh, S. (1992). Surviving childhood cancer, social support, and parents' psychological adjustment. *Journal of Pediatric Psychology, 17,* 15–31.

Spinetta, J., Murphy, J., Vik, P., Day, J., & Mott, M. (1988). Long-term adjustment in families of children with cancer. *Journal of Psychosocial Oncology, 6,* 179–191.

Spirito, A., Stark, L., Cobiella, C., Drigan, R., Androkites, A., Hewett, K. (1990). Social adjustment of children successfully treated for cancer. *Journal of Pediatric Psychology, 15,* 359–371.

Stuber, M., Nader, K., Yasuda, P., Pynoos, R., & Cohen, S. (1991). Stress responses after pediatric bone marrow transplantation: Preliminary results of a prospective longitudinal study. *Journal of the American Academy of Child and Adolescent Psychiatry, 30,* 952–957.

Tebbi, C., & Mallon, J. (1987). Long-term psychosocial outcome among cancer amputees in adolescence and early adulthood. *Journal of Psychosocial Oncology, 5,* 69–82.

Terr, L. (1989). *A proposal for an overall DSM-IV category, Post-traumatic stress.* Paper prepared for the DSM-IV Workgroup on Post-traumatic Stress Disorder, Washington, DC.

Teta, M., Po, M., Kasl, S., Meigs, J., Myers, M., & Mulvihill, J. (1986). Psychosocial consequences of childhood and adolescent cancer survival. *Journal of Chronic Diseases, 39,* 751–759.

Tyc, V. (1992). Psychosocial adaptation of children and adolescents with limb deficiencies: A review. *Clinical Psychology Review, 12,* 275–292.

Van Eys, J. (1987). Living beyond cure: Transcending survival. *American Journal of Pediatric Hematology/Oncology, 9,* 114–118.

Wallace, M., Reiter, P., & Pendergrass, T. (1987). Parents of long-term survivors of childhood cancer: A preliminary survey to characterize concerns and needs. *Oncology Nursing Forum, 14,* 39–43.

Wallander, J., Feldman, W., & Varni, J. (1989). Physical status of psychosocial adjustment in children with spina bifida. *Journal of Pediatric Psychology, 14,* 89–102.

Wallander, J., Varni, J., Babani, L., Banis, H., & Wilcox, K. (1989). Family resources as resistance factors for psychological maladjustment in chronically ill and handicapped children. *Journal of Pediatric Psychology, 14,* 157–174.

Wasserman, A., Thompson, E., Wilimas, J., & Fairclough, D. (1987). The psychological status of survivors of childhood/adolescent Hodgkin's disease. *American Journal of Diseases of Childhood, 141,* 626–631.

Williams, K., Ochs, J., Williams, M., & Mulhern, R. (1991). Parental report of everyday cognitive abilities among children treated for acute lymphoblastic leukemia. *Journal of Pediatric Psychology, 16,* 13–26.

Zee, P., & Chen, C. (1986). Prevalence of obesity in children after therapy for acute lymphoblastic leukemia. *American Journal of Pediatric Hematology/Oncology, 8,* 294–299.

9

Care of the Dying Child
and the Bereaved

IDA M. MARTINSON AND DANAI PAPADATOU

This chapter discusses the principles of children's hospice care and describes some of the existing programs that provide services to dying children and bereaved families. The major studies that address issues related to the dying process in children and the bereavement experienced by parents and siblings following the death of a child are also discussed and suggestions are offered concerning the development of further research and applications of models of care.

Hospice Philosophy and Hospice Care

The concept of hospice refers not to a facility or institution but rather to a philosophy of care (Corr & Corr, 1983). It is an approach focused on comfort when cure is no longer a reasonable expectation. Hospice care addresses the physical, psychosocial, and spiritual needs of the dying individual and provides support to family members during the illness and after the death of the patient. The goal is to "maximize present quality of living" (National Hospice Organization, 1987) by promoting a way of living rather than a way of dying.

The philosophy of hospice care applies both to adults and to children, but the services provided differ. First of all, children requiring hospice care suffer from different diseases than adults, although childhood cancer is the most common cause of death of children presently involved in pediatric hospice. During the terminal phase, families are more directly involved in caring for the child. Parents derive satisfaction from being the primary caregivers but require a lot of support and guidance in meeting the complex needs of the child and other family members. Furthermore, the death of a child affects a great number of individuals of various ages (parents, siblings, peers, grandparents) who are often in need of support. The grief experienced by relatives is thought to be more intense, compli-

193

cated, and long lasting than the grief experienced after the death of an adult patient, and it requires bereavement services for longer periods of time. Finally, caregivers need to acquire in-depth knowledge of the developmental needs of children, the family's dynamics, and the coping patterns used throughout the illness and the child's death. Caregivers also need specific skills that will help them communicate with children on a direct, indirect, and symbolic level, and they need to use appropriate methods of intervention to help families cope with the insistent psychosocial problems they face during the terminal phase and after the child's death.

According to Children's Hospice International (1989), hospice care is "both a concept for caring and a system of comprehensive, interdisciplinary services." Its goal is the enhancement of quality of life as defined by each child-and-family unit. It considers the child and family in the decision-making process about services and treatment choices to the fullest degree that is possible and desired. It addresses, in a comprehensive and consistent way, the physical, social, and spiritual needs and issues of children and families through an individualized plan of care. Finally, it ensures continuity and consistency of care in all settings where hospice services are provided. The International Work Group on Death, Dying and Bereavement (in press) has published a statement pertaining to the principles of palliative care for children which can serve as guidelines in developing hospice services across cultures.

Child Hospice Movement

In the United States approximately 100,000 children die each year. The most recent statistics indicate that 937 per 100,000 children are infants who die within the first year of their lives due to birth defects, sudden infant death syndrome, and problems related to pregnancy, childbirth, or complications following birth. Death rates fall to 44 per 100,000 children for those aged 1 to 4, the leading cause of death being accidental injury. There are 24 deaths per 100,000 children aged 5 to 14, the leading cause of death being accidents (National Center for Health Statistics, 1990).

The rate of death from pediatric cancers has decreased dramatically during recent years and now accounts for 1800 per year in the United States. Before the advent of chemotherapy, children died from leukemia within a very few months. Table 9.1 presents the data on children's deaths, including cancer.

Until the early part of the twentieth century, children in developing countries died at home. Because hospitals were not common, the process of dying as well as the death of any family member, including a child, took place within the home. Between the 1930s and the 1960s in the United States, services for dying children became increasingly centered in the hospital. If a child was terminally ill, he or she became a patient in an acute, cure-oriented, technology-based system. This practice continued into the early 1970s, when dying children were still being admitted to the hospital for care.

In 1972 Ida Martinson became involved in providing home-care services to a

Table 9.1. Estimated Number of Deaths where
Hospice Clinical Services Might Have Been
Utilized, 1988

Up to 1 year	
Congenital anomalies (birth defects)	8,244
1–4 years	
Congenital anomalies (birth defects)	913
Cancer, leukemia	542
Heart disease	352
Human immunodeficiency virus (HIV)	114
Subtotal	1,921
5–14 years	
Cancer, leukemia	1,096
Congenital anomalies (birth defects)	499
Heart disease	324
Asthma and other pulmonary disease	103
Carcinoma and other tumors	103
Cerebrovascular diseases (stroke)	72
Subtotal	2,197
15–19 years	
Cancer, leukemia	947
Heart disease	545
Human immunodeficiency virus infections	267
Congenital anomalies (birth defects)	237
Cerebrovascular diseases	133
Asthma and other pulmonary diseases	89
Subtotal	2,218
Total:	14,580

Source: Data adapted from advanced report of Final Death
Statistics, 1990. Reprinted by permission of W.B. Saunders,
Journal of Pediatric Oncology Nursing, July 1993.

dying child with cancer whose pediatric oncologist was frustrated because he had to admit the boy to the hospital solely because he was dying. Martinson's response was immediate: "Why admit a dying child to a hospital when the child would most likely want to be at home?" This question and many more regarding the death of a child from cancer became the basis for a major research program, *Home Care for the Child with Cancer* (Martinson, Moldow, & Henry, 1980). The research project served as a model of pediatric hospice care. It examined the feasibility and desirability of the home as an alternative to hospitalization for children dying of cancer.

When the study began in the early 1970s seriously ill children were admitted to the hospital to die. Each of the 58 families who participated in the study presented a new opportunity to refine the model of home care for dying children. Findings indicated that the families' responses to caring for their dying children at home was encouraging and the tremendous strength with which they dealt with the crisis of the death of their own children encouraged Martinson to tell their stories.

One value of Martinson's research has been the use of families' stories to illustrate and make more meaningful the objective data. For example, Martinson reported the remarkable story of an adolescent boy who knew he was going to die and who wished to be cared for at home. He had fallen in the bathroom and had fractured both hips. The pediatric oncologist and the pediatric surgeon made home visits to ascertain the situation and when the family discovered that the surgeon would not perform surgery, they requested that the child be permitted to remain at home. This request dismayed Martinson, who felt that the child should be in the hospital. Home care and pediatric hospice care at that time did not consider it appropriate for a child with two fractured hips to be cared for at home, and Martinson initially considered using this case to illustrate conditions for which home care would not be appropriate and hospitalization would be necessary. However, in the meantime, the parents provided superb care for their child at home, going so far as to use their best china dishes and their sterling silver when feeding him. The nurse who supported the family in all their efforts thought the boy's death at home was "outstanding." When Martinson's team interviewed the boy's mother 1 month postdeath, the mother revealed that "the day before he died, he said to me, 'I never used to like you but I sure love you now.' " That statement helped Martinson realize that what her project was really about was creating an environment in which communication could be reestablished and relationships strengthened within the family. What greater challenges could health-care providers have?

There are numerous published reports of various aspects of this study (Martinson, 1976; Martinson, Birenbaum, Martin, Lauer, & Eng, 1991; Martinson, Davies, & McClowry, 1987; Martinson, Kersey, & Nesbitt, 1987; Martinson & Martinson, 1983; Martinson, Nesbit, & Kersey, 1985; Martinson et al., 1978, 1980, 1982, 1986; Moldow, Armstrong, Henry, & Martinson, 1982; Moldow & Martinson, 1980, 1991). This same sample also was used in articles by Edwardson (1983, 1984, 1985). Since then, there have been several other studies of alternatives to hospitalization (Lauer & Camitta, 1980; Lauer & Mulhern, 1984; Lauer, Mulhern, Bohne, & Camitta, 1985; Lauer, Mulhern, Hoffman, & Camitta, 1986; Lauer, Mulhern, Wallskog, & Camitta, 1983; Martin, 1986). While Martinson's study examined care for children dying of cancer, more recent studies have included care for children with other kinds of terminal conditions.

Home-Care Programs

Mary Lauer developed a home-care program at Children's Hospital in Milwaukee, Wisconsin, based on the model provided by Martinson. In January 1976 an eight-bed chemotherapy unit was opened, and for 2 years pediatric oncology patients received comprehensive care, including terminal care, in that unit. In June 1978 the nursing staff initiated home-care services and began collecting data on the experiences derived from the first year of the home-care program. This program has since expanded from children who have cancer to any child with a terminal illness. Research publications from this group have focused on family adjustment following a child's death at home (Lauer et al., 1983; Mulhern, Lauer, & Hoffman, 1983). They found that multiple factors influenced the positive adjustment of siblings who participated in home care. The siblings expressed their desire to be involved in the care of the dying child, and findings suggest increased family intimacy and communication.

In 1980, two years after the Milwaukee initiative, a home-care program was started at Children's Hospital of Los Angeles. From the beginning, this program was designed to serve children with any terminal illness. This program was funded in 1985 by the Maternal and Child Health Program as a Pediatric Hospice Demonstration Model Project to conduct a retrospective chart review and also to conduct a prospective study. The study team identified 167 patients who had received services from August 1980 to May 1981 and located 114 primary caretakers (68.3 percent of the sample population) to be part of the retrospective study. The prospective study included 59 additional patients and families participating in the home-care program from mid-1985 to February 1988, and included 46 (78.0 percent of the sample population) of the primary caretakers. Although more children died in the hospital than at home (54.5 percent vs. 45.5 percent), more than two-thirds of the total time that children spent in the hospice program was spent at home. While most of the children died from cancer (72.2 percent), other diagnoses included neonatal deaths (14 percent) and deaths related to AIDS (4.6 percent) (Martin, 1989). Families were able to provide home care with the assistance of nursing personnel.

Among currently active hospice and home-care programs, one was developed at Johns Hopkins Hospital in Baltimore and another at Memorial Sloan Kettering Cancer Center in New York. Two institutions that provide beds specifically for pediatric hospice care are St. Mary's Hospital for Children in Bayside, New York, and San Diego Hospice in San Diego, California. Adult hospices are increasingly including children in their programs, and children's hospitals are providing more hospice services to their families.

Programs also have been developed outside the United States. In 1982, in Melbourne, Australia, the district nursing service of a hospital's hematology/oncology pediatric unit expanded its role to provide a 24-hour on-call service for the families of children dying from cancer. In a 15-month period, 21 children, aged 2 to 18 years, were included in the Pediatric Palliative Care Project. All but 3 died at home. According to Norman and Bennett (1986), in Australia, home is a viable alternative to hospitalization for the terminally ill child until the time of death. They concluded that ''it is both feasible and desirable for parents who wish to assume responsibility for total care of their child to do so with the support and guidance of a team of health care professionals who are available 24 hours a day.''

Similar programs are appearing in Asia. The Childhood Cancer Foundation in Taiwan provides support for nurses to assist Chinese families caring for their dying children at home. In 1992 Dr. Susie Kim, a nurse and dean of the Ewha Womans University in Seoul, South Korea, established a pediatric hospice. Other adult-focused hospices in Korea also care for dying children at home. The Tianjin Hospice Program in China cares for children dying from cancer at home. To date, however, there are no known pediatric hospice programs in Japan or Hong Kong.

In England, home care for dying children developed later than hospice care for adults. Dr. Cecily Saunders, founder of St. Christopher's Hospice, chose not to include children in her original hospice model because the number of dying children was relatively small and she did not believe she had the appropriate background in pediatrics. Today, however, home care for dying children is more widely available in England. In the early 1980s a respite facility in Oxford, Helen House, provided respite care primarily for families with long-term chronically ill children (Dominica 1982, 1987). At the Great Ormand Street Children's Hospital (London) home care for children dying of cancer is provided from the time of diagnosis through the terminal stage of the illness, including bereavement follow-up services.

A home-based palliative program for children initiated in 1984 at the Hospital for Sick Children in Toronto, Canada, provided care to 29 children, most of whom had central nervous system tumors. All but 1 of the 29 children died at home (Duffy, Pollock, Levy, Budd, Caulfield, & Koran 1990; Levy et al., 1990).

In Greece, the Nursing School of the University of Athens, with partial funding from the European Economic Community, developed a home-based palliative program for children with cancer. During the first phase, a feasibility study was conducted and the findings suggested that home care was both feasible and desirable for families who, despite the lack of home-care services, preferred caring for their child at home during the terminal phase of the disease (Papadatou, Yfantopoulos, Vassilatou-Kosmidis, & Maistros, 1992). Semistructured interviews were conducted with 15 families who lived in the area of Athens and whose children had died. The study confirmed a significant need for families to care for their children at home during the terminal period, a choice which generally was reinforced by the children's requests. In 87 percent of the cases, children chose to return home as they became aware that they were dying. They expressed their choices directly, indirectly, or symbolically. Findings indicated that the experience at home was perceived as "very positive" by 40 percent and "positive" by 60 percent of the 10 families who chose to care for their children at home. All of the mothers were involved in their children's care and were helped mostly by spouses, other children, and relatives. The mothers, however, reported a greater need for support and guidance by members of the health-care team and, in particular, by physicians.

The second phase of the project, which currently is under way, involves an intensive training program of 600 hours that is being offered to health professionals who are interested in providing home-care services to children with cancer and their families. In 1993, following the completion of the training program, an ongoing program of clinical care and research in pediatric hospice-home care will be in place.

Other kinds of environments in which hospice services have been provided to children include "houses" located close to hospitals. These facilities offer professional nursing services for a limited period of time and can be an appropriate adjunct to hospice-home care. A homelike environment is made available that is close to the acute-care hospital. Terminally ill children who are unable to return home or families who need respite can be referred to such a houses. Such a project currently is under way in Vancouver, Canada.

The development of the pediatric hospice movement has been influenced by the Children's Hospice International, founded in 1983 by Ann Armstrong-Dailey. She had worked in the National Hospice Organization and believed that a separate organization for children was necessary. Through articles and conferences, this organization has raised the consciousness of both health-care professionals and the public to the tragedy of the death of a child (Dailey, 1986). A major portion of the above historical perspective was published in *Journal of Pediatric Oncology Nursing,* July 1993.

Studies on Psychosocial Issues Related to the Dying Process

There is very little research concerning the circumstances surrounding the death of a child and the dying process as it is experienced by children, parents, siblings, and health professionals. Most accounts remain anecdotal and provide insights or suggestions for clinical interventions. One reason for the lack of research on terminal care is the increased rate of cure for childhood cancers, which has led to greater emphasis on studies of coping patterns and the adjustment of families to this chronic illness (see Kupst, Chapter 2, this volume). The absence of a widely accepted definition of the "terminal phase" and the lack of specific criteria establishing when a child is considered to be "dying" or "terminally ill" also hinder research on terminal care.

Our definition of dying refers to the end stage of an illness, when disease is beyond the present-day management of a medical goal of a cure. The goal then is to comfort the child. This definition does not include respite care for chronically ill children with life-threatening illnesses.

Studies of Dying Children

The first studies of dying children were conducted in the 1950s by psychiatrists who were consulted by pediatricians confronting psychological problems among leukemic children (Bozeman, Orbach, & Sutherland, 1955; Cobbs, 1956; Richmond & Waisman, 1955; Solnit & Green, 1959). These studies were followed by two studies conducted by French psychoanalytically oriented physicians and psychologists (Alby & Alby, 1971; Alby, Alby, & Chassigneux, 1967; Bernard & Alby, 1956). The purpose of these studies was to examine the reactions of children with leukemia, of their parents (particularly mothers), and of the physicians and nurses who were confronted with the diagnosis, the short remissions, the relapses, and the impending and actual death of the children. Clinical data were collected using semistructured interviews with children and their parents and nonstructured interviews with members of the treatement teams who shared their frustrations and difficulties in caring for the child and the family. Although these studies presented methodological problems, they provided rich data and clinical insights in explaining the relationships and interactions established among children, parents, and hospital staff.

A major concern in these early studies was whether children were aware of the seriousness of their condition and their impending death. Natterson and Knudson (1960) and Morrissey (1963a, 1963b) studied children's understanding of death, based on parents' accounts and hospital staffs' observations. Their approach was criticized for relying on parents' and staffs' observations of children with cancer who were hospitalized instead of the children themselves and for not having a control group that would allow a comparison with children who had chronic but nonfatal illness. Other studies focused on the communication patterns among dying children, their parents, and health professionals (Karon & Vernick, 1968; Kikuchi, 1972; Solnit & Green, 1963; Vernick & Karon, 1965).

Waechter (1971, 1987a, 1987b, 1987c) worked directly with dying children and, using projective techniques, found that children with cancer were preoccupied with their future and told stories relating to death. From her studies, it became apparent that the dilemma of whether clinicians should or should not inform a child that he or she has a potentially fatal illness was meaningless because the child was already intimately concerned and aware. Waechter's research provided a major impetus for advocating a more open approach with children, for encouraging them to express their concerns, and for having their questions answered honestly.

Studies by Spinetta and colleagues supported Waechter's conclusions (Spinetta, 1974; Spinetta & Maloney, 1975; Spinetta, Rigler, & Karon, 1973, 1974). He found that terminally ill children had a hightened awareness of the hospital experience, personnel, and procedures. In contrast to other chronically ill children, patients with leukemia expressed more hospital and nonhospital anxiety.

Bluebond-Langner (1978) reported an anthropological study of a pediatric oncology ward that demonstrated how children knew that they were dying. According to Bluebond-Langner, they acquired this knowledge in five consecutive stages. Regardless of their ages, children in the first stage realized the seriousness of their illness. In the second stage they learned, from personal experience, the side effects of treatment. In the third stage they understood the purpose of the procedures and treatment. During the fourth stage, and as their condition deteriorated, children became aware of the cycles of relapses and remissions of their disease, but they did not yet perceive that they were going to die. It was only when they learned about the death of another child on their unit that they realized they too could die. Children accumulated information about their disease through their personal experiences and they progressively came to understand their disease and its prognosis.

These three researchers, Waechter, Spinetta, and Bluebond-Langner, provided the research base for policies advocating improved communication between health-care professionals, the family, and the dying child. Today it is ironic that many children may be at risk for believing they are dying or they are going to die when indeed they are not. This situation is created by the increased complexity of treatment regimes which, in effect, bring many children close to death and then medically rescue them from death in an effort to cure them.

A French psychoanalyst, Raimbault, described the concerns, feelings, and anxieties expressed by children with life-threatening diseases regarding their death. However, she believed that death was not the children's only concern and that it did not necessarily prevent them from enjoying life, provided that there were people close to them who were willing and able to listen to them without lying or inducing false hopes. According to Raimbault (1975), children who openly expressed themselves, regardless of their age, developed the same images and conclusions about death as adults did. She believed that there was no special knowledge about death that children ought to be taught but that children had beliefs, concerns, and feelings that had to be expressed and heard. The challenge for parents and health professionals was how to listen to dying children talk about their concerns (Raimbault, 1991).

Clinical reports of the management of the dying child from cancer also included concerns for their families (Evans & Edin, 1968; Geis, 1965; Green, 1967; Howell, 1967; Knudson & Natterson, 1960; Singher, 1974). Clinical studies of the care of the dying child also included reports of pain management (Burne, 1988; Burne & Hunt, 1987; Chapman & Goodall, 1980; Hunt, 1990; Martinson et al., 1982). Foley & Whittan (1991) published a review of the care of the dying child from cancer and the concerns of family members. Studies of home versus hospital care for the dying child continued to encourage the home-care alternative (Dufour, 1989; Hutter, Farrell, & Meltzer, 1991). Wilson (1982) discussed the establishment of a pediatric hospice and Corr and Corr (1992) reiterated the concept of pediatric hospice care.

Studies of Parents of Dying Children

Several attempts have been made to examine the reactions of parents in response to the awareness of their children's impending death. Although a process of "anticipatory grief" has been described in the literature, questions have been raised about whether this term is a misnomer of a phenomenon that is more complex than grieving only in anticipation of a child's death. For example, Rando (1986) found that parental mourning included grief responses over past losses (e.g., a mother may grieve over the dreams she once had for her healthy child), present losses (e.g., a father may grieve over the actual deterioration of the child's condition), and future losses (e.g., parents may grieve over the losses that will occur in the family as a result of the child's death). Grieving over these losses evoked feelings of intense anxiety, anger, depression, and guilt. Often parents experienced a process of "decathexis," not from their child, but from the hopes, dreams, and expectations they once held for him or her.

Some of the early studies conducted in the 1960s, when most children with cancer died of the illness, attempted to describe parents' reactions from the time of diagnosis to the inevitable death of their child. Natterson and Knudson (1960) described three phases experienced by mothers who learn that their child has cancer: (1) initial shock and denial that progressively give way to an intellectual acceptance of the reality, (2) a period when energy is directed to activities that offer hope, but during which a relapse of the disease triggers a process of anticipatory grief; and (3) a period of detachment and philosophical resignation about the death of the child. However, our clinical experience led us to conclude that parents' detachment from their dying children was rare.

Other studies focused on the terminal phase in an attempt to examine the phenomenon of anticipatory grief. Rando (1983) found that among parents of children who had cancer, "too much" anticipatory grief, experienced for a long period of time (over 18 months), compromised the parents' ability to care for and interact with their dying children, who consequently were left feeling abandoned and emotionally isolated. On the other hand, "too little" or an absence of anticipatory grief, due to the short length of a terminal illness (less than 6 months), resulted in intense grief reactions at the time of death and predisposed family members to poor bereavement outcomes. Rando concluded that there is an "optimum" degree of anticipatory grief that is therapeutic and associated with fewer atypical grief responses following the death of a child, and she stressed the need for further research to determine more precisely when anticipatory grief has greater therapeutic value.

There are conflicting findings regarding the value of anticipatory grief on adjustment following the death of a child. Some researchers believe it may have a positive effect on the postdeath experience (e.g., Alby, Alby, & Chassigneux, 1967; Binger et al., 1969; Friedman, Chodoff, Mason, & Hamburg, 1963; Futterman, Hoffman, & Sabshin, 1972; Natterson & Knudson, 1960), while others believe that grieving in anticipation is unrelated to bereavement outcomes (e.g., Benfield, Leib, & Reuter, 1976; Kennell, Sltyter, & Klaus, 1970; Spinetta, Swarner, & Sheposh, 1981). Rosenblatt (1983) postulated that anticipatory grief can make postdeath grief problematic because the person who anticipates the death of a loved one invests more energy in the care of the dying patient and therefore suffers more as he or she has to disengage from additional memories and emotional experiences after the death.

It may be more important to consider the duration and circumstances with which grieving over the impending death of a child occurs than the various forms by which grief responses are experienced, expressed, and handled within a family during the terminal period. The grieving process that may develop in response to a child's impending death does not minimize the pain over the loss of the child and it is qualitatively different from postdeath grief. Parents who have been grieving during the terminal period may have less intense grief reactions at the time of death, but their responses should not discourage health-care professionals from providing them extensive support during their period of bereavement. According to Miles (1985), these parents may need even more support than parents who lose their child due to a sudden death. In addition, special attention should be directed to the differences in the grieving patterns used by mothers and fathers. Rando (1983) found that although fathers did not always participate in the child's care during hospitalization, they nevertheless experienced anticipatory grief that was equal to, or more intense than mothers'.

Finally, some studies (Lauer et al., 1983; Mulhern et al., 1983) assessed how the circumstances of the terminal care that is provided to dying children affect parental bereavement. Lauer et al. (1983) interviewed parents between 3 and 28 months after the death of their children. They compared 24 sets of parents who cared for their dying children at home to 13 whose children died in the hospital and found more favorable outcomes among the home-care parents. Home-care parents had less guilt, fewer regrets, and more positive views of themselves and their marriages than did hospital-care parents.

Professionals Involved in the Care of Dying Children

Contrary to the popular belief that professionalism involves an attitude of "detached concern," effective terminal care presupposes emotional investment on the part of health professionals. As a result, caregivers who are involved in caring for dying children and bereaved families may be at risk for developing chronic stress and burnout. Several studies have discussed the kinds of stressors encountered by members of the health-care team who care for children with life-threatening diseases in general (Lattanzi, 1985; Lattanzi-Licht, 1991; Raimbault, 1975) and, more particularly, with childhood cancer (Alby & Alby, 1971; Goodell, 1980; Koocher, 1980; Papadatou, 1991; Rothenberg, 1967; Sahler, McAnarney, & Friedman, 1981). Some of the studies provided suggestions for staff support and consultation (Gronseth, Martinson, Kersey, & Nesbit, 1981; Koocher, Sourkes, & Kean, 1979; Maloney & Ange, 1982). For example, Vachon and Pakes (1984) described the specific stressors that are encountered in various pediatric settings that provide care to critically and terminally ill children and the mediating factors that either increased or decreased a caregiver's vulnerability to stress. They recommended prevention and coping strategies that reduce stress.

Some of the occupational factors which are specific to the care of childhood cancer include (1) the chronic nature of the disease and the uncertainty of its development; (2) the emotional impact of the long-term involvement with children and families, which may lead to overinvolvement with a specific child or parent; (3) the witnessing of the suffering of dying children who struggle to maintain a sense of control over a premature death; (4) the occurrence of multiple deaths within a short period with no available time for grieving; (5) the grief experienced over the death of a child, which leads to chronic levels of stress when it not recognized and expressed; (6) the role ambiguity that ensues when the goal of intervention becomes one of caring instead of curing; and (7) the social stigma and isolation that sometimes are experienced by team members who care for the dying child with cancer and the bereaved family. Several of these stressors may increase a sense of helplessness and powerlessness among health-care providers, who need to acknowledge the potentially damaging effects of their work and to develop positive coping strategies. Chiriboga, Jenkins, and Bailey (1983) found that hospice nurses who coped best with the difficulties of terminal care expressed emotional responses to job-related stresses and resorted to more cognitive and rational kinds of coping strategies. In other words, they were able to acknowledge how their work affected them and they were able to put their experiences in a cognitive framework that helped them give meaning to caring for dying patients and bereaved families. This finding may explain how this highly demanding and stressful kind of work can be very rewarding for those caregivers who are involved.

Studies of Bereavement
Parents' Response to the Death of a Child

The death of a child is one of the most painful experiences for any parent. Schmidt (1987) discussed how the death of a child reverses the natural order of life in that parents expect to grow old and see their children into adulthood. It is significant that there is no culturally approved term that describes the state of a parent who has experienced the death of a child. The term "widow" or "widower" refers to a spouse who has lost a mate, and "orphan" to a child who has lost his or her parents. According to Schmidt, these kinds of deaths are more culturally acceptable than a parent's loss of his or her child as evidenced by the availability of terms to refer to the former kinds of loss and not to the latter. A parent's experience of the death of a child has been described as the most difficult and intensive of all grief experiences (Fischoff & O'Brien, 1976; Miles, 1985; Sanders, 1979–80; Tietz, McSherry, & Britt, 1972; Videka-Sherman, 1982). Despite this, little is known of the actual impact of the death, the length of time needed for resolution, or the variables that influence the particular outcomes achieved.

A classic study by Lindemann (1944) suggested that grief should be resolved in a matter of weeks. However, more recent studies indicated that a much longer time frame, including a great degree of individual variability, is more realistic. McClowry, Davies, May, Kulenkamp, and Martinson (1987) investigated families 7 to 9 years after the death of a child and found that grieving may last that long. They identified three different kinds of grieving patterns used by parents: (1) getting over it by accepting and giving some meaning or explanation to the death; (2) filling the emptiness by keeping busy and involved in various projects and activities; and (3) maintaining the connection by integrating the "empty space" caused by the child's death into everyday living and cherishing recollections of the child. It was evident that grief did not follow a timetable but rather seemed to be an individual journey. Other studies reported that parents may still experience intense symptoms 2 to 3 years after the death of their children (Miles, 1985; Moore, Gilliss, & Martinson, 1988; Spinetta et al., 1981).

McHorney and Mor (1988) studied predictors of bereavement and its related costs to the health-care system. They concluded that bereavement may have a significant impact on the health-care system in terms of increased physician visits. In the case of somatic symptoms, there could be an increased burden to the health-care system with unnecessary medical testing and hospitalization for the bereaved, which typically was related to their depression.

Some studies have reported high rates of marital discord and family dysfunction (Kaplan, Smith, Grobstein, & Fischman, 1973), although others have reported that while parents experience symptoms of grief, they generally were able to adjust in the postdeath period (Lansky, Cairns, Hussanein, Wehr, & Lowman,

1978; Lansky & Lowman, 1974). Lascari and Stebhens (1973) reported that only 1 of 20 parents in their sample had difficulty with emotional crying episodes by the second year following the death of their child. Futterman and Hoffman (1973) also found that most of the parents they sampled did well following the death of their leukemic child.

Stebhens and Lascari (1974), in a retrospective study conducted with families between 6 months and 3 years after their children's death, reported that 33 percent of the parents experienced guilt feelings about their children's illness at the time of diagnosis, and that during the terminal phase 65 percent reported sleeping difficulties and 50 percent, a loss of appetite. No consistent pattern of pre- and postdeath symptomatology was found.

Little has been written about what characterizes those parents who are successful in adjusting to their children's death. Spinetta, Swarner, and Sheposh (1981) interviewed parents during the postdeath period and concluded that those who adjusted best had a consistent philosophy guiding them through the illness; had ongoing support, which included a spouse; and had good communication with their children during the course of the illness.

Rando (1983) investigated the influence of personal characteristics, time factors, and parental experience during the illness on grief and adaptation among parents following the death of their children from cancer. Data were collected on three dependent measures: the Grief Experience Inventory, developed by Sanders (1985); a structured interview; and the Parental Experience Inventory, developed by Rando. She found that previous loss experiences were associated with poorer bereavement outcomes. Rando concluded that direct involvement in the child's care may not be as important to the resolution of the loss as had been theoretically postulated.

The relationship between the parents' symptoms and the length of the illness of their children is not clear. Moore, Gilliss, and Martinson (1988) and Martinson, Davies, and McClowry (1987) found no relationship between the length of the children's illnesses and the severity of their parents' symptoms. Miles (1985) also found that there was no difference in physical symptoms between parents who experienced the sudden death of a child and those who experienced the death of a child from a chronic illness.

Siblings' Response to the Death of a Child

Studies of the immediate or long-term effects of the death of a child from cancer on the surviving healthy siblings are limited. Approximately 50 percent of the siblings in a study by Binger and his colleagues (1969) had significant behavioral difficulties. Specific problems included school phobia, poor school performance, depression, headaches, and severe separation anxiety. In approximately 50 percent of the families studied, these symptoms were significant enough to have required psychiatric help.

Wald and Townes (1969) found that, according to parents' reports, 42 percent of the siblings were considered to be at risk for adjustment problems. In each of the families interviewed, one or more siblings were identified as having actual or potential adjustment problems. The ordinal position of the surviving sibling was found to be significant, with the oldest or the closest in age to the dying child being at greatest risk. In addition, certain personality patterns were associated with siblings at risk. These included aggression in males and withdrawal in females.

Illes (1979) conducted a small pilot study to explore what siblings of seriously ill children experience during various phases of the illness. The most pervasive theme was one of unanticipated change for which there was little preparation. Disruption of interpersonal relationships with family members and peers, absence of parents from the home environment, and parental substitutes were experienced at all stages of the illness. The siblings also were affected by physical changes in the ill child and by disturbances in family routines.

In a larger and more sophisticated study, Lansky et al. (1978) studied the impact and adaptation of siblings to childhood cancer. Their findings indicated that siblings experienced a great deal of distress and fear for their own health. These concerns often were manifested as physical symptoms similar to those of the ill child. Feelings of isolation from parents, other family members, and friends also were common.

Later work by Balk (1983a, 1983b) examined the relationship between post-death adolescent sibling functioning and family closeness. Although family closeness was not significantly related to adolescents' self-concept, it was significantly and positively related to their school performance and personal maturity. Approximately 50 percent of the adolescents experienced grief reactions of confusion, anger, depression, and guilt.

Although siblings often developed academic, psychological, or social problems after the death of a brother or sister, these problems usually decreased with time. Two studies (Hogan, 1988; Hogan & Greenfield, 1991), however, reported that the siblings' problems continued for a long time. Davies (1988, 1991) studied siblings' bereavement up to 3 years postdeath and found that 50 percent of the siblings were nervous, unhappy, sad, depressed, or liked to be alone. The internalizing scores from the Child Behavior Checklist also reflected a turning inward and the social competency scores decreased with time. These findings indicate the need for caregivers to monitor the reactions of bereaved siblings.

The literature is mixed on the self-concept of bereaved adolescent siblings. Balk (1983a, 1983b) and Martinson, Davies, and McClowry (1987) found that bereaved siblings had self-concept scores that were the same as or higher than normal subjects. Hogan and Greenfield (1991), however, found that the level of bereavement intensity was a significant factor among siblings more than 18 months bereaved. Siblings who had mild levels of bereavement intensity had high levels of self-concept, but siblings who had moderate or severe levels of bereavement intensity had low levels of self-concept.

Factors found to be associated with positive responses and coping methods among siblings included good communication in the family, ability to share the death experience with others, expression of pleasure in the surviving siblings' social relationships, and reliance on the family for support after death (Balk, 1983a, 1983b; Martinson & Campos, 1992). In the Martinson and Campos (1992) study, four out of five bereaved adolescents did not have long-term negative effects. Although religion assumed increasing importance during bereavement, it did not make coping necessarily easier (Balk, 1991).

Several studies compared parents' and siblings' bereavement. According to Demi and Gilbert (1978), siblings' grief patterns were different from those of their parents in that siblings tended to react behaviorally rather than emotionally. Mothers thought that their children had stronger self-concepts and that they were struggling more with grief than did the siblings themselves and their fathers (Hogan & Balk, 1990). Other studies have considered how parents and siblings communicate with one another and how it affects how they cope with the death (Adams & Deveau, 1987, Birenbaum, 1989, Birenbaum, Robinson, Phillips, Stewart, & McCown, 1989).

Conclusion

In the past decade, there has been an increasing interest in the concept of quality of life and a significant number of researchers have attempted to design instruments that assess aspects of the quality of life among adult cancer patients. However, most of the existing instruments are not appropriate for patients who are terminally ill (Cohen & Mount, 1992), and none are applicable to dying children and adolescents. There is an urgent need to design instruments that assess the quality of life among terminally ill children since the essential purpose of any hospice intervention is the enhancement of quality of life. While adult patients are often able to articulate their concerns regarding quality of life during the terminal stages of their illness, children rely more on indirect and symbolic ways to express their concerns and feelings. Thus in designing instruments, researchers need to be sensitive to children's modes of communicating at different times in their development in order to assess their experience of "living until they die." Research also needs to consider the quality of life of parents, siblings, and health professionals involved in caring for terminally ill children. Concepts such as "anticipatory grief" need to be reconsidered and examined in new ways that take account of the multidimensional aspects and the complexities of the grief experience for families and health professionals as well as the dying child.

There also is a need to systematically assess the effectiveness of services provided to children and families according to various models of hospice care. To date, a random clinical trial has never been done on pediatric hospice. Another promising area of research is parental mourning. It is crucial to delineate a model of mourning appropriate for bereaved parents and to establish new criteria for what consitutes normal and pathological mourning, since their intense and complicated grief cannot be understood within the existing theories on bereavement. Longitudinal studies are needed to focus on how marital, parent-child, and family relationships evolve over time as a result of the loss of a child, and how the family's grief may be affected by their experiences throughout the illness and terminal care.

Some initial findings have suggested that the family's philosophy on death, the members' involvement in the care of the dying child, family relationships, family functioning, openness in communication, and the existence of social support before and after the death of the child influence bereavement outcomes (Davies, Spinetta, Martinson, McClowry, & Kulenkamp, 1986). However, most of the existing studies on parental and sibling bereavement are purely descriptive and are not based on any theoretical framework. Because the loss of a child leads to an intense and complicated process of mourning that is likely to cause physical, psychological, and emotional problems to bereaved parents, siblings, and grandparents, new approaches are needed to understand families' responses to the death of a child from cancer.

Finally, the stress experienced by caregivers who provide hospice services to dying children and bereaved families needs to be better understood so that preventive measures and interventions can be designed and implemented to help these people in their work. The hospice philosophy suggests that in addition to the needs of children and families, equally important are the needs for education, ongoing support, and supervision of the health professionals who provide hospice services. One of the greatest challenges for health professionals is to learn how to care for themselves and to maximize the quality of living for themselves as well as their patients.

References

Adams, D. W., & Deveau, E. J. (1987). When a brother or sister is dying of cancer: The vulnerability of the adolescent sibling. *Death Studies, 11,* 279–295.

Alby, N., & Alby, J. M. (1971). L'enfant malade et le silence [the Infants' silence during Illness]. *Perspectives Psychiatriques, 34,* 51–57.

Alby, N., Alby, J. M., & Chassigneux, J. (1967). Aspects psychologiques de l'évolution et du traitement des leucemiques, enfants et jeunes adultes, dans un Centre Spécialise [The psychological aspects resulting from treatment changes in childhood cancer]. *Nouvelle Revue Française d'Hematologie, 7,* 577–588.

Balk, D. (1983a). Adolescents' grief reactions and self-concept perceptions following sibling death: A study of 33 teenagers. *Journal of Youth and Adolescence, 12,* 137–161.

Balk, D. (1983b). Effects of sibling death on teenagers. *Journal of Public Health, 53,* 14–18.

Balk, D. (1991). Death and adolescent bereavement: Current research and future directions. *Journal of Adolescent Research, 6,* 7–27.

Benfield, D. G., Leib, S. A., & Reuter, J. (1976). Grief responses of parents after referral of the critically ill newborn to a regional center. *New England Journal of Medicine, 294,* 975–978.

Bernard, J., & Alby, J. M. (1956). Incidences psychologiques de la leucemie aigue de l'enfant et de son traitement [Incidences of psychological behaviors during treatment of childhood leukemia]. *Hygiene Mentale, 3,* 241–255.

Binger, C., Ablin, A., Feuerstein, R., Kushner, J., Zoger, S., & Mikkelen, C. (1969). Childhood leukemia: Emotional impact on the family. *New England Journal of Medicine, 280,* 414–418.

Birenbaum, L. K. (1989). The relationship between parent-siblings' communication and siblings' coping with death experience. *Journal of Pediatric Oncology Nurses, 6,* 213–228.

Birenbaum, L. K., Robinson, M. A., Phillips, O. S., Stewart, B. J., & McCown, D. (1989). The response of children to the dying and death of a sibling. *Omega: Journal of Death and Dying, 20,* 213–228.

Bluebond-Langner, M. (1978). *The private worlds of dying children.* Princeton, NJ: Princeton University Press.

Bozeman, M., Orbach, G., & Sutherland, A. (1955). The adaptation of mothers to the threatened loss of their children through leukemia. Part I. *Cancer, 8,* 1–19.

Burne, R. (1988). Terminal care in children. *Maternal and Child Health, 13,* 284–287.

Burne, R., & Hunt, A. (1987). Use of opiates in terminally ill children. *Palliative Medicine, 1,* 27–30.

Chapman, J. A., & Goodall, J. (1980). Helping a child to live whilst dying. *Lancet, 1,* 753–756.

Children's Hospice International. (1989). Children's hospice definition. Alexandria, VA: Author.

Chiriboga, D. A., Jenkins, G., & Bailey, J. (1983). Stress and coping among hospice nurses: Test of an analytic model. *Nursing Research, 32,* 294–299.

Cobbs, B. (1956). Psychological impact of long-term illness and death of a child on the family circle. *Journal of Pediatrics, 49,* 746–751.

Cohen, S., & Mount, B. B. (1992). Quality of life in terminal illness: Defining and measuring subjective well-being in the dying. *Journal of Palliative Care, 8,* 40–45.

Corr, C. A., & Corr, D. M. (1992). Children's hospice care. *Death Studies, 16,* 431–449.

Corr, C. A., & Corr, D. M. (Eds.). (1983). *Hospice care principles and practice.* New York: Springer.

Dailey, A. A. (1986). The pain of loneliness: Children's hospice international. *Caring, 5,* 9–10.

Davies, B. (1988). Shared life space and sibling bereavement responses. *Cancer Nursing, 11,* 339–347.

Davies, B. (1991). Long-term outcome of adolescent sibling bereavement. *Journal of Adolescent Research, 6,* 83–96.

Davies, B., Spinetta, J., Martinson, I., McClowry, S., & Kulenkamp, E. (1986). Manifestations of levels of functioning in grieving families. *Journal of Family Issues, 7,* 297–319.

Demi, A. S., & Gilbert, C. M. (1987). Relationship of parental grief to sibling grief. *Archives of Psychiatric Nursing, 1,* 385–391.

Dominica, F. (1982). Helen House: A hospice for children. *Maternal Child Health Journal, 7,* 355–359.

Dominica, F. (1987). The role of the hospice for the dying child. *British Journal of Hospital Medicine, 38,* 334–343.

Duffy, C. M., Pollock, P., Levy, M., et al. Budd, E., Caulfield, L., & Koren, G. (1990). Home-based palliative care for children: 2. The benefits of an established program. *Journal of Palliative Care, 6,* 8–14.

Dufour, D. F. (1989). Home or hospital care for the child with end-stage cancer: Effects on the family. *Issues in Comprehensive Pediatric Nursing, 12,* 371–383.

Edwardson, S. R. (1983). The choice between hospital and home care for terminally ill children. *Nursing Research, 2,* 29–34.

Edwardson, S. R. (1984). Using research in practice: Factors associated with the adoption of a nursing innovation: Home care as an alternative to hospital for children terminally ill. *Western Journal of Nursing Research, 6,* 141–143.

Edwardson, S. R. (1985). Physician acceptance of home care for terminally ill children. *Health Services Research, 20,* 83–101.

Evans, A. E., & Edin, S. (1968). If a child must die. *New England Journal of Medicine, 278,* 138–142.

Fischoff, J., & O'Brien, N. (1976). After the child dies. *Journal of Pediatrics, 88,* 140–146.

Foley, G. V., & Whittam, E. H. (1991). Care of the child dying of cancer. *Ca—A Cancer Journal for Clinicians, 41,* 52–60.

Friedman, S. B., Chodoff, P., Mason, J. W., & Hamburg, D. A. (1963). Behavioral observations on parents anticipating the death of a child. *Pediatrics, 32,* 610–625.

Futterman, E., & Hoffman, I. (1973). Crisis and adaptation in the families of fatally ill children. In E. J. Anthony & C. Koupernik (Eds.), *The child and his family: The impact of disease and death.* New York: Wiley.

Futterman, E. H., Hoffman, J., & Sabshin, M. (1972). Parental anticipatory mourning. In B. Schoenberg, A. C. Carr, D. Peretz, & C. Kutscher (Eds.), *Psychosocial aspects of terminal care* (pp. 243–272). New York: Columbia University Press.

Geis, D. P. (1965). Mothers' perceptions of care given their dying children. *American Journal of Nursing, 65,* 105–107.

Goodell, A. S. (1980). Responses of nurses to the stresses of caring for pediatric oncology patients. *Issues in Comprehensive Pediatric Nursing, 4,* 2–6.

Green, M. (1967). Care of the dying child. *Pediatrics, 40,* 492–497.

Gronseth, E., Martinson, I., Kersey, J., & Nesbit, M. (1981). Support system of health professionals as observed in the project of home care for the child with cancer. *Death Education, 5,* 37–50.

Hofer, M., Wolff, C., Friedman, S., & Mason, J. (1972). A psychoendocrine study of bereavement: I. 17 hydroxycorticosteroid excretion rates of parents following death of their children from leukemia. *Psychosomatic Medicine, 34,* 481–502.

Hogan, N. S. (1988). The effects of time on the adolescent sibling bereavement process. *Pediatric Nursing, 14,* 333–335.

Hogan, N. S., & Balk, D. E. (1990). Adolescent reactions to sibling death: Perceptions of mothers, fathers and teenagers. *Nursing Research, 39,* 103–106.

Hogan, N. S., & Greenfield, D. B. (1991). Adolescent sibling bereavement symptomatology in a large community sample. *Journal of Adolescent Research, 6,* 97–112.

Howell, D. A. (1967). A child dies. *Hospital Topics, 45,* 93.

Hunt, A. M. (1990). A survey of signs, symptoms and symptom control in 30 terminally ill children. *Developmental Medicine and Child Neurology, 32,* 341–346.

Hutter, J. J., Farrell, F. Z., & Meltzer, P. S. (1991). Care of the child dying from cancer: Home vs. hospital. In D. Papadatou & C. Papadatos (Eds.), *Children and death* (pp. 197–208). Washington, DC: Hemisphere.

Illes, P. (1979). Children with cancer: Healthy siblings perceptions during the illness experience. *Cancer Nursing, 2,* 371–377.

International Work Group on Death, Dying and Bereavement. (in press). Position statement: Palliative care for children. In *Death studies.* Washington, DC: Hemisphere.

Kaplan, D., Smith, A., Grobstein, R., & Fischman, S. (1973). Family mediation of stress. *Social Casework, 18,* 60–69.

Karon, M., & Vernick, J. (1968). Approaches to emotional support of fatally ill children. *Clinical Pediatrics, 7,* 274–280.

Kennell, J. H., Slyter, H., & Klaus, M. H. (1970). The mourning response of patients to the death of a newborn infant. *New England Journal of Medicine, 283,* 344–349.

Kikuchi, J. (1972). A leukemic adolescent's verbalizations about dying. *Maternal Child Nursing Journal, 1,* 259–264.

Knudson, A., & Natterson, J. (1960). Participation of parents in the hospital care of their fatally ill children. *Pediatrics, 26,* 482–490.

Koocher, G. P. (1980). Pediatric cancer: Psychosocial problems and the high costs of helping. *Journal of Clinical Child Psychology, 9,* 2–5.

Koocher, G. P., Sourkes, B. M., & Keane, W. M. (1979). Pediatric oncology consultations: A generalizable model for medical settings. *Professional Psychology, 10*, 467–474.

Lansky, S., Cairns, N., Hussanein, R., Wehr, B., & Lowman, J. (1978). Childhood cancer: Parental discord and divorce. *Pediatrics, 62*, 184–188.

Lansky, S., & Lowman, J. (1974). Childhood malignancy. *Journal of Kansas Medical Society, 75*, 91–94.

Lascari, A., & Stebhens, J. (1973). The reaction of families to childhood leukemia. *Clinical Pediatrics, 12*, 210–214.

Lattanzi, M. E. (1985). An approach to caring: Caregiver concerns. In C. A. Corr & D. M. Corr (Eds.), *Hospice approaches to pediatric care* (pp. 261–277). New York: Springer.

Lattanzi-Licht, M. E. (1991). Professional stress: Creating a context for caring. In D. Papadatou & C. Papadatou (Eds.), *Children and death* (pp. 293–302). Washington, DC: Hemisphere.

Lauer, M. E., & Camitta, B. M. (1980). Home care for dying children: A nursing model. *Journal of Pediatrics, 97*, 1032–1035.

Lauer, M. E., & Mulhern, R. K. (1984). Parental self-selection versus psychosocial predictors of capability in home care referral: A case study. *American Journal of Hospice Care, 1*, 35–38.

Lauer, M. E., Mulhern, R. K., Bohne, J. M., & Camitta, B. M. (1985). Children's perceptions of their sibling's death at home or hospital: The precursors of differential adjustment. *Cancer Nursing, 8*, 21–27.

Lauer, M. E., Mulhern, R. K., Hoffman, R. G., & Camitta, B. M. (1986). Utilization of hospice/home care in pediatric oncology: A national survey. *Cancer Nursing, 9*, 102–107.

Lauer, M. E., Mulhern, R. K., Wallskog, J. M., & Camitta, B. M. (1983). A comparison study of parental adaptation following a child's death at home or in the hospital. *Pediatrics, 1*, 107–112.

Levy, M., Duffy, C. M., Pollock, P., Budd, E., Caulfield, L., & Koren, G. (1990). Home-based palliative care for children: 1. The institution of a program. *Journal of Palliative Care, 6*, 11–15.

Lindemann, E. (1944). Symptomatology and management of acute grief. *American Journal of Psychiatry, 101*, 141–148.

Maloney, M. J., & Ange, C. (1982). Group consultation with highly stressed medical personnel to avoid burnout. *Journal of the American Academy of Child Psychiatry, 21*, 481–485.

Martin, B. B. (1986). Pediatric hospice care: An update. *Caring, 5*, 5–6.

Martin, B. B. (1989). *Implementation of a hospital-based pediatric hospice care program.* Final Report to the Maternal and Child Health Program, Department of Health Resources & Service Administration Health and Human Services. Children's Hospital of Los Angeles, California.

Martinson, I. M. (1976). Why don't we let them die at home? *Registered Nurse, 39*, 57–65.

Martinson, I. M. Pediatric Hospice: Past, Present & Future (1993). *Journal of Pediatric Oncology Nursing*, July 1993.

Martinson, I. M., Armstrong, G. D., Geis, D. P., Anglim, M. A., Gronseth, E., MacInnis, H., Kersey, J. H., & Nesbit, M. E. (1978). Home care for children dying of cancer. *Pediatrics, 62*, 106–113.

Martinson, I., Birenbaum, L., Martin, B., Lauer, M., & Eng, B. (1991). *Hospice/home care: A nurses' manual for management for children.* Alexandria, VA: Children's Hospice International.

Martinson, I. M., & Campos, R. G. (1992). Adolescent bereavement: Long term responses to a sibling's death from cancer. *Journal of Adolescent Research, 6,* 54–69.

Martinson, I. M., Davies, E. B., & McClowry, S. G. (1987). The long-term effects of sibling death on self-concept. *Journal of Pediatric Nursing, 2,* 227–235.

Martinson, I. M., & Henry, W. F. (1980). Some possible societal consequences of changing the way in which we care for dying children. *Hastings Center Report, 10,* 5–8.

Martinson, I., Kersey, J., & Nesbitt, M. (1987). Children's adjustment to the death of a sibling from cancer. *Advances in Thanatology, 6,* 1–7.

Martinson, I. M., & Martinson, P. V. (1983). Developing theory from practice: Alternative models of nursing care. In A. Miller, S. R. Epstein, & J. O'Brien (Eds.), *Behavioral science and nursing theory* (pp. 119–139). St. Louis: Mosby.

Martinson, I. M., Moldow, D. G., Armstrong, G. D., Henry, W. F., Nesbit, M. E., & Kersey, J. H. (1986). Home care for children dying of cancer. *Research in Nursing and Health, 9,* 11–16.

Martinson, I. M., Moldow, G., & Henry, W. F. (1980). *Home care for the child with cancer.* Final Report, National Cancer Institute, University of Minnesota, Minneapolis, Minnesota.

Martinson, I., Nesbit, M., & Kersey, J. (1985). Physician's role in home care for children with cancer. *Death Studies, 9,* 283–293.

Martinson, I. M., Nixon, S., Geis, D., YaDeau, R., Nesbit, M., & Kersey, J. (1982). Nursing care in childhood cancer: Methadone. *American Journal of Nursing, 82,* 432–435.

McClowry, S. G., Davies, E. B., May, K. A., Kulenkamp, E. J., & Martinson, I. M. (1987). The empty space phenomenon: The process of grief in the bereaved family. *Death Studies, 11,* 361–374.

McHorney, C. A. & Mor, V. (1988). Predictors of bereavement depression and its health services consequences. *Medical Care, 26,* 882–893.

Miles, M. (1985). Emotional symptoms and physical health in bereaved parents. *Nursing Research, 34,* 76–81.

Moldow, D. G., Armstrong, G. D., Henry, W. F., & Martinson, I. M. (1982). The cost of home care for dying children. *Medical Care, 20,* 1114–1160.

Moldow, D. G., & Martinson, I. M. (1980). From research to reality: Home care for the dying child. *MCN: The American Journal of Maternal Child Nursing, 51,* 159–166.

Moldow, D. G., & Martinson, I. (1991). *Parents manual for seriously ill children at home.* Alexandria, VA: Children's Home International.

Moore, I. M., Gilliss, C. L., & Martinson, I. M. (1988). Psychosomatic manifestations of bereavement in parents two years after the death of a child with cancer. *Nursing Research, 37,* 104–107.

Morrissey, J. R. (1963a). Children's adaptations to fatal illness. *Social Work, 8,* 81–88.

Morrissey, J. R. (1963b). A note on interviews with children facing imminent death. *Social Casework, 44,* 343–345.

Mulhern, R. K., Lauer, M. E., & Hoffmann, R. G. (1983). Death of a child at home or in the hospital: Subsequent psychological adjustment of the family. *Pediatrics, 71,* 743–747.

National Center for Health Statistics. (1990). Advanced report of final mortality statistics, 1989. In *Monthly Vital Statistics Report* (Vol. 39, p. 13). Hyattsville, MD: Public Health Service.

National Hospice Organization. (1987). *Meeting the challenge for a special kind of caring: Standards of a hospice program of care recommended by the National Hospice Organization.* Unpublished manuscript.

Natterson, J. M., & Knudson, A. G., Jr. (1960). Observations concerning fear of death in fatally ill children and their mothers. *Psychosomatic Medicine, 22,* 456–465.

Norman, R., & Bennett, M. (1986). Care of the dying child at home: A unique cooperative relationship. *Austrian Journal of Advanced Nursing, 3,* 3–16.

Papadatou, D. (1991). Working with dying children: A professional's personal journey. In D. Papadatou & C. Papadatos (Eds.), *Children and death* (pp. 285–292). Washington, DC: Hemisphere.

Papadatou, D., Yfantopoulos, J., Vassilatou-Kosmidis, E., & Maistros, Y. (1992). *Feasibility study: Home based palliative care for children with cancer.* Final report to Europe Against Cancer, European Economic Communities, University of Athens, Athens, Greece.

Raimbault, G. (1975). *L'enfant et la mort.* Paris: Éditions Privat, Brussels, Belgium.

Raimbault, G. (1991). The seriously ill child: Management of family and medical surroundings. In D. Papadatou & C. Papadatos (Eds.), *Children and death* (pp. 177–187). Washington, DC: Hemisphere.

Rando, T. (1983). An investigation of grief and adaptation in parents whose children have died from cancer. *Journal of Pediatric Psychology, 8,* 3–20.

Rando, T. A. (1986). A comprehensive analysis of anticipatory grief: Perspectives, processes, promises and problems. In T. A. Rando (Ed.), *Loss and anticipatory grief* (pp. 3–38). Lexington, MA: Lexington Books.

Richmond, J. B., & Waisman, H. A. (1955). Psychologic aspects of management of children with malignant disease. *American Journal of Diseases of Children, 89,* 42–47.

Rosenblatt, P. (1983). Bitter, bitter tears: Nineteenth-century diarists and twentieth-century grief theories. Minneapolis: University of Minnesota Press.

Rothenberg, M. F. (1967). Reactions of those who treat children with cancer. *Pediatrics, 40,* 507–519.

Sahler, O. J., McAnarney, E. R., & Friedman, S. B. (1981). Factors influencing pediatric interns' relationships with dying children and their parents. *Pediatrics, 67,* 207–216.

Sanders, C. (1979–80). A comparison of adult bereavement in the death of a spouse, child and parent. *Omega, 10,* 303–332.

Sanders, C. (1985). The grief experience inventory. Palo Alto, CA: Consulting Psychologists Press.

Schmidt, L. (1987). Working with bereaved parents. In T. Krulik, B. Holaday, & I. M. Martinson (Eds.), *The child and family facing life-threatening illness* (pp. 327–344). Philadelphia: Lippincott.

Singher, L. J. (1974). The slowly dying child. *Clinical Pediatrics, 13,* 861–866.

Solnit, A. J., & Green, M. (1959). Psychologic considerations in the management of deaths on pediatric hospital services. *Pediatrics, 24,* 106–112.

Solnit, A. J., & Green, M. (1963). The pediatric management of the dying child: II. The child's reaction to the fear of dying. In A. Solnit & S. Provence (Eds.), *Modern perspectives in child development.* New York: International Universities Press.

Spinetta, J. J. (1974). The dying child's awareness of death. *Psychological Bulletin, 4,* 256–260.

Spinetta, J. J., & Maloney, L. J. (1975). Death anxiety in the outpatient leukemic child. *Pediatrics, 56,* 1034–1037.

Spinetta, J. J., Rigler, D., & Karon, M. (1973). Anxiety in the dying child. *Pediatrics, 52,* 127–131.

Spinetta, J. J., Rigler, D., & Karon, M. (1974). Personal space as a measure of a dying child's sense of isolation. *Journal of Counseling and Clinical Psychology, 42,* 751–756.

Spinetta, J. J., Swarner, J. A., & Sheposh, J. P. (1981). Effective parental coping following the death of a child from cancer. *Journal of Pediatric Psychology, 6,* 251–263.

Stebhens, J., & Lascari, A. (1974). Psychological follow-up of families with childhood cancer. *Journal of Clinical Psychology, 30,* 393–397.

Tietz, W., McSherry, L., & Britt, B. (1972). Family sequelae after a child's death due to cancer. *American Journal of Psychotherapy, 26,* 417–425.

Vachon, M. L., & Pakes, E. (1984). Staff stress in the care of the critically ill and dying child. In H. Wass & C. A. Corr (Eds.), *Childhood and death* (pp. 151–182). Washington, DC: Hemisphere.

Vernick, J., & Karon, M. (1965). Who's afraid of death on a leukemia ward? *American Journal of Diseases of Children, 109,* 393–397.

Videka-Sherman, L. (1982). Coping with the death of a child: A study over time. *American Journal of Orthopsychiatry, 52,* 688–698.

Waechter, E. H. (1971). Children's awareness of fatal illness. *American Journal of Nursing, 71,* 1168–1172.

Waechter, E. H. (1987a). Children's reactions to fatal illness. In T. Krulik, B. Holaday, & I. M. Martinson (Eds.), *The child and family facing life-threatening illness* (pp. 108–119). Philadelphia: Lippincott.

Waechter, E. H. (1987b). Dying children: Patterns of coping. In T. Krulik, B. Holaday, & I. M. Martinson (Eds.), *The child and family facing life-threatening illness* (pp. 293–312). Philadelphia: Lippincott.

Waechter, E. H. (1987c). Working with parents of children with life-threatening illness. In T. Krulik, B. Holaday, & I. M. Martinson (Eds.), *The child and family facing life-threatening illness* (pp. 246–257). Philadelphia: Lippincott.

Wald, D., & Townes, B. (1969). The adjustment of siblings to childhood leukemia. *Family Coordinator, 18,* 155–160.

Wilson, D. C. (1982). The viability of pediatric hospices: A case study. *Death Education, 6,* 205–212.

10

Future Directions in
Pediatric Psychooncology

RAYMOND K. MULHERN AND DAVID J. BEARISON

A spectrum of psychological research among children with cancer and their families has been discussed in this book. In the present chapter we will review some themes emerging from previous chapters to chart a possible course for research in pediatric psychooncology. Before considering specific chapter topics we discuss the current state of findings in pediatric psychooncology on two conceptual dimensions of research: medically driven versus psychologically driven research and epidemiological versus intervention research.

Conceptual Dimensions of Psychooncology Research
Medically Driven versus Psychologically Driven Research

According to many psychosocial investigators in pediatric oncology, their research is necessarily dependent upon, and a reaction to, new medical developments. Their research may be motivated less by psychological theory than by the technical needs of pediatric oncologists. For example, medically driven psychosocial research may be in response to the need to evaluate acute and chronic psychological toxicity of a new therapy so that the efficacy/toxicity ratio can be compared to the clinical standard. There is nothing wrong with this type of research, and significant contributions to our scientific knowledge have come from it. Examples found in this book include studies of neuropsychological toxicity associated with different treatments for childhood cancer. The positive impact on patient care from such studies is indirect in that medical treatment protocols are subsequently modified to reduce toxicity while retaining efficacy. Another example of indirect benefit comes from studies on compliance with medication and improving cure rates by enhancing compliance behavior. Despite the value of the medically driven ap-

215

proach, some investigators feel that it is the work of technical assistants rather than independent investigators, and it limits the scope of their research to those topics of interest to oncologists.

At the other pole of the medically versus psychologically driven dimension are investigators who believe that psychological studies in pediatric oncology should use psychological theories to define the importance of scientific questions. In this book Kazak as well as Carpenter and LaVant argue for using psychological models to guide the study of patient and family adaptation. This approach often samples patients (subjects) across medically relevant variables and seeks common behavioral patterns among patients. The psychologically driven approach yields findings that have more direct and general applicability to children with cancer and their families. For example, styles of coping with life-threatening disease may depend more on child and family demographics than on a specific type of cancer.

From our experience, the ideal approach lies more to the center of this dimension; that is, psychological data valuable to the oncologist's research objectives can be obtained concurrent with data that are derived from psychological models. To achieve this goal, a strong collaborative relationship between oncologists and behavioral scientists is essential.

Epidemiology versus Intervention Research

The research discussed in this text also can be considered, in general terms, as having either epidemiology or intervention as its primary objective. Epidemiological research defines the incidence of phenomena associated with the experience of childhood cancer, the variables that place children and/or their families at risk for adverse psychological outcomes, and the variables that appear to play a protective role in preventing adverse consequences of the disease and its treatment. These studies are important because they identify groups of children requiring more intensive surveillance and early intervention and variables that are salient for prevention. Examples in this book include discussions of children who are more vulnerable to pain, those more susceptible to noncompliance with medications, and those more likely to suffer brain damage as a consequence of their treatment.

Less common are studies that compare the effectiveness of different types of psychosocial interventions. Intervention studies are labor-intensive and require extended time periods within a longitudinal design to obtain sufficient follow-up data. Yet they constitute the most direct path to our goal of reducing human suffering associated with childhood cancers. It is a testimony to the perseverance of a select number of psychooncologists and their colleagues, such as Kupst, Martinson, and Zeltzer, that clinical practice has benefited from their intervention studies of facilitating family coping, reducing problems in the terminal care process, and better management of pain and anxiety.

Some of the salient variables in epidemiological research (e.g., age, gender, family structure) cannot be modified. However, when variables are identified that are modifiable, studies should be designed to test the effects of manipulating one or more of them as independent variables in reducing adverse outcomes among children and their families. Future efforts in pediatric psychooncology should concentrate on further translating the results of epidemiologic studies into comparative trials of different types of intervention techniques.

Selective Discussion of Chapter Topics
Neuropsychological Late Effects

A basic understanding of medical variables (e.g., cranial irradiation) and demographic variables (e.g., young age at treatment) that place children at risk for cognitive delays as a result of their cancer or its treatment has now been established. The ability to quantitatively compare chronic neurotoxicities associated with different therapies, and to use these findings to define the risk/benefit ratios for different therapeutic approaches, is critical to advancements in this area. A major impediment to this kind of research, however, is that we must wait until the child is a long-term survivor in order to infer any conclusions about chronic neuropsychological toxicities.

A primary direction for future research in this area is the development of methods of cognitive assessment that, if used early in the child's treatment, will predict later outcomes. Computerized administration of psychological tasks and integration of results with concurrent electrophysiological recordings from the brain (e.g., cognitive evoked potentials) or real-time imaging of the functioning brain (e.g., positron emission tomography or magnetic resonance imaging spectroscopy) (PET or MRI-SPECT) will be increasingly used to define the relationship between acute and chronic neuropsychological toxicities.

A second major area of needed research is intervention. Cognitive rehabilitation methods found to be useful in other settings with brain-damaged children and adults (e.g., learning disabilities, attention deficit disorders) need to be evaluated for their efficacy with children who manifest neuropsychological abnormalities as a result of their cancer experience.

Coping and Adaptation

The term "coping," as Kazak and Carpenter and LaVant illustrate, is used to define several different areas of psychooncology research. In general, research on coping and adaptation has moved beyond initial concerns with psychopathology and now seeks to further understanding of how individuals or family systems react to the stress of pediatric cancer. Several complementary models for conceptualizing this process, such as those by Lazarus and McCubbin, were discussed. These models generate useful hypotheses that require further validation among children with cancer.

This area of research is moving in the direction of intervention studies that yield prescriptives that are responsive to the individual qualities of a given child-patient, family, or family system. These approaches emphasize positive adaptation as opposed to the mere absence of psychopathology in defining adjustment. However, in the absence of psychopathology, it may be difficult for investigators to justify the expense of these interventions. Therefore, the salutary effects of interventions in social and economic terms (better school or job attendance or performance, fewer doctor visits, etc.) should be considered as outcome measures in future studies.

Terminal Care and Bereavement

Although extraordinary advances have been made in the cure rates for many types of childhood cancer, there is still a need for empathic methods of helping children die unafraid and with dignity. The psychological interventions necessary for comprehensive terminal home-care programs already exist. But as Martinson and Papadatou discussed, there remain major obstacles in operationally defining successful interventions, even when their benefits are obvious to the caregivers and the family. They and others have emphasized the need for a valid ''quality of life'' measure suitable for children receiving terminal care in different settings. The international dissemination of pediatric terminal care programs raises the question of whether such measures can be made culture-free, and this issue deserves further investigation.

Oftentimes ignored are the long-term survivors of the terminal care experience—the child's friends and family members. Continued research on the adjustment of family members and complications of bereavement should be conducted, and these outcomes need to be associated with the circumstances of the child's death and the quality of his or her terminal care. Research in this area is difficult because of the sensitive nature of the questions that need to be asked and the strong emotions they evoke.

Compliance with Prescribed Treatments

Psychological factors may directly interfere with the successful application of curative anticancer therapies. It is not clear why an otherwise rational person with a life-threatening disease would not adhere to the prescribed course of treatment or why parents would not comply with the treatment prescribed for their child. Bearison's chapter uncovers multiple problems with how compliance is assessed and the limited progress in identifying variables that target patients at high risk for noncompliance. Seemingly simple and intuitive relationships, such as the relationship between severity of medication side effects and noncompliance, have not been confirmed by empirical findings. Despite an increasing body of descriptive data documenting a substantial incidence of noncompliance among pediatric cancer patients, compliance issues have not been routinely considered when evaluating treatment protocol efficacy.

Because child or parent noncompliance with prescribed treatment may be only one manifestation of a more pervasive psychological dysfunction, clinical referrals for noncompliance would seem to warrant a complete look at how the child and family adjust to the illness, as well as the psychological history antedating the child's diagnosis of cancer.

Cognitive-behavioral research on the principles of reinforcement, approach-avoidance conflicts, delay of gratification, and self-control behaviors has not been adequately applied to adherence issues in pediatric oncology. Principles derived from other areas of human behavior such as weight loss, smoking cessation, and unprotected sexual activities should be considered in developing a conceptual model to explain noncompliance in pediatric oncology and to develop intervention programs to reduce the incidence of noncompliant behaviors.

Pain Management

Greater advocacy by psychologists and other psychosocial practitioners for children experiencing pain is needed because of frequent undermedication. Zeltzer's chapter provides a wealth of information regarding state-of-the-art methods of clinical assessment and alternative psychological and pharmacological interventions.

Future research in this area will define the relationship between biological (genetic and constitutional) and experiential (pain chronicity, subjective interpretation) factors that affect pain tolerance in children. Attempts to define the ''pain-vulnerable'' child by using highly controlled experimental pain paradigms, such as the cold pressor procedure of Fanurik and Zeltzer, hold promise for a better understanding of the experience of children with cancer undergoing painful medical procedures. These authors are developing and testing different cognitive pain-control strategies based on the experimental pain model. Further research is needed to determine how well these findings apply to children with cancer.

Bone Marrow Transplantation

Bone marrow transplantation incorporates important aspects of all of the foregoing topic areas. It is difficult to imagine a more medically and psychologically challenging experience for the child, family, and involved professionals. Because bone marrow transplantation will be more frequently used in the future for treating pediatric cancer, as well as other diseases such as sickle cell anemia, it is important to better understand the acute and chronic psychological risks associated with this procedure. The current literature is limited to descriptive and correlational analyses. As Phipps points out, bone marrow transplantation also provides fertile ground for needed investigations of ethical issues involving informed consent, compliance, psychopharmacology, late effects among long-term survivors, and effects of stress on medical staff members.

Emerging Areas of Pediatric Psychooncology

There are several emerging areas in pediatric psychooncology research that have not yet developed a sufficient body of literature to warrant individual chapters in this volume. However, we perceive them to be important in the future development of the field.

Psychoimmunology

The relationship between psychological health and immunological competence continues to be a controversial area within psychology and oncology. Well-controlled empirical studies have been infrequent in the adult oncology literature and, to our knowledge, absent from the pediatric oncology literature. The existing adult oncology studies are equivocal on balance, although at least some suggestion of a relationship between mood and length of survival has been shown.

One limitation of this area has been the multitude of sometimes discrepant laboratory methods for measuring immunocompetence. Recent research with HIV-positive patients can help remedy some of the immunocompetence measurement issues for oncology. There is a need for longitudinal research with pediatric oncology patients in this area. Such studies should control for premorbid levels of stress and adjustment in the child and family before attempting to associate disease outcome with psychological adjustment.

School Intervention Programs

Innovative methods of helping children with cancer maintain their academic progress while they receive therapy are badly needed, and studies comparing the effectiveness of different methods of school intervention should be conducted. With the increased effectiveness of antiemetic drugs and other drugs that stimulate recovery of immune function following chemotherapy, children may miss fewer days of school in the future. However, school absences for inpatient admissions and outpatient clinic visits will continue to be a problem that will require intervention. Children with cancer also are frequently absent from school because of treatment and its side effects. Even among patients with normal intellectual abilities, the frequency of repeated grades because of school absence is higher than among healthy children. Services provided by the treating institutions and community school systems to these children vary substantially, depending upon geographic region and financial resources.

Quality-of-Life Instrumentation

Valid quality-of-life measures for children with cancer and with other chronic or life-threatening childhood diseases are not currently available. If such measures were developed, they would enable comparisons between outcomes from different cancer treatment protocols and longitudinal analysis of single cases as well as comparisons with diseases other than cancer. Comparisons of the relative toxicity of different diseases and therapies in terms of the child's functional level (motor, sensory, pain, cognitive, school, mood, relationships, etc.) would be available from quality-of-life measures. Developmental changes in defining what is considered to be normal at different ages makes this a more difficult task than in the adult population. Large samples of children will be needed to validate quality-of-life scales, but the effort is clearly justified.

Closing Comments

A senior pediatric oncologist noted that childhood cancer was the "perfect" disease for psychosocial researchers because "it has everything." He meant by this statement that cancer encompasses more medical and psychological components than any other pediatric disease: it potentially affects all organ systems, so one can investigate diverse topics such as amputation, sensory deficits, and brain damage; it involves periods of acute illness that occur in the context of a chronic disease, so one can investigate mechanisms of coping with symptoms, school absence, and family relationships over time; it is curable, so one can study hopefulness and adjustment among long-term survivors; it is fatal, so one can investigate issues involving terminal care; and it may be associated with acute and chronic pain syndromes, so one can study the effectiveness of different pain interventions.

These characteristics have made childhood cancer an especially useful model for those interested in the relationship between medical and psychological health of children. This may explain Eiser's observation, cited in the introduction, that the amount of psychosocial research in pediatric cancer is disproportionately high given its incidence. Future efforts, therefore, should extend the results of pediatric psychooncology research beyond the confines of childhood cancer.

Author Index

Subject Index

235